AIDS Care at Home

Also by Judith Greif

The No-Hysterectomy Option: Your Body—Your Choice
(with Herbert Goldfarb, M.D.)

AIDS Care at Home

A GUIDE FOR CAREGIVERS, LOVED ONES, AND PEOPLE WITH AIDS

Judith Greif, M.S., R.N.C., F.N.P.
Beth Ann Golden, M.S.N., R.N.C., A.N.P.

John Wiley & Sons, Inc.
New York ■ Chichester ■ Brisbane ■ Toronto ■ Singapore

Illustrations on pages 56, 78, 114, 115, 165, 290, 291, and 292 by Brian Pendley.

This book is printed on acid-free paper.

Copyright © 1994 by Judith Greif and Beth Ann Golden.
Published by John Wiley & Sons, Inc.

ISBN 0-471-58468-1

Printed in the United States of America

10 9 8 7 6 5 4 3 2 1

To Our Families

To my parents, Myra and David Golden, for their never ending support, patience, encouragement, and most of all for their love. I am who I am because of you.

To my brother, Jeffrey, and sister-in-law, Jodi (who is a sister in every way): You always stand by me, make me laugh, give me a push, love me, and—just like Wubby and Dabid—drive me crazy.

To Jason and Lucas, my nephews, for the sticky kisses I can never get enough of. They're worth moving to Florida for.

Thank you all. I love you.

—Beth

To the Two Most Important Men in My Life

To the memory of my father, Sy Greif, who died of cancer over a decade ago, but who taught me things and left me a legacy of wonderful memories that are with me every day of my life. You taught me what it was like to be a caregiver for the terminally ill. You taught me how to live and die with humor, with courage, and with dignity.

To my husband, Joe, who never stops encouraging me to be the best I can be every day of my life. I cannot imagine a better partner in every facet of my life. You are a world-class husband, father, professional writer and editor, and the most romantic and caring man I've ever known.

—Judi

Special Dedication

This book would never have come to be if the need for it had not been identified and expressed by people with AIDS and their caregivers and significant others. It is our deepest wish that the information contained here will be helpful, thought-provoking, and reassuring to those who read it. All who are helped by this book owe a debt of gratitude to those who came before them for planting the seed of an idea and for persevering.

This book is dedicated to all caregivers and receivers; to those people with AIDS past, present, and future; and to their loved ones—never have we seen soldiers so brave in the face of a battle so fierce.

Acknowledgments

The authors acknowledge and thank Peter Canavan, R.N., for writing the perfect foreword and J. R. Rich and Lary Campbell, R.N., for opening up their hearts and sharing their emotions and their thoughts on caregiving. We also express our gratitude to Antonia Bongiardina, a great AIDS dietitian and friend; to Malinda (Lindi) Dunn, senior occupational therapist extraordinaire; to Joyce Anastasi, Ph.D., R.N., for providing information and encouragement and for always asking how it was going. Thanks to the entire staff of the Roosevelt Hospital AIDS unit for being the best examples of what caregivers should be. Our gratitude also goes to the staff of Rutgers Student Health Service, who were always there with words of encouragement, and especially to Khyati Gokli, M.D., Edward Lifshitz, M.D., William Newrock, M.D., and Barbara Cannon, medical technologist, for sharing their medical expertise.

The authors are grateful to Brian Pendley for doing his usual great job in preparing the illustrations for this book.

We also commend and acknowledge the staff at John Wiley & Sons—most especially PJ Dempsey, Chris Jackson, and Ruth Greif—for their assistance in making this book a reality.

In conclusion, we would like to extend a very special acknowledgment to Joseph Pedreiro, for his invaluable assistance throughout this entire project in preparing the manuscript—for his expertise as a production editor, for his honest appraisals, and for just being wonderful. We are in your debt.

As the old man walked the beach at dawn, he noticed a young man ahead of him picking up starfish and flinging them into the sea. Finally catching up with the youth, he asked him why he was doing this. The answer was that the stranded starfish would die if left until the morning sun.

"But the beach goes on for miles and there are millions of starfish," countered the other. "How can your effort make any difference?"

The young man looked at the starfish in his hand and then threw it to safety in the waves.

"It makes a difference to this one," he said.

—Anonymous

Foreword

By Peter Canavan, R.N.

A friend of mine, a fellow nurse who works with me on the AIDS unit, recently told her four-year-old daughter that she did not own a VCR when she was a little girl. The child was amazed. Her world was defined by *Beauty and the Beast* and *The Little Mermaid,* and she could not believe that a world without video cassettes could exist. Had she caught her mother in another one of those "mother jokes"? She asked her mother, "Then how did you play your tapes?"

The revolution of modern technology has changed the world in which this little girl lives, and the way she views the world. The impact of technology and its ability to transform human lives have been nowhere more evident than in the AIDS community—those people whose lives have been affected by AIDS/HIV, either directly through infection, or because of their involvement and concern for people who have been infected. For myself, for a majority of gay men, and for the millions of people affected by AIDS/HIV, the world has been completely transformed. AIDS/HIV has become the central concern of our lives and the principal organizing characteristic.

Laypeople in some segments of the AIDS community have developed a knowledge base so sophisticated it includes skills and information that 15 years ago were either unknown or in the hands of only the most specialized scientists. Discussions of T-cell ratios and drug interactions sound like they are taking place in a medical classroom or laboratory. Advances in medicine and technology define the AIDS/HIV world, and it has become implausible for many individuals to consider a world without these essential innovations. It is difficult for some of us to imagine a world without the most recent antifungal medication or central venous catheters. Confronted with the possibility of a world without central venous catheters, the sophisticated child, born in the post-AIDS generation, could challenge her mother, "then how did you infuse your T.P.N.?" (T.P.N. stands for total parenteral nutrition, a nutritional supplement administered intravenously through a central venous access device.)

The last time I sat down to write about the gay community was in 1975. I was working as an assistant to the regional sociologist of the National Park Service. The federal government had made a commitment to urban recreation, and I was hired to study patterns of nude bathing at the newly acquired Jacob Riis Park in New York City. The community that I documented at that time, less than 20 years ago, was marked by levity and festivity. It had a truly "gay" atmosphere. It was a community organized around patterns of recreation and conspicuous consumption. The party atmosphere was pervasive. A stratification system emerged based on where people went to party, with whom, with what, and what they were wearing. The settings in which gay people expressed themselves were typically leisure settings, segregated from the larger society, and outside the constraints of traditional business and family values. Excluded from participation in the dominant institutions of our society, gay people created their own community outside the mainstream, where they could associate voluntarily and define their own cultural standards. This resulted in a recreational community that extolled the private pursuit of pleasure, was loosely bound, usually apolitical, light-hearted—often lightweight. It frequently avoided serious issues, emphasizing style over substance, beauty over character—sometimes appearing frivolous or flamboyant.

The community I described less than 20 years ago has completely disappeared. The reality for those individuals from that era who were fortunate enough to have survived is totally transformed. The almost paralyzing fear of aging among gay men has been replaced by the almost paralyzing fear of *not* aging. The center of the gay community has shifted from the bars and the beaches, and other leisure settings, to the medical centers and the supporting organizations. When I went through the volunteer orientation for the Gay Men's Health Crisis 6 years ago, a gay man stood up. He said that 20 years earlier he had asked himself, "Where is it happening? Where is the heart of the gay community?" His answer was, The Tea Dance at the Pines in Fire Island. That's where he was, and that's where he wanted to be. Ten years later, in answer to the same question, he decided it was The Saint, an exclusive gay male disco in New York's Greenwich Village. Again, he was a part of the scene. When this man asked himself, in 1986, "Where is it happening? Where do I want to be?" His answer was, "Here. Helping out. Giving back to my people."

AIDS has changed the gay community in positive ways, increasing social concern and responsibility. Members of the gay community have matured and learned, through their own mortality and illness, to support one another through life's major crises while at the same time to appreciate and cherish the experience of the present. Let's be glad we're all together while we're here.

AIDS has changed reality for many in the AIDS/HIV community. The new reality makes new demands and requires increasing levels of knowledge to function effectively. This book attempts to fill one of the major gaps in the information system. By providing caregivers with the basic skills and facts, the authors hope to build the confidence that will enable readers to provide care for the person with AIDS in the home. This is important for two reasons. The first is that hospital discharges are most commonly delayed because patients do not have anyone in the home who can provide them with basic nursing care. If a relative or significant other is willing to take responsibility and learn the necessary skills, it can greatly expedite the patient's discharge from the hospital. The home is such a warm and familiar setting compared to the hospital. It is many patients' foremost wish that they just go home. Mastery of the information in this book can help the reader to make a patient's dream come true.

Second, this book can be of critical importance for those patients who wish to die at home. The ability to be at home, among one's family members and friends, surrounded by the objects of one's life, at the time of one's death, is a blessing not available to many, because so few people have had the skills to support the dying at home, or the willingness to do so.

Those of you who make the supreme sacrifice to provide care in the home for people who are sick and dying with AIDS are already blessed. Your decision is noble and empowering and will help to restore the dignity and humanity of the person for whom you are caring.

I wish you Godspeed in your endeavor and offer you the knowledge that when you begin to provide care for people with AIDS in the home or in the community, you are joining a larger circle of individuals who have made a similar commitment to people with AIDS. Try to get in touch with other caregivers in your community. They may provide you with the much needed support to continue your work.

Contents

Part V: *Appendixes*

AIDS Care at Home

Introduction

In 1986, five years after the first case of *acquired immunodeficiency syndrome (AIDS)* was identified in this country, Dr. Peter Selwyn, Assistant Professor of Epidemiology at the Albert Einstein College of Medicine, wrote a treatise on what was known about this disease at the time. In this now classic article ("AIDS: What Is Now Known," *Hospital Practice,* Volume 21, issue 5), he said,

> Few physicians will find their practices untouched by this epidemic: few communities will be spared from the disease. The difficult decisions ahead, involving not only individual patient care but also public policy, must be made with reason, compassion, and a sober understanding of the reality of this devastating illness.

The statistics are stark. When Dr. Selwyn wrote these tragically prophetic words, 19,181 cases had been reported, with 10,152 lives lost. Today, AIDS has become the second leading cause of death among young men and the fifth leading cause of death in young women. It is the number one cause of death of children in some areas. AIDS will claim the lives of more men aged 25 to 44 than heart disease, cancer, suicide, and homicide.

As compared with only seven years ago, there have now been a total of 718,894 documented AIDS cases (with estimates as high as 2.5 million). More than half have died. The World Health Organization estimates that 13 to 14 million adults and 1 million children worldwide are infected with the *human immunodeficiency virus (HIV)* and that by the year 2000, that figure will more likely be 40 million. Each one of these infected persons has the potential to someday manifest the full-blown disease.

These frightening statistics emphasize the critical need for a practical, hands-on manual on the subject of home care for people with AIDS (*PWA*s), all of whom at some point in their illness will be sent home with or without a friend, a lover, or a family member, to cope with their diagnosis and with their symptoms.

At the time of this writing, Beth Ann Golden had been a registered nurse at the bedside of hundreds of patients, working on the AIDS unit at St. Luke's-Roosevelt Hospital since it opened its doors in 1987. I am a family nurse practitioner who first met Beth during the course of my teaching responsibilities as a member of the faculty at the Columbia University Graduate School of Nursing.

We began to share our varied experiences both as writers and nurses. Soon the idea for a home care book aimed directly at PWAs and their caregivers began to take shape, in part because of an identified need—a need by people involved with this disease to know more; a need to have specific questions answered about how to survive at home with AIDS.

These needs were identified by visitors of AIDS patients and by the PWAs themselves on the Roosevelt Hospital AIDS unit. Many of those visitors had been and knew that they would again become caregivers upon discharge of the patient from the hospital. In an informal poll of all AIDS patients and their caregivers at Roosevelt Hospital, 20 of 25 identified areas of concern. The response most often expressed was the need for one piece of written material that would discuss subjects concerning the provision of home care to a person with AIDS. Questions repeatedly arose on subjects such as what to do about loss of fluid due to diarrhea, how to help a person with AIDS maintain weight, and issues related to sexuality and displaying affection.

One mother of an AIDS patient interviewed was asked how she had been handling the soiled sheets from her son who had been vomiting repeatedly before being admitted to the hospital. She replied that she had been burning them! Despite the lack of knowledge, the insecurity, and the outright fear that many who are directly involved with PWAs feel, and despite the fact that scores of books have been written about AIDS, we have found that not one book specifically tackles home care in any great detail. Yet every day, hundreds of people with AIDS are sent home with their caregivers (and sometimes without) to confront this situation—often feeling very alone and very afraid.

We hope that our book will allay some of the fears and bolster the confidence of PWAs and caregivers who often do the right things because common sense dictates what they should do. Indeed, many of the recommendations in this book are simple and drawn from common sense. They are often so simple that a person outside the AIDS crisis might wonder why a written guide such as this is needed at all. PWAs and caregivers, however, point out how overwhelming it is to be responsible 24 hours a day, 7 days a week, for the care of another human being. Caregivers we have interviewed emphasize the emotional aspects of caregiving, their own fears of illness and death, and the physical toll on their bodies as reasons why simple recommendations need to be in print before them. Many caregivers liken themselves to new parents reaching for their copies of Dr. Spock's book. Emotional involvement and exhaustion often prevent caregivers from calmly thinking through a problem and arriving at a solution themselves.

In addition, it is always reassuring to see the solution you arrived at in print. And this book is about reassurance, about comfort, about care. It is also a reminder. It reminds PWAs that where there's life there's hope, and it strives to help people with AIDS to help themselves to the maximum extent possible for as long as possible. It reminds caregivers that they too need to be taken care of from time to time; to be good to themselves and their bodies; to laugh now and then. Caregivers should never lose sight of how much they are appreciated—even if their charge is too ill or too distracted to outwardly say so.

In short, this book is for people with AIDS and about people with AIDS. And the words of Dr. Peter Selwyn will serve to sum up what we hope we have accomplished with this work—that is, a home care book that deals with the everyday issues and questions "with reason, compassion, and a sober understanding of the reality of this devastating illness."

J. G.

How to Use This Book

This book is a guide for adult people with AIDS (PWAs) and their caregivers. Thus no attempt is made to discuss the special needs or issues that arise when caring for a child or adolescent with AIDS.

We suggest that you skim through the book, familiarizing yourself with its content and reading chapters you find pertinent to your current circumstances (it is not intended to be read straight through). Then, in the future, you may consult other sections as the need arises.

We have organized the book around specific *subjects* (like dressing changes for venous access devices) and *symptoms*—not disease entities—so that you do not have to diagnose a problem to be able to decide how to deal with it. For example, if you are grappling with a cough, you do not need to decide whether to look under "pneumonia" versus "cardiac disease" or "asthma"—all of which can cause coughing. Simply look for the portion of Chapter 14 dedicated to "cough" to ascertain what other symptoms to look for as well as what to do, what not to do, and when to consult your doctor.

Chapter 1 offers a basic overview of the disease and its assault on the immune system, including how it comes to cause the multitude of opportunistic infections and cancers that it does. Look through Chapter 2 for a "how-to" guide concerning setting up your home to be safe and comfortable for the PWA. It includes a list of equipment you will need. Later chapters include special sections on such issues as what is safe to share, when you need to wear gloves, and how to disinfect contaminated items. Other chapters and appendixes are devoted to how to move people safely, preparing for hospitalization, dealing with legal issues, holistic and other adjunct therapies, laboratory tests, medications, where to seek additional help from organized groups, and further reading.

A glossary gives definitions for terms used throughout the book that you may not be familiar with. The first time one of these words is used, it is defined and set in *italics*. Throughout the book, all vital material is highlighted in **bold,** and special instructions are set off in boxes.

A few words about the conventions used in this book: For brevity's sake, we use the initialism "PWA" to refer to the person with AIDS. We use the word "doctor" to mean the health care professional who is your primary health care provider. And the terms "he" and "she" are meant to be interchangeable when referring to PWAs, caregivers, and health care professionals. We also wish to acknowledge that the caregiver is often the PWA himself or herself. Thus, some sections of this book necessarily address the PWA directly and at other times are aimed at a second person (the caregiver).

What Is a Caregiver?

by J. R. Rich

When I was approached and asked to write about being a caregiver, I was surprised at how little I had thought about this subject. And yet, I am a natural caregiver and acquired my caregiving role by default. It was an automatic reaction for me—as a woman and a by-product of growing up in a highly disfunctional home, where the children were adults early, and by circumstances were thrust into the caregiver role. So I pondered awhile and realized that my only reference point on being a caregiver was to discuss what I had learned about myself through my own experiences.

I learned my first major lesson while taking care of Thom, my first friend with AIDS: There is a huge difference between being a "caretaker" and a "caregiver."

With Thom, I soon began to unravel the confusion my childhood had instilled in me about taking care of people. As a child, I had assumed the role of taking care of people for my own survival. The outside world looks upon people such as I was as saviors, but underneath, the behaviors are based on purely selfish motivations. This communicates a sense of your being a martyr to the person you are taking care of and actually creates in the person guilt about being sick. Thom helped me begin to see the subtle but profound differences in the joy of giving from the heart as opposed to giving to fill a space that feels empty in a person's personality.

At first, I was overwhelmed with feelings of responsibility toward Thom and went to the hospital every day for four months. I began to lose my own sense of self and felt as if my life were temporarily on hold until Thom's journey was complete. I refused to attend support meetings set up for people like me, because I felt I was fine. So, the support team—Ron, head of volunteers, and Beth and Peter, who were nurses—came to me. They each individually counseled me and taught me the great value for Thom in taking care of myself. I saw that if I didn't take care of myself first, I was useless to Thom as a friend and a caregiver. As I began to negotiate the balance of taking care of myself and Thom, my life took on new colors. I felt the deep satisfaction of really loving my friend, and the desire to be there deepened because I felt like I was not giving up anything to care for Thom—only bringing more meaningful experiences into my life.

I next learned the lesson of reaching out and asking for help—something I had never been good at. One year during that time, Christmas was approaching, and I had planned to go home to Atlanta. But Thom was still in the hospital. He was heading more in the direction of dying than living, and I was torn about what I should do. I decided that I had to go home because that was what I needed. I asked my friends who were also supporting Thom and myself to take over during the holidays. I realized that by taking total charge over Thom, I had not only limited my own support but had inadvertently limited their experiences with Thom. I learned the value of getting out of the way and allowing him the support of many instead of the dependency on one.

The greatest gift Thom gave me was the ability to retain my sense of humor during what feels like deep tragedy. Thom had a terrific dry wit and sarcastic humor, which he maintained until our final moments together. He taught me to greet life's challenges with as much laughter as you can muster even with tears of grief streaming down your cheeks.

There was a stage in Thom's illness where he truly despised food of any sort. This was a dramatic challenge for us to deal with, because through most of Thom's illness, he had retained an enormous appetite. He was a huge, strapping man of about 230 pounds. He was a dancer and his hobby was body building. The restaurant we both worked at willingly provided for any food requests he made, which were generally for filet mignon or sirloin steaks with all the trimmings. So, in the later part of his illness with his appetite diminishing, a lot of pressure was placed on Thom to eat.

I arrived at the hospital one day to find Thom staring at his plate with a look of despair in his eyes. As I walked in, he voiced his anger and frustration about everyone's energy being focused on controlling his eating. He was very frightened of the disapproving looks and tones of voices that the food technicians would use as they took away the untouched food trays. His fear was taking the form of anger. Basically, what he said was, "I'm going to belt the next person who tells me to eat. . . . She's going to be back here any minute yelling at me and forcing me to eat." He had tears in his eyes and I closed my eyes and prayed. Within seconds, I found myself raking the food into napkins and hiding the bundles in the bottom of the trash cans—much to Thom's delight. He joined in, and we crowed over our apparent victory. I, of course, told the nurses that Thom did not eat his dinner, but I also stressed that I did not want Thom shamed or reprimanded for his choice not to eat.

I guess Thom still carried some shame, however, about his inability to eat. For the next two weeks, the nurses told me Thom's appetite had increased and he was eating. One Sunday, my friend Suzanne and I were visiting. We decided to look in Thom's bottom drawer for some cassettes. As Suzanne went over to open the drawer, Thom said in a very serious tone, "I wouldn't do that if I were you." Suzanne opened the drawer slowly to find two weeks of food shoveled into the secret hiding place! Suzanne and I stared at each other in silent disbelief. We looked at Thom, who was lying in bed, hands folded under his chin, and he said, "I told you not to do that." At this point, we all broke out in laughter. It felt as if all the emotions we had ever felt during this time—the fear, the grief, the love—had all been given a life in the form of side-splitting laughter. We laughed until we cried, and we continued to laugh even beyond the tears. We knew then, as we always had, in the words of our dear friend, Thom, "I am running this show, so get over it."

There is a level of control that is loving, but control in the form of taking away a person's rights is *not* loving. I saw Thom needed to exercise his right to say no, and I realized the importance of allowing Thom to have a choice in as many situations as possible. People lose a lot of this luxury in a hospital setting: They have no choice in when to eat, very limited choice in what to eat, no choice in who is going to be a roommmate, who is going to drop in and when they visit, and so on. Patients also basically lose the right to privacy simply by virtue of the circumstances. So I began to consciously give Thom as many choices as possible, even simple ones such as whether he would prefer the door to his room to be left open or closed. He struggled with the loss of his independence, but then regained it with direct honesty.

The most beautiful gift Thom gave me was to allow me to witness his personal growth through his experience and blossoming. I began to blossom also. We had many of the same lessons and issues to confront within ourselves. He was not only my friend and my care receiver, he was also my teacher. I feel strongly that there are no accidents in life. Despite the heartbreak and despair that is ever present in dealing with a life-challenging illness, I feel there is a higher purpose present in our experiences with it.

With Thom's death, I moved into a deeper place within myself. Thom is present in that deepness. Though we may not physically continue to walk hand in hand on this earth, we still remain connected in that depth. His presence is felt in the energy of my laughter, my grief, and my continuing growth. It would appear that without the presence of his body, the relationship is still and quiet.

Since Thom's death, I have become a volunteer in caring for AIDS patients. The difference between entering the room of a person with whom you have already established a relationship and a stranger's has given me many insights. For example, I noticed that I spent a lot of time in caregiving activities and "doing" and was uncomfortable and uneasy in just "being." I placed pressure on myself as I entered each patient's room to *do* something, *say* something— to fill up the space with anything other than just standing there and being there. This pressure translated itself into an uncomfortable energy in the room.

I also began to notice my own fears: fear of illness, fear of people, fear of rejection. I noticed how my fears created a defensiveness. I was truly not present with the person in front of me. It was as if I were in a state of unconsciousness, oblivious to my surroundings. It reminded me of my younger days when I would meet someone to whom I was attracted. Nervousness would bubble up into mindless chatter aimed at impressing and above all else at avoiding a quiet place or a lull in conversation. Later, with sanity restored, I would not even be able to recall the conversation. I would think, "Who was that and what was that about?"

My greatest insight, however, has been that I must learn to receive in order to go deeper as a caregiver. In my most complete and satisfying visits with someone, there was a mutual energy exchange of giving and receiving. I began to practice acting like I was relaxed even if I was in total fear. Through prayer and meditation, I began to uncover the reasons for my fearful behavior. I continue to delve deeper into these issues, to observe myself and grow. I still become afraid and nervous. It would only be my ego that would think I am a caregiver because I am so giving and together.

As I said earlier, I don't believe in accidents. I know for me, being a caregiver is a mutual exchange. Someone once said, "God will use whatever he can get his hands on." I see now that the universe has taken an unhealthy caretaker and has begun to transform her into a caregiver. Through this process, my own wounds are being healed at the same time as others' needs are being met. To me, caregiving is a journey to self, and truly, is there any other place to go?

PART I

What Is AIDS?

CHAPTER 1

Understanding the Human Immunodeficiency Virus

Stan's parents sat in overstuffed leather chairs, their faces frozen, their minds racing. Across the desk was the doctor. He might just as easily have been a judge who had just passed sentence upon their son. They grappled to understand the meaning of his words and how this would change all of their lives.

Stan's mother's mind wandered. She was thinking back to happier times, like the day she found out that she was pregnant. Stan had been a child who was very much wanted. Max and Esther had tried for five years to have a child. In those days, people did not discuss infertility. Little was understood about the causes. Less still was understood about the cures. You just had to keep trying and in the meantime face the inevitable, embarrassing questions. Questions such as: "So when am I going to be a grandmother?" or, "You two are such a lovely couple. Why don't you have any children?"

Esther rushed home to make the announcement to Max over his favorite dinner. They spent the next nine months with their heads in the clouds. When Stan was born, he was immediately the star of the family.

Through the years, Stan never failed to live up to expectations. He was an A student. He played the piano and baseball with equal precision and skill. Later, Stan attended law school in San Francisco and moved to Los Angeles to join a major film studio as an entertainment lawyer.

Meanwhile, no one back home in the East knew of Stan's "secret life." It didn't seem odd that Stan, still single, would have a male roommate. Stan could not bring himself to tell his parents that this man was his lover.

Max, Esther, and Stan were such a close family. Stan was as devoted to them as they were to him. He knew they would never understand. He believed that they would somehow feel guilty—blame themselves for "bringing him up wrong."

And now they sat across from this doctor trying to listen to his words, but not hearing them. Stan's roommate had called them when Stan was hospitalized. Stan had probably contracted AIDS while a student in San Francisco. There was no widespread knowledge of the disease then and Stan was leading the carefree life of someone who at last felt liberated from a lifetime of secrets. Little did he suspect that the newfound freedoms of his student days would become the cruel prison of today.

In many ways, Stan is luckier than many people with AIDS. Max and Esther still love him and want to do all that they can to help. But as they sat in the doctor's office with a million questions on their minds, none was formulated on their lips. There was too much to understand all at once. What was this disease? What did it mean? How did they feel about it? About Stan's homosexuality? Could they take care of him themselves when he came out of the hospital? What would this entail? Should they allow his roommate to be involved? What did Stan want? What did they want? And last, if not least . . . what had happened?

The Origins and Spread of AIDS

The *virus* that causes AIDS was discovered separately in mid-1984 by three different scientific teams (led by Drs. Gallo, Montagnier, and Levy, respectively). It was given various names through the years, but the one finally settled upon by an international committee in 1986 is HIV, which stands for *human immunodeficiency virus.* HIV is somewhat unique among human viruses because of the type of genetic material it possesses and the way in which it destroys the immune system. Because of its unusual behavior, HIV poses many challenges to scientists. They must race against its seemingly endless ability to mutate as well as the speed with which it is taking over the cells of more and more individuals every day.

As of the writing of this book, a total of 718,894 cases of AIDS has been reported worldwide, with 315,390 of those cases originating in the United States. However, the World Health Organization, the Centers for Disease Control and Prevention (CDC) in Atlanta, and Dr. Louis Sullivan, the Secretary of the U.S. Department of Health and Human Services, all believe that reported cases are just the tip of the iceberg. It is more likely that at least 2.5 million people, in 186 countries, have AIDS and that another 14 million are infected with the virus but are yet to display any symptoms of the disease. The World Health Organization projects that 30 to 40 million people will be infected with HIV by the year 2000. Researchers fear that a quarter to a third of HIV positive people will come down with a full-blown case of AIDS by seven years post-infection and that all of them will die of its ravages eventually if a cure is not discovered. Thus far, 194,334 people have succumbed to the infection since the disease began to be tracked in the United States in June of 1981. According to sources at the Centers for Disease Control and Prevention National AIDS Clearinghouse, one person dies every 13 minutes from AIDS.

Tracking the Epidemic

Theories abound as to where the virus originated and how it infiltrated the U.S. population. Some theorize that it was brought into this country by people who had visited areas in Africa or the Caribbean where HIV had previously taken hold. Others say that it is a mutant strain of a virus that was already present in animals similar to ourselves. One final theory of particular interest is that it is a *mutation* of a harmless virus isolated from healthy prostitutes in

Senegal, West Africa. This related virus, isolated by Dr. Max Essex of the Harvard School of Public Health and named HIV Type 2 or HTLV-IV, may hold the key to developing a vaccine against the lethal HIV strain.

AIDS appeared on the medical horizon rather abruptly in a short report in the June 5, 1981, issue of a then somewhat obscure pamphlet published by the Centers for Disease Control and Prevention, entitled *The Morbidity and Mortality Weekly Report.* In this particular issue of *MMWR,* doctors in California described a cluster of cases of a rare pneumonia called *Pneumocystis carinii (PCP)* among *homosexual* men. About a month later, another report discussed the appearance—again, among young homosexual men—of a cancer called *Kaposi's sarcoma (KS),* which usually afflicts older men. Soon the CDC began tracking all cases of PCP and KS. The hunt was on to try to solve the enigma of this syndrome of rare and *opportunistic infections* and *malignancies.* It was in 1982 that the CDC officially adopted the name acquired immunodeficiency syndrome, or AIDS, for short.

Epidemiologists hypothesize that the first case of AIDS in the Western Hemisphere probably occurred between 1976 and 1978 and that the disease probably appeared even earlier in central Africa. Originally, it was believed to be linked to butyl or amyl nitrate "poppers" used by homosexual men for their alleged *aphrodisiac* properties. When this was ruled out as a cause, the frequenting of gay bathhouses—where homosexual men had sexual encounters with many different partners—was investigated.

Then in 1986 Dr.Gerald Friedland of Montefiore Medical Center in the Bronx, New York, appeared in a *Newsweek* cover story that shocked the country with the news that AIDS was not strictly a disease of gay, promiscuous men. He had uncovered multiple cases among *heterosexuals,* both male and female, who were also intravenous drug users.

If the world was not frightened and dismayed enough to learn that AIDS could infect those with rather atypical lifestyles, the news really hit home as report after report identified new at-risk groups (*hemophiliacs* and blood transfusion recipients, among others), until we reached the reality that confronts us today: Just about anyone and everyone is at risk. You might be a teenager, a college student, a yuppie, or a retiree. You might be male, female, black, white, or Asian. It is not your age, the color of your skin, or your ethnicity that determines your risk. Instead, it is your lifestyle and your behavior.

By the mid-1980s AIDS had been definitely determined to be a *sexually transmitted disease*—a blood and body fluid–borne virus. However, it is still hypothesized by some that other factors, "cofactors," may determine why some people carry HIV without manifesting AIDS and others quickly succumb to the full syndrome. Some of the cofactors known to suppress the immune system include: use of recreational drugs; repeated infections with diseases such as *herpes simplex, cytomegalovirus,* and *Epstein-Barr virus;* and the direct entry of sperm into the bloodstream through small tears made in the rectal lining during anal *intercourse.* Of course, other environmental conditions (heavy drinking, stress, poor nutrition) may also play a role.

An Assault on the Immune System

Microbes and Opportunistic Infections

From the moment of birth, each human being is exposed to a multitude of substances produced by the world around us. There are *microbes* and chemicals in the birth canal we must make our way through, in the air we must breathe, and in the food and water we must drink to survive. The embrace of a friend, the kiss of a lover, the first juicy bite of a summer peach—all of these and more present substances to us that our bodies must process. We must determine if these materials are foreign or a part of us. And if they are foreign, it then must be determined whether or not these chemicals pose a threat to our survival. The cells of our immune system make these determinations for us and are primarily responsible for defending us against any harmful invaders once they are identified.

Microbes are everywhere. If you could put this page under a microscope, you would see it teeming with a world normally unseen by us. Indeed, there are thousands of microbes on the surface of our skin and inside our bodies all the time. *Microbiologists* consider us the "hosts" to these numerous bacteria, viruses, and *fungi*. Most microbes are harmless to a healthy person with an intact immune system. They can even be beneficial. Some produce as by-products of their chemical reactions certain vitamins and other substances we need and don't make ourselves. Others protect us from their harmful counterparts simply by being present and altering the environment in such a way that *pathogenic* strains cannot survive.

Only about 3 percent of all the different varieties of microorganisms on earth are capable of producing disease in humans. They are prevented from doing so by a complex system of mechanical barriers (the skin and mucous membranes, for example) as well as chemical substances that destroy them before they damage our cells.

Another 10 percent are "opportunistic" pathogens. It is this group that is of particular interest in AIDS. As the name implies, opportunistic microorganisms may be of little consequence to people unless something occurs in the body to afford them the opportunity to wreak havoc. A certain type of bacterium may live innocuously in the mouth, for example. But if that bacterium is permitted to enter the bloodstream through a human bite, it can cause a life-threatening infection of the blood called *septicemia*.

Invasion by harmful "outsiders" is one way to disrupt the normal balance between host and microbial flora. Think of it this way. We as humans are the landlord in a huge housing complex. Some microbes are invited guests or rent-paying tenants. They don't trouble us and may even help us out. Along come squatters in the form of pathogenic bacteria, fungi, or viruses. They disrupt the harmony of the household and may even cause some of the usually peaceful tenants to start trouble.

Other circumstances permit opportunistic infections to flourish in a healthy person. These may include: nutritional deficiencies, stress, hormonal changes, or the introduction of a new chemical or drug. A common example of this last circumstance occurs when a woman takes an *antibiotic* to cure a sore throat. The drug is not selective; that is, it not only kills off the harmful bacteria present in her throat but it also may kill off much of the bacteria that live in harmony with her body while leaving fungi unaffected. This then permits the overgrowth of a normally innocuous fungus in her vagina called *Candida albicans*. This fungus, usually held in check by bacteria, is now left unopposed and can proliferate to the point of causing annoying symptoms such as vaginal discharge, itching, and odor—the classic yeast infection.

The Normal Immune System

AIDS is an *immunodeficiency* disease. This means that the normal harmony and checks and balances under which we coexist with microbes is disrupted by a defect in the body's defenses. Although the complexities of immunology are far beyond the scope or purpose of this book, a fundamental understanding of how the normal immune system keeps microbes in check is essential to understand what goes wrong when the body is infected with the human immunodeficiency virus.

Our *bone marrow* is the birthplace of the immune system. Within the bone marrow, immature blood cells develop into various components of the immune system. Some are called *leukocytes,* or *white blood cells.* There are leukocytes whose primary responsibility is to surround or engulf a foreign invader and chemically digest it in a process called *phagocytosis.* Others contain special chemicals that attack and destroy molecules (usually proteins) that the body recognizes as foreign. These foreign molecules are known as *antigens.* Antigens trigger the production by the immune system of substances called *antibodies,* designed to oppose them.

Of all the different leukocyte types, probably the most important ones— key to the proper functioning of the immune system—are the *lymphocytes.* The lymphocytes are to the immune system what the brain is to the rest of the body. Constituting about a third of all immune system cells, lymphocytes turn on, turn off, and regulate the functioning of all of the remaining 60 percent of leukocytes involved in immunity.

Lymphocytes are divided into three main types: *B cells, T cells,* and *null cells* (which are neither B nor T). Each B cell produces an antibody to only one specific antigen. Once the antibody comes in contact with the antigen, they fit together like a key into a lock. The antibody effectively neutralizes the harmful effects of that antigen by forming with it into an inactive complex that may then be destroyed by other elements of the immune system (collectively called *complement*) in a series of steps known as the *complement cascade.*

This works very well against simple bacteria. However, when the body is confronted with a more complex enemy, such as a virus or a poison (a *toxin*) produced by a bacterium or a virus, B cells require assistance from a particular subgroup of T cells called *T helper cells.* In essence, they help the antibody-antigen reaction. T helper cells also play a role in activating other T cells, such as those involved in fighting cancers.

When the antigen has been effectively eradicated, *T suppressor cells* stop any further production of antibody. T helper and T suppressor cells are also named *T4* and *T8* lymphocytes, respectively, according to chemical markers on their surfaces that are used to identify them.

Not much is understood about the third and final subset of T lymphocytes, the null cells. They appear to secrete toxic chemicals capable of killing aberrant cells of the body that have been adulterated by mutations or viruses. Thus, the most prominent of the null cells are commonly called *natural killer cells* or *NK cells.*

The body has a variety of different methods of locating, attacking, and eliminating pathogens. During phagocytosis, special types of white blood cells called *macrophages* migrate to the site of invasion. They are systematically attracted there by special chemicals produced either by the microbe itself or the cells of the body. Once there, the invader becomes attached to the surface of the macrophage, which then extends itself to completely surround and trap the microbe inside. Once the microbe is so trapped, the macrophage (or phagocyte) secretes chemicals to kill and digest it. This is how the body rids itself not only of bacteria but also of old blood, dead tissues, and other debris, and renegade cells that cause cancer.

In another scenario, primarily involving viruses, *parasites,* fungi, and cancers, macrophages release antigens as by-products of the destruction of these invaders. These antigens whip the T lymphocytes into action. Clones of T cells form—some are T helper cells; some are T suppressor cells; others are killer T cells. The T helper cells activate the B lymphocytes to produce antibodies specific to that antigen. Binding to the antigen, the antibody immobilizes and inactivates it until it is eliminated by complement. Meanwhile, any enemy cells that have slipped through will be sought out and destroyed by the killer T cells.

After the troublesome pathogen has been effectively eradicated, T suppressor cells signal the B cells that antibody production specific to that antigen is no longer needed, and that aspect of the immune system shuts down. In time, all but a few *memory* T and B cells will remain, ready to multiply rapidly should the body ever encounter this particular enemy again.

In summary, the normal immune system consists of a complicated series of steps including:

- Phagocytosis by macrophages with the presentation of antigens as a by-product,
- T and B cell–mediated antibody production,
- Complement cascade, and
- Destruction of any elusive infected cells by killer T cells.

HIV Infection and the Destruction of the Immune System

HIV, like any other virus, is mainly a core of genetic material (called either *RNA* or *DNA*) surrounded by a protein coat. Viruses differ from other microorganisms in that they are like the stripped-down model of a car: only the absolute essentials are there, with no added options or frills. Thus, viruses are equipped with only the genetic material necessary to allow them to reproduce. They accomplish this by taking over the nerve center of another living thing (its *nucleus*) and directing it to stop whatever function it was performing and start making virus. Viruses are incapable of surviving outside of a host. Once the virus has altered the nucleus and directed it to replicate more virus, the infected cell is then destroyed, or breached, to permit the newly formed viral particles to be released and dispersed throughout the body. This permits the virus to spread (and continue to reproduce itself) within the host and/or from person to person to ensure the virus's continued survival.

In the case of HIV, the virus begins by attaching itself to susceptible cells via a protein on its surface called *gp-120*. Certain cells in the human body contain a compatible protein on their surfaces called *CD4*. Specifically, the cells that contain the surface antigen CD4, and thus become infected with AIDS, include many of the cells of the immune system as well as those of the brain, lungs, and intestinal tract.

Once gp-120 and CD4 link up, yet another viral protein permits the virus (now attached to the surface of the human cell) to penetrate and become incorporated into the host's cell. As was mentioned earlier, a virus contains genetic material within its core. Genetic material is one of only two types: RNA or DNA. Human cells "understand" the commands of DNA, which contain the codes for producing more of the cells specific to each and every one of our bodies. With the exception of identical twins, all humans have a unique DNA composition that makes us who we are.

HIV is a *retrovirus*, meaning that it contains RNA instead of the DNA contained in most of the viruses that ordinarily infect humans. Retroviruses are a relatively rare and new enemy to humans. An RNA-containing virus ordinarily would not be compatible with human cells, because the RNA codes would be gibberish to the cell nuclei that are used to following the commands of DNA. HIV can reproduce in our bodies, however, because it contains a vital chemical called *reverse transcriptase*. Reverse transcriptase translates RNA into DNA, thus making it comprehensible to the nuclei of human cells.

Using reverse transcriptase, the viral particles become integrated into the cell, and its genetic code becomes indistinguishable from the body's own DNA. Infected cells start to manufacture the AIDS virus to the exclusion of their own vital functions. When this happens, the body begins to break down and disease ensues.

Specifically, it is theorized that the large-scale release of virions (viral particles) from the human cells ruptures their cell membranes, killing cells en masse. In addition, the AIDS virus may cause human body cells to stick together, bonding them into a useless mass of tissue unable to function and survive.

Because HIV has the ability to mutate as fast as antibodies are produced against it, and because CD4 is present on the surface of many cells involved in immunity (T4 cells, in particular), the immune system itself is extremely vulnerable to the AIDS virus and is helpless to defend itself or the rest of the body against it.

The body is thus unable to fight against either HIV or any other threat. In other words, with so many immune cells out of commission (remember: T4 cells regulate not only other T cells but antibody-producing B cells as well), the body cannot defend itself against *any* pathogens. Nor can it destroy its own mutated cells, which then go on to cause cancers if left unchecked. And finally, the opportunistic microbes that live within our bodies begin to overgrow and cause disease. The result is what we see in a full-blown case of AIDS: overwhelming opportunistic infections and cancers.

Defining AIDS

The CDC Definition of AIDS

On December 18, 1992, the Centers for Disease Control and Prevention in Atlanta issued a revised classification system for HIV infection and an expanded definition of what constitutes a case of acquired immunodeficiency syndrome. To understand the new criteria, it's important to first understand the old definition.

In 1987, the CDC stated that "a case of AIDS is defined as an illness characterized by one or more 'indicator' diseases" even if there had been no conclusively positive HIV test. At the time, according to the CDC, (*MMWR* 36, Supp. no. 1S (1987):3S–15S), the indicator diseases included the following for adults and adolescents (pediatric definitions have been omitted for the purpose of this book):

1. *candidiasis* of the *esophagus, trachea, bronchi,* or lungs
2. *cryptococcosis,* extrapulmonary [outside of the lungs]
3. *cryptosporidiosis* with diarrhea persisting [for more than] one month
4. cytomegalovirus disease of an organ other than the liver, spleen or lymph nodes in a patient [older than] 1 month
5. herpes simplex virus infection causing a mucocutaneous ulcer [a sore of the skin or mucous membranes] that persists longer than 1 month; or bronchitis, or esophagitis [inflammations of the lungs or esophagus] for any duration affecting a patient [more than] 1 month of age
6. Kaposi's sarcoma affecting a patient [less than] 60 years of age
7. *lymphoma* [cancer of the lymphatic tissue or lymph glands] of the brain . . . affecting a patient [less than] 60 years of age
8. *Mycobacterium avium* complex or *M. kansasii* disease, disseminated [spread to] . . . a site other than or in addition to lungs, skin, or cervical or hilar [lung] lymph nodes
9. *Pneumocystis carinii* pneumonia
10. *progressive multifocal leukoencephalopathy* [a rare, rapidly progressive and usually fatal disease of the central nervous system caused by an infection with a "slow" virus]
11. *toxoplasmosis* of the brain affecting a patient [more than] 1 month of age

In a person who had tested positive for HIV, the presence of certain other indicator diseases was considered to indicate a definite diagnosis of AIDS. These included brain infections collectively called "AIDS dementia," *lympho-*

mas and other cancers, *tuberculosis*-related diseases, *salmonella* blood poisoning, cytomegalovirus retinitis–related blindness, and "HIV wasting syndrome," among others.

Many of these diseases have the same or similar symptoms, all of which will be addressed in the chapters that follow. These include: generalized weakness or fatigue, unexplained weight loss, poor appetite, swollen glands, persistent fevers, *anemia, thrush,* skin rashes, mental or behavioral changes, chronic diarrhea, cough, and shortness of breath.

The recent changes in the classification system and case definition include all HIV-infected persons who have less than a certain percentage of their lymphocytes as T-lymphocytes or who have an absolute number—that is, less than 200—of so-called CD4+ T-lymphocytes (T helper cells). (In Appendix A, we discuss how T-lymphocyte, or CD4, counts are conducted.) These criteria were added, according to the CDC, because:

> The CD4+ T-lymphocyte is the primary target for HIV infection because of the affinity [attraction] of the virus for the CD4 surface marker. The CD4+ T-lymphocyte [T helper cell] coordinates a number of important immunologic functions, and a loss of these functions results in progressive impairment of the immune response. . . . Studies of the natural history of HIV infection have documented a wide spectrum of disease manifestations, ranging from *asymptomatic* infection [HIV positive and well] to life-threatening conditions characterized by severe immunodeficiency, serious opportunistic infections, and cancers. Other studies have shown a strong association between the development of life-threatening opportunistic illnesses and the absolute number . . . or percentage of the CD4+ T-lymphocytes . . . *As the number of CD4+ T-lymphocytes decreases, the risk and severity of opportunistic illnesses increase . . .*

Whereas back in 1987, CD4+ T-lymphocyte cell counts (CD4 counts) were not as widely used or available, today they are commonly employed not only as a means of identifying a case of AIDS, but also to attempt to define what stage the person is in and to track the severity and progression of illness. Scientists have discovered that initiating treatment (such as giving the medication *AZT*) when individuals' tests reveal CD4 counts of certain amounts can in some cases prevent the onset of particular opportunistic infections. In short, according to the CDC, "measures of CD4+ T-lymphocytes are used to guide clinical and therapeutic management of HIV-infected persons."

At present, a person is considered to have AIDS if he is HIV positive and has a CD4 count of less than 200. Furthermore, the definition of AIDS has been expanded to include three more indicator diseases: pulmonary tuberculosis (TB of the lung), recurrent pneumonia, and invasive cervical cancer (cancer of the lowermost portion of the uterus that has spread beyond its initial location). This does not mean that every person who contracts TB or cervical cancer, or has pneumonia more than once, has AIDS! These conditions indicate a diagnosis of full-blown AIDS in HIV positive people only.

The Hierarchy of Illness

Since 1987 the definition of AIDS has covered a broad spectrum of signs and symptoms, from little or no evidence of active disease to severe, debilitating, and even life-threatening illness. Scientists have designated a hierarchy for classifying the disease. Some like to compare HIV infection with a pyramid (see Figure 1.1). At the base of the pyramid are millions of individuals worldwide who have been exposed to and infected with the virus. Often, such a person will have a brief flulike or mononucleosislike illness, which will resolve itself; the person will then feel well, although be a carrier of HIV. These individuals are "asymptomatic and HIV positive." As you make your way up the pyramid, there are individuals who, again, feel well but have chronically swollen lymph nodes throughout their bodies. They are said to have "persistent generalized *lymphadenopathy.*"

Next come those who experience signs and symptoms of AIDS to varying degrees. They may manifest fever, weakness, diarrhea, and wasting. They may suffer from memory loss, attention deficits, psychological problems, difficulties with maintaining balance, even seizures and paralysis. Others may develop rashes, mouth lesions, vaginitis, pelvic infections, or abnormal *PAP smears.* Yet they do not have any of the specific opportunistic infections that the CDC expressly lists in their new "surveillance case definition." These groups used to be said to have *"AIDS-related complex (ARC),"* but that term is no longer sanctioned by the CDC. Since 1987, the CDC has decided to classify everyone who is HIV positive as falling somewhere along the spectrum of acquired immunodeficiency syndrome rather than considering ARC and AIDS as two separate and distinct entities. This permits better surveillance of the AIDS epi-

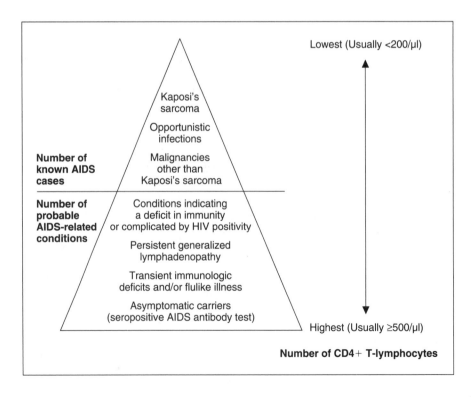

FIGURE 1.1
Pyramid of HIV-Related Illnesses

TABLE 1.1   *Rate of Progression to AIDS with Each Passing Year*

Years from Seroconversion	Rate of Progression
1	0%
2	Less than 1%
3	3%
4	6%
5	12%
6	20%
7	27%
8	36%
9	45%
10	53%

From "1992–93 Recommendations for the Medical Care of Persons with HIV Infection." The Johns Hopkins School of Medicine, 1992. Reprinted with permission.

demic and ensures better care and financial benefits for all who are infected with the virus whatever their symptoms.

Finally, as you approach the apex of the pyramid, a small percentage of HIV positive people suffer the full-blown syndrome, including immunodeficiency-induced opportunistic infections and cancers.

Tables 1.1 and 1.2 illustrate the chance of progressing from the base of the pyramid to its apex with each passing year once a person is discovered to be HIV positive and according to CD4 counts. Table 1.3 is a summary of the new classifications, according to CD4+ T-lymphocyte categories and clinical categories.

TABLE 1.2   *Probability of AIDS within 18 Months Based on CD4 Cell Count*

CD4 Cell Count	Probability of AIDS
100 per cubic millimeter	60%
200 per cubic millimeter	30%
300 per cubic millimeter	15%
400 per cubic millimeter	8%
500 per cubic millimeter	3%

From "1992–93 Recommendations for the Medical Care of Persons with HIV Infection." The Johns Hopkins School of Medicine, 1992. Reprinted with permission.

TABLE 1.3 **The New CDC Classification Systems for HIV and AIDS**

CD4+ T-Lymphocyte Categories
Category 1: Greater than or equal to 500 cells per microliter
Category 2: 200–499 cells per microliter
Category 3: Less than 200 cells per microliter

(Note: The CDC states that HIV-infected persons should be classified using the lowest accurate, but not necessarily the most recent, CD4 count.)

Clinical Categories
Category A
- Asymptomatic HIV infection (HIV positive with no evidence of illness)
- Persistent generalized lymphadenopathy (chronically swollen glands)
- Acute (primary) HIV infection with accompanying illness or history of acute HIV infection (HIV positive with flulike illness)

Category B
Conditions with symptoms not included in the Category C List, but that occur in any HIV positive person and are attributed to HIV infection, are indicative of a defect in immunity or are considered by physicians to have a clinical course or to require management that is complicated by the presence of infection by the HIV virus. Examples of Category B illnesses include: thrush (a yeast infection of the mouth), early (noninvasive) cervical cancer, fever, or chronic diarrhea.

Category C
HIV positive persons who have or who have had any of the following conditions.

- Candidiasis of bronchi, trachea, or lungs
- Candidiasis, esophageal
- Cervical cancer, invasive*
- Coccidioidomycosis, disseminated or extrapulmonary
- Cryptococcosis, extrapulmonary
- Cryptosporidiosis, chronic intestinal (>1 month's duration)
- Cytomegalovirus disease (other than liver, spleen, or nodes)
- Cytomegalovirus retinitis (with loss of vision)
- Encephalopathy, HIV-related
- Herpes simplex: chronic ulcer(s) (>1 month's duration); or bronchitis, pneumonitis, or esophagitis
- Histoplasmosis, disseminated or extrapulmonary
- Isosporiasis, chronic intestinal (>1 month's duration)
- Kaposi's sarcoma
- Lymphoma, Burkitt's (or equivalent term)
- Lymphoma, immunoblastic (or equivalent term)
- Lymphoma, primary, of brain
- *Mycobacterium avium* complex or *M. kansasii*, disseminated or extrapulmonary
- *Mycobacterium tuberculosis*, any site (pulmonary* or extrapulmonary)

(continued)

TABLE 1.3   *(continued)*

- *Mycobacterium,* other species or unidentified species, disseminated or extrapulmonary
- *Pneumocystis carinii* pneumonia
- Pneumonia, recurrent*
- Progressive multifocal leukoencephalopathy
- *Salmonella* septicemia, recurrent
- Toxoplasmosis of brain
- Wasting syndrome due to HIV

*Added in the 1993 expansion of the AIDS surveillance case definition.

The Signs and Symptoms of HIV- and AIDS-Related Diseases

The diseases that afflict people with AIDS are primarily opportunistic infections or cancers. This section provides brief explanations of the conditions you may be dealing with. The information contained here is by no means comprehensive. It should, however, provide a foundation for understanding this disease so that you can better digest and utilize the information in the rest of the book.

Opportunistic Infections

Approximately 20 to 25 different viruses, bacteria, parasites, and fungi have been known to cause opportunistic infections in people with AIDS. The common ones are briefly explained here, along with the symptoms they cause and how they are diagnosed and treated.

Candidiasis

Candidiasis is an infection from a fungus called *Candida albicans* and commonly known as yeast. Yeast is a normal inhabitant of our intestinal tract; under conditions of immunodeficiency, however, it can overgrow and spread to areas where it isn't generally welcome.

In women with AIDS, yeast can cause vaginal itching, burning, redness, and discharge. And in all HIV positive individuals, *Candida* infection of the mouth (called oral thrush) is often the first sign of AIDS illness.

Candida causes patchy white plaque to form in the mouth, on the tongue, and sometimes in the *esophagus,* brain, or lung tissue. Though it is more annoying than life-threatening and is reasonably responsive to antifungal medications (e.g., ketoconazole or amphotericin B), candidiasis may be a sign of worse things to come. In addition, lifelong treatment is usually needed because the yeast commonly returns once medication is withdrawn.

Coccidioidomycosis

Known most commonly as a fungus that is present in areas of the southwestern United States (e.g., southern California and Arizona), *coccidioides immitus* can infect both HIV positive and non-HIV positive people. In nonimmunocompromised hosts, it rarely even causes symptoms; at most, it may cause a self-limited respiratory illness. Even in PWAs, coccidioidomycosis is not common. However, when it does occur (primarily among those who live in areas where the fungus is most prevalent), the infection spreads beyond the lungs (its usual initial site of infection) to the blood, bone marrow, urinary tract, liver, spleen, brain, thyroid, lymph nodes, bones, and skin. It may cause fever, weakness, weight loss, and cough. Currently, the disease is diagnosed by *bronchoscopy* (see Appendix A) and/or cultures of various potential sites of infection (like the blood), and treatment involves lifelong antifungal medications.

Cryptococcosis

Cryptococcus neoformans is the fungus that causes *cryptococcal meningitis,* an inflammation and infection of the membranes that line the brain and spinal cord. Meningitis causes fever, headache, nausea, and vomiting in PWAs so afflicted; however, only a third also experience the usually commonplace symptoms found in non-AIDS patients of stiff neck, seizures, light sensitivity, and changes affecting the *retina* of the eye.

PWAs have been known to have cryptococcosis of other systems of the body, including the skin, heart, joints, eyes, lungs, and intestines. Cryptococcus has been isolated from the brain, lymph nodes, adrenal glands, kidney, spleen, liver, bone marrow, and thyroid as well.

Cryptococcosis may be diagnosed by taking a small sampling of the affected tissue (called a *biopsy*) and analyzing it. There are also blood tests to detect the cryptococcal antigen. Cryptococcosis is primarily treated with an antibiotic called amphotericin B. Since the recurrence rate is generally high, lifelong therapy may be attempted if the PWA is able to tolerate amphotericin's side effects.

Cryptosporidiosis

The microbe that causes cryptosporidiosis is a *protozoan,* a tiny parasitic animal. Although this microbe has been known for many years to cause diseases in calves and other animals, the first human case of cryptosporidiosis was reported only about 15 years ago. When healthy individuals contract cryptosporidiosis (as has happened, for example, with veterinarians and slaughterhouse workers), it causes only a mild diarrheal illness that goes away on its own after a few days.

By contrast, AIDS-related cryptosporidiosis can cause severe bouts of diarrhea. PWAs with the disease may have 10 to 20 watery stools every day for months on end. Such a situation frequently results in wasting and *malnutrition.* In addition, they may suffer from abdominal cramping, nausea, mild fever, and occasional vomiting.

To date, there are experimental therapies, but no definitively effective drugs to cure this condition. PWAs are given treatments to help control the diarrhea and replace depleted essential body fluids and nutrients.

Isosporiasis, caused by another protozoan, *Isospora belli,* is very similar to cryptosporidiosis in terms of signs and symptoms, with one important exception: Isosporiasis responds well to antibiotic therapy with *Bactrim* (trimethoprim and sulfamethoxazole).

Cytomegalovirus Disease

Cytomegalovirus (CMV) is related to the *herpes*virus family. Other herpesviruses are responsible for causing chicken pox, shingles, fever blisters, and genital sores. Nearly half of all well adults show evidence in their blood of having been exposed to this virus. In PWAs, virtually all have positive blood tests for CMV. In these individuals, CMV has been known to cause pneumonias and gastrointestinal disorders, including inflammations of the esophagus and the small and large intestines. The most frightening of its effects is to produce severe damage to the retina, leading to blindness.

A drug called ganciclovir (DHPG) has been proven effective in fighting CMV infections. The drug improves vision by reducing swelling and inflammation of the retina; areas that have already been scarred, however, will never recover, so some blindness may be permanent. An unfortunate aspect of ganciclovir therapy is that it is rarely used when AZT is also being taken. Together, the drugs could cause life-threatening bone marrow suppression.

Herpes Simplex Virus Infection

Most people have heard of herpes simplex virus in relation to its role as a sexually transmitted disease that causes painful genital sores and, occasionally, mouth sores. In PWAs, the most common sites of these ulcers are in and around the rectum. Here, they may cause pain, itching, and bleeding. Because of the suppression of the immune system in PWAs, herpes infections can also sometimes spread beyond the genital and rectal areas to the brain, heart, and esophagus, although it is unusual for them to do so. Herpes simplex responds well to a drug called Zovirax (acyclovir). Like most HIV-related conditions, once treatment is stopped, the infection returns. Therefore, lifelong maintenance therapy is necessary to prevent a resurgence of the illness.

Histoplasmosis

Histoplasma capsulatum is a fungus native to the central and southern portions of the United States. Yet it rarely causes any disease symptoms in healthy people who carry the fungus. When PWAs develop *histoplasmosis,* they come down with a disseminated illness (i.e., one that spreads throughout the PWA's system) characterized by fever, chills, sweats, nausea, vomiting, diarrhea, and weight loss. They may also have skin rashes, pneumonia, and swollen glands. Liver disease is also not uncommon. The diagnosis is sometimes made by attempting to isolate the fungus from blood and body tissues.

Once a diagnosis of histoplasmosis has been established, the infection is usually treated with antifungal medications such as ketoconazole or amphotericin B.

Mycobacterium Tuberculosis and Mycobacterium Avium Intracellulare Complex

For many years, tuberculosis was on the decline in the United States. It conjured up images of bleak sanatoriums, where people used to be confined to slowly succumb to *consumption,* as it was then called. The disease would literally consume a person because no effective therapies existed to cure or control it. It makes for an interesting comparison to AIDS today. And it is especially ironic that virulent and drug-resistant forms of tuberculosis are making a comeback as they find a niche among *immunocompromised* individuals.

Mycobacterium avium intracellulare (MAI) is an exotic relative of *Mycobacterium tuberculosis,* the microbe that was responsible for virtually all the cases of TB that sent people to sanatoriums earlier in this century. *Mycobacterium avium intracellulare, Mycobacterium tuberculosis,* and other strains inhabit the bodies of people with AIDS. But unlike most opportunistic diseases and cancers that afflict those with AIDS, tuberculosis is capable of spreading beyond the "borders," so to speak, of this population to people with intact immune systems. Therefore, all caretakers (medical personnel and laypersons) should be screened for TB using the *Mantoux test* (see Appendix A).

Precautions must be taken to safeguard caregivers and others against TB infection. PWAs with tuberculosis are on respiratory isolation in the hospital and they are not released until their sputum specimens indicate that they are no longer capable of infecting others. Masks are worn to protect health care workers, caregivers, and others from contracting TB, which is spread when someone inhales an infected droplet from the air. TB droplets are capable of remaining suspended in the air for an indefinite period. Thus, whenever anyone enters the room of a PWA with tuberculosis, she must put on a mask, and whenever the PWA ventures out into public areas (e.g., going to the x-ray department), *he* must wear a mask.

Once it gains a foothold within the human body, MAI and other atypical incarnations of TB spread throughout the system. In the case of MAI, *Mycobacterium avium intracellulare complex (MAC)* is the term used to describe the cluster of symptoms associated with this infection. MAI has been isolated from the organs of PWAs with fever, weight loss, swollen glands, cough, and diarrhea who have no other known pathogens that could be causing their symptoms. Doctors and researchers have presumed that MAI is the cause of these symptoms, but this has not been proven. Nor is there an effective cure. Unlike its cousin *M. tuberculosis,* MAI does not seem susceptible to antibiotic treatments, although most of the drugs used to treat tuberculosis are tried.

Pneumocystic Carinii

If there can be a disease made "famous" by AIDS, *Pneumocystis carinii pneumonia (PCP)* is it. Few people who watch television, read newspapers, or listen to the radio have not heard of PCP. The first identified and probably still the most common consequence of getting AIDS is infection with this opportunistic protozoan. In *AIDS: Etiology, Diagnosis, Treatment and Prevention,* Second Edition (DeVito, Vincent, et al. J. B. Lippincott, 1988), Drs. Joseph A. Kovacs and Henry Masur of the National Institutes of Health write:

> Pneumocystic pneumonia is the initial AIDS-defining process (infection or tumor) in 65% of HIV-infected patients and ultimately occurs in at least 80% of patients. Because of the frequency and lethality of this opportunistic infection, its diagnosis, therapy, and prevention are major issues in the management of an HIV-infected patient. (p. 203)

It appears that *Pneumocystic carinii* protozoans infect all humans from an early age, but they never cause disease until the immune system is severely challenged. Then, pneumocystis causes a pneumonia (infection of the lungs) that is similar in symptoms to a dozen other types of respiratory infections, making it very difficult to diagnose. PCP causes chest pain, cough, fever, and shortness of breath. Sometimes it will reveal itself on an ordinary chest X ray, but just as often, it may be absent. There are no simple diagnostic tests to confirm PCP. Most PWAs ultimately require a bronchoscopy to obtain a sample of lung tissue that can be tested to see if this *parasite* is present.

Two primary drugs are currently available for treating PCP: trimethoprim-sulfa and pentamidine. Both effectively clear the infection in 70 to 80 percent of people after about three weeks. Cure rates are slightly higher in PWAs experiencing their first bout of PCP and slightly lower in repeat infections. Many PWAs are placed on long-term antibiotic therapy to prevent a relapse, and those PWAs who are taking AZT at the time of PCP infection actually double their predicted life span from 9 to 18 months. In more severe cases, a traditional anticancer drug combination of trimetrexate with a leucovorin rescue has been used to attempt to enhance the effects of antibiotic drugs. The drug trimetrexate doesn't distinguish between healthy white cells and damaged white cells. The leukovorin rescue is given to help protect the healthy white cells from attack by the anticancer medicine.

The problem is that these drugs have serious side effects when taken in the high doses and for the long terms required to deal with HIV infections. Pentamidine is given in aerosol form to PWAs with mild infections and those needing preventative therapy in the hope of minimizing these adverse reactions.

Salmonella

Salmonella encompasses many bacterial species that cause intestinal diseases in humans. Few individuals in the world have not at some point in their lives succumbed temporarily to the uncomfortable, even debilitating, effects of eating chicken that was improperly prepared or mayonnaise left out too long at the company picnic.

PWAs also get severe diarrhea and cramping, fever, weakness, and loss of appetite from salmonella. The difference is that their symptoms often persist for weeks. And, though food poisoning rarely leads to blood poisoning (septicemia) in healthy individuals, this is a common consequence for people with AIDS.

Salmonella is isolated from the blood and stool of infected individuals, and it is curable using standard antibiotics such as ampicillin.

Toxoplasmosis

Toxoplasma gondii is a protozoan carried by cats. It can be transmitted to humans through contact with cat feces, as can occur when changing a litter box. Although it can cause fetal illness, toxoplasmosis is harmless to most people. Some studies reveal that as many as 9 out of 10 people possess antibodies to toxoplasmosis, meaning that they have been infected at some point in their lives.

For reasons yet unknown, some HIV positive individuals reactivate an old toxoplasmosis infection that has been dormant for years and subsequently develop an inflammation of the brain called *toxoplasmosis gondii encephalitis*. When this occurs, PWAs develop neurologic disease marked by headaches, fever, vision changes, and, later, *seizures* and partial paralysis. A two-drug combination of sulfadiazine and pyrimethamine often clears the infection, but relapses are common.

Cancers

Cancer occurs when the cell's normal replicating mechanism somehow goes awry and abnormal cells begin to grow and develop. Usually these aberrant cells are targeted and destroyed by the lymphocytes of the immune system. When a person has AIDS, his lymphocytes are incapable of acting upon these damaging cells.

Left to their own devices, these mutated cells multiply at an astounding rate until they overgrow the normal tissue in the affected area. But, because these cells are defective, they are unable to carry out the normal functions of the body that are necessary to its survival. Illness ensues because the cancerous cells use the body's resources in a counterproductive manner, essentially draining it of nutrients and energy so that nothing is left for use by the remaining healthy tissues. Furthermore, cancerous cells may produce substances that are toxic to the body.

Cancer as a consequence of an infectious disease is a relatively new and frightening concept. Most of us don't think of cancer as something that we can "catch." Yet, in 1992, the Centers for Disease Control and Prevention documented 5,908 cases of AIDS-related cancers, including Kaposi's sarcoma and various B cell lymphomas. These individuals "caught" cancer in the sense that they were infected with a virus that suppressed the cells in their immune system that are responsible for ridding the body of its abnormal cells.

Kaposi's Sarcoma

Kaposi's sarcoma (KS) was identified more than 100 years ago by an Austro-Hungarian dermatologist named Moritz Kaposi. However, until AIDS came on the scene, KS was an exceedingly rare and relatively *benign* form of skin cancer that primarily affected elderly men of Mediterranean or Eastern European Jewish descent. People rarely died of it because it grew so slowly; it was mainly a cosmetic worry, since it causes ugly blue or purplish spots to appear on the extremities. Initially, it may resemble a bruise, because it is a tumor of the wall of the blood vessel. Unlike a bruise, however, KS will fail to heal after a week or two.

In association with AIDS, a much more virulent, aggressive, and damaging form of Kaposi's sarcoma has happened upon the scene. It has been dubbed *epidemic Kaposi's sarcoma*. Today, 96 percent of all cases of KS in the United States occur among homosexual or bisexual men with AIDS. Kaposi's sarcoma continues to afflict the elderly and the immunocompromised from other causes (such as renal transplant patients on immunosuppressive medications to prevent tissue rejection), but in much smaller numbers. Interestingly, KS seems to have a favorite host even among people with AIDS. More than a quarter of all gay men with AIDS will eventually develop Kaposi's sarcoma, whereas only 3 percent of *intravenous* drug users with AIDS, 3 percent of blood transfusion recipients with AIDS, 3 percent of women with AIDS, and 1 percent of hemophiliacs with AIDS have KS as a manifestation of their disease.

Some scientists have theorized that other cofactors more specific to the homosexual population may assist KS in gaining a foothold. For example, it seems that PWAs with KS commonly also have had a number of different sexually transmitted diseases, have been exposed to certain viruses (e.g., Epstein-Barr, cytomegalovirus, *hepatitis,* and herpes), and have used various recreational drugs, any or all of which may have served as cofactors.

Whatever the cause, KS riddles the body with blue, brown, or purple tumors. They may grow on the skin or infiltrate various internal organs, including the brain, lungs, intestines, and lymph nodes. Because the lesions become so widespread, surgery is usually not an option to eliminate the tumors. Instead, a combination of drugs to boost the immune system (such as interferon or Interleukin-2) and kill the cancer cells (vinblastine, etoposide, vincristine, and bleomycin) may be used in conjunction with radiation therapy.

PWAs rarely succumb to Kaposi's sarcoma alone. Indeed, 80 percent live for an average of two years after diagnosis with KS. By comparison, survival rates drop to 20 percent when opportunistic infections are also present. Tragically, the very same agents necessary to kill the cancer cells in KS cause immunosuppression as a side effect and therefore act as an open invitation to opportunistic diseases.

Non-Hodgkin's or B Cell Lymphomas

Lymphoma refers to a type of cancer that affects the lymphocytes. Lymphomas may be of two types, *Hodgkin's disease* or *non-Hodgkin's lymphoma.* The latter term classifies all cancers of the white blood cells that do not have the characteristic appearance under the microscope of a specific type of cell called a Sternberg-Reed cell. Although PWAs are at risk for developing both types of lymphomas, most get the non-Hodgkin's type. Furthermore, unlike other groups at risk for this disease (mainly immunocompromised children), PWAs seem to have tumors in atypical sites, such as the brain and the bowel.

Like Kaposi's sarcoma, B cell lymphomas seem to be afflictions of homosexual PWAs in particular. Again, a connection can be made with the Epstein-Barr virus. In the United States, EBV infections most commonly cause the disease known as infectious mononucleosis, which is a flulike malady. Infectious mononucleosis causes swollen glands, an inflamed liver and spleen, weakness, and fatigue that may linger for days or weeks before it resolves on its own. By contrast, in both Africa and Asia, EBV virus has been linked to various forms of cancer. In Africa in particular, the Epstein-Barr virus causes *Burkitt's lymphoma,* a malignancy that bears a remarkable resemblance to AIDS-related lymphomas in the United States. This has led some researchers to say that the combination of HIV and EBV is what causes the activation of lymphoma in susceptible PWAs.

Lymphomas are rampant forms of cancer for PWAs. Various combinations of chemotherapeutic agents are used to combat the malignancy, but the remission rate is only about 50 percent.

Invasive Cervical Cancer

The *cervix* is the lowermost portion of the uterus or womb, which is the organ of a woman's body that houses and nourishes a developing fetus. Certain sexually transmitted diseases, including herpes, human papilloma virus (HPV or genital warts), and now HIV, may predispose a woman to develop cervical cancer and cellular abnormalities that are considered to be precancerous. This is because these viruses direct the cells located there to mutate and begin to grow in the wild and erratic manner typical of cancer.

Under the influence of the AIDS virus, cancerous tissue may then invade the main body of the uterus beyond the cervix. Rates of cervical cancer and of all precancerous lesions (called *cervical dysplasia*) have been found to be higher among HIV positive women than among noninfected women, thus prompting the CDC to begin considering cervical cancer in its case definition of AIDS. But because this is so recent a change (tracking began in January 1993), only 41 cases of AIDS-related invasive cervical cancer have been reported as of this writing. Experts predict, however, that the addition of cervical cancer to the list of AIDS-related cancers will have a tremendous impact on the number of AIDS cases identified, and that this will help women to receive better medical care and financial aid for their care than in the past, when AIDS cases were more commonly defined in terms of male-oriented diagnoses.

Cervical dysplasias and cancers in the early stages (noninvasive) have a good cure rate. Treatment is usually accomplished through various surgical techniques, including the following: cryosurgery (freezing the malignant area), laser surgery (excising the tissue with the intense light of a laser beam that cuts and/or burns away the cancer), or in more extensive cases, the removal of a cone-shaped section of tissue from the center of the cervix (conization or cone biopsy). Hysterectomy (surgical removal of the uterus and sometimes its associated structures—such as the ovaries and lymph nodes) is necessary when there is invasive cervical cancer.

PART II

Getting Organized

Goals of Caregiving

1. Maximize autonomy, both for the PWA and for yourself. Whenever possible, encourage the PWA to be as self-sufficient as possible, assisting only when necessary. **Remember: PWAs can cook, clean, drive a car, socialize, travel, go to public places (i.e., bathrooms, pools, cinemas), and so on, as long as they feel able to and their doctor approves.**

2. Promote an environment where the values, customs, and lifestyles of both the PWA and yourself can be respected. Try to understand each other and agree to compromise when necessary.

3. Help the PWA explore and decide who should and should not know the details of the illness and why. Respect the PWA's decision.

4. Learn about and educate others in subjects such as infection control practices, safe sex, and personal care.

5. Maintain the best quality of life for both yourself and the PWA as defined by your own individual wants, needs, and desires.

6. Keep an open mind to the many treatments, ways of relieving pain and stress, experimental *protocols,* thoughts, and opinions you will encounter regarding this unique disease.

CHAPTER **2**

Setting Up a Safe and Comfortable Environment

Household Safety Precautions

After the initial diagnosis of AIDS is made, most people can return home without needing to change anything in the home or introduce any safety measures. However, with the passage of time and the onset of various opportunistic infections, PWAs often become weaker, may have periods of confusion or memory loss, and may experience reduced eyesight, shortness of breath, diarrhea, decreased mobility, or periods of fatigue. Once a PWA has any of these symptoms, it is essential to institute safety precautions in the household to prevent accidents that can cause life-threatening injuries. In addition, a safe, comfortable home environment can make the PWA feel better psychologically as well as physically.

What to Do

- Keep a list of vital telephone numbers handy at all times (see box, page 36).
- Replace all throw rugs, mats, plastic runners, and area rugs with wall-to-wall carpet. If this is too expensive, remove all floor coverings and leave the floors uncovered and unwaxed. This will decrease the possibility of falls due to slipping.
- Make sure carpet does not have worn patches or areas where loose nails may protrude. Keep stairs in good repair. If uncarpeted, install rubber mats, treads, or runners to prevent falls. Place securely anchored handrails on *both* sides of any stairs.
- Remove all loose wires and electrical cords from high-traffic areas. Tack or tape and cover any wires that cannot be removed.
- Maintain good lighting, especially in high-traffic areas, such as the path from the bedroom to the bathroom. Use night-lights throughout the house to light a path from room to room and along staircases.
- Keep floors unobstructed, especially in narrow passageways. Remove from the floor any items such as decorative sculptures, potted plants, hassocks, or throw pillows.

Vital Telephone Numbers

Make a list of the telephone numbers of vital persons and services in your locale. Keep a copy of the list near the telephone; in addition, both the PWA and the caregiver should keep a copy in their wallet or purse. The list should include the numbers of the following:

> PWA (home and work numbers)
> Caregiver (home and work numbers)
> Neighbor
> Physician
> AIDS clinic
> Hospital
> Emergency ambulance service
> Poison control center
> Suicide/Psychiatric emergency/Crisis intervention hotline
> Substance abuse hotline
> Police
> Fire

- Place a nonskid mat on the bottom of the bathtub or shower. Handrails for the bathtub, shower, and commode are a good idea, if you can afford to buy or rent them.
- Consider installing a toilet seat extender. This raises the seat to facilitate the use of the commode and also decreases the chances of falling due to loss of balance.
- Install window guards to prevent falls due to dizziness or confusion.
- Be sure all locks, especially the one on the front door, can be operated from both sides of the door. Give a spare key to a trusted neighbor, close friend, or family member who can be reached at any time. This is to safeguard the PWA in case he accidentally locks himself in or out of the house. It also permits access to the home in case of an emergency.
- Install childproof locks on cabinets and drawers to prevent a confused PWA from gaining access to liquor, cleaning supplies, and other household poisons.

What Not to Do

- **Never leave household cleansers or other potential poisons in unmarked containers or store them near medications or food.**
- Do not move furniture or household items without the PWA's knowledge and consent. Unexpected changes in surroundings can cause confusion, disorientation, and injury if the person trips and falls.

To the PWA: Personal Safety Precautions at Home

- Always wear rubber-soled shoes or slippers; never walk around the house barefoot or in just socks or stockings.
- Be sure bathrobe, pajama pants, and nightgown are no longer than ankle-length and that belts for these items are not long enough to trip over.
- Make sure you have a way to call out for help, especially if you are unable to speak loudly. Consider using an intercom system with a mobile receiver. Baby monitors, which cost about 30 dollars, are excellent for this purpose. A simple, inexpensive solution is to ring a bell or bang on a metal pot with a spoon.
- Keep items that are used often within reach to help preserve energy. Place items such as tissues, the television remote control, and the telephone on a table beside a favorite chair or on a nightstand beside the bed.
- Purchase a cordless telephone or install additional extensions in frequently used rooms to prevent rushing from one room to another when the phone rings. This also enables you to quickly call for assistance in an emergency. Purchase extralong telephone cords so that phones can be placed next to you. Remember to secure long cords to prevent tripping.
- Keep clocks with large numbers in each room. Try to use one that indicates A.M. and P.M. Keep calendars in the most frequented rooms and mark off each day to help recall date and time.
- Wear identification at all times. Medic Alert bracelets or necklaces with your name and address are sold in many drugstores. There is no need to state on the tag that you have AIDS—the tag is strictly for identification in case of confusion or memory loss. Tags inside clothing as well as a wallet identification card are also advisable.

Equipment for the Care of the PWA

There are hundreds of items on the market today for use at home in the care of someone who is chronically ill. Some of these items are an absolute necessity for every home with a PWA in residence. Others are expensive luxuries; that is, they are nice to have but not essential. Buy what you feel you really need and be creative about the rest—a homemade substitute can often work as well as a store-bought product. You can also place an ad in a local paper to see if someone is selling what you need or is willing to donate it, or call local support groups (see Appendix G) for help. Remember: Prices vary, so shop around for the best possible deal.

Essential Equipment

- **Disposable latex gloves.** These gloves *do not* need to be sterile (unless you are using them to change a sterile dressing—see Chapter 10). **These gloves are worn once and then thrown away.**

- **Disposable plastic-lined pads** or washable absorbent pads, often called *chucks*. These are used to protect sheets and furniture from fecal or urinary soiling. Always buy the largest size. They are available from surgical supply stores.
- **Protective apron.** This is worn by the caregiver to cover clothing. It can be disposable or reusable, but in either case **must be fluid resistant**, like plastic or vinyl.
- **Urinal and bedpan.** These are available in aluminum or plastic. Most people prefer plastic because it does not feel cold against the skin.
- **Adult disposable diapers.** These are used for fecal and/or urinary incontinence and are especially useful in cases of diarrhea.
- **Nonskid mats** for bathtub and/or shower floors.
- **Hand-held shower nozzle.** This device makes giving a bath or shower much faster and easier.
- **Laundry bags or containers.** Any store-bought laundry bag, plastic bag, or container is fine. You will need to keep separate bags for all laundry soiled with the PWA's blood or body fluids. *Dry* contaminated laundry can be placed in a cloth bag; anything wet and soiled, however, must be put in a plastic bag.

Useful but Nonessential Equipment

- **Hospital bed.** This is helpful for the person who is not very mobile, since it changes positions to allow for sitting and can be raised and lowered mechanically to protect the caregiver's back. Hospital beds can be purchased or rented at a surgical supply store.
- **Foot or bed cradle.** This C-shaped aluminum object, one curve of which is placed under the mattress beneath the bed linens, curves up over the bottom of the bed and forms a tent of the linens to keep them off the PWA's legs and feet.
- **Safety rails** (also called "grab bars"). These are used on beds, bathtubs, toilets, showers, and hallways. Rails are helpful to the person who has an unsteady gait, because they allow safe passage down a hallway and provide stability when getting in or out of a bath or bed. Safety rails can be bought or rented.
- **Wheelchair.** This can be an absolute necessity, but it is a luxury if the PWA can walk. Be sure the wheelchair is foldable or collapsible for easy storage and transport in a car and that it has good brakes and comfortable footrests. Try to get one that has removable armrests to allow the person to slide from the bed or chair to the wheelchair and vice versa rather than needing to stand and pivot or take a few steps. Wheelchairs may be rented or bought and range dramatically in price. They come with high or low backs and may be manual or battery-operated.
- **Hemi-walker or quad cane.** These devices are useful for persons who can still walk but need extra support to help maintain their balance. They are adjustable to suit the height of the user.

- **Bedside commode.** Generally made of a plastic or an aluminum frame with a removable basin or bedpan inside, commodes resemble chairs and are helpful for people who are not strong enough to walk to the bathroom. A good substitute is a bedpan placed on a sturdy chair at the bedside, with a disposable absorbent pad ("chuck") under the bedpan to protect the chair from becoming soiled.

- **Texas catheters** (also called "condom catheters"). These consist of a rubber sleeve that is slipped over the penis like a *condom.* A drainage tube attached to one end of the *catheter* leads to a collection bag that can be easily emptied into the commode. The drainage bag is also measured off to allow you to monitor urinary output when necessary. Texas catheters prevent the wetting of sheets, clothing, and furniture. They are available in a variety of sizes. These devices must be changed daily so the skin can be washed and assessed for rashes or sores.

- **Toilet seat extender.** This device raises the level of the seat and prevents the weakened person from bending so low that he cannot get back into a standing position.

- **Shower or bathtub chair/bench.** This facilitates washing in cases where the PWA can't stand for very long or can't bend low enough to sit in the tub.

- **Shampoo tray.** This facilitates hairwashing if a PWA is confined to bed.

- **Toothettes.** These small sponge-tipped sticks are soaked in water or mouthwash to clean the teeth and refresh the mouth (without toothpaste) of a person who cannot do so himself. A good substitute is a piece of gauze, or a strip of terrycloth cut from a towel or washcloth, wrapped around a popsicle stick or a child's soft-bristled toothbrush.

- **Special utensils, cookware, dishes, and glasses.** These are only to be used in cases where the PWA requires implements with special handles, as in the case of a PWA with a neuropathy who has lost his ability to grip and perform fine motor tasks. Utensil extenders are made of rubber, foam, or plastic and they fit onto the handle of a spoon, fork, or knife, enlarging its circumference to make it easier to hold. Otherwise, regular household items are fine as long as they are properly washed and dried between uses.

- **Disposable masks and safety goggles.** These are necessary for the caregiver to wear only in rare instances, such as when suctioning a PWA.

CHAPTER 3

Preventing the Transmission of Infection to and from the Person with AIDS

Protecting the PWA against Infections

As we discussed in Chapter 1, AIDS interferes with the body's ability to mount an immune response. An immune response is the reaction of the body to any substance that it sees as foreign—specifically, it is the body's attempt to rid itself of the invader. Therefore, when invaded by microorganisms such as viruses, bacteria, fungi, rickettsia, or parasites, the body of a PWA is often unable to effectively fight back against these invaders. Illness ensues and medical attention must be sought. To avoid illness, the PWA must be protected from infection and from further damage to the immune system.

Remember: The PWA is much more likely to become ill from exposure to people without AIDS who are sick than they are to contract AIDS from him. Therefore, it's vital to protect the PWA at all times.

What to Do

- Avoid anyone who has recently been near another person who was sick. Remember that many infections are *contagious* during their incubation period, the time when an infected person has not yet shown any symptoms of the disease.
- Stay away from households where there is illness—even those of friends and family members.
- Avoid high-risk environments such as hospitals or schools.
- Ensure that the PWA wears a mask in the presence of a person with a respiratory illness or when in a high-risk environment, such as a doctor's waiting room.
- Avoid having the PWA sit for long periods in the doctor's waiting room. If possible, arrange to have the first or last appointment of the day, or call ahead to see if the appointments are running on time so the PWA can adjust her schedule so as not to have to wait more than a few minutes.

- Help the PWA to maintain her health. Keep all appointments with the doctor and dentist, even those for routine checkups. Have blood work and other tests done in a timely fashion. Prevention of illness is easier than treatment.
- Urge the PWA to receive immunizations, such as pneumovax and influenza vaccines. Discuss these with the doctor.
- Encourage those around the PWA at home to cover their noses and mouths when coughing or sneezing.
- Use and encourage others to use good handwashing technique and gloves when coming in contact with the PWA to prevent the spread of infection.
- Prevent damage to the PWA's natural barriers against infection by taking care not to cut or abrade the skin, covering any cuts or open wounds to keep germs out, and wearing a mask when it's called for.
- Maintain proper nutrition (see Chapter 15).
- Make sure the PWA gets adequate rest and sleep. Fatigue lowers a person's resistance to disease, as does stress.
- Ensure that medications are taken as prescribed: on time and in the correct amounts.
- Make sure the PWA practices only safe sex (see Chapter 17).
- Avoid recreational drugs and alcoholic beverages, which increase susceptibility to illness and impair judgment. While under the influence of mind-altering substances, the PWA may be unsure of what is a safe practice and what is not. If the PWA is an IV drug user, she should not share her "works"—needles, syringes, spoons—even if they've been cleaned with chlorine bleach.

Preventing the Transmission of HIV

Body Fluids— What Is Contagious?

At this time, HIV and AIDS are thought to be transmitted only through an exchange of infected body fluids. This occurs primarily in two ways: (1) by exposure to semen and/or vaginal secretions, as during sexual intercourse (penile-vaginal, penile-anal, and oral sex with ejaculation); and (2) by direct blood-to-blood contact, such as when an IV drug user shares a "dirty" (blood-tinged) needle. Bloodborne transmission can also occur by means of a transfusion of infected blood or blood products, such as *platelets* or Factor Eight, a substance given to hemophiliacs to help them clot their blood. However, the nation's blood supply is now screened for HIV contamination and is considered to be safe.

HIV can be transmitted both directly and indirectly. Direct exposure occurs during sexual intercourse, whereas indirect exposure occurs by means of an object that has infected body fluids on it. For example, a vibrator or *dildo* can transfer the virus from the host to another person if it has been soiled with the host's blood, semen, or other body fluids. This can be avoided by keeping separate sexual toys for each person's exclusive use. If such an item is to be shared (**not recommended**), it must first be properly disinfected with a 10 percent chlorine bleach solution (see box, page 46).

As of this writing, there is no evidence that the virus is transmitted by the airborne route or by handling objects that were touched by an infected person. And although HIV has been isolated from saliva, stool, urine, mucus, sweat, and tears, thus far no evidence demonstrates transmission by means of these substances. It is still strongly recommended, however, that precautions be taken when coming into contact with these body fluids. It is absolutely essential to wear gloves and to follow proper handwashing procedure.

Using Gloves

Direct contact with blood or body fluids must be avoided to decrease the risk of transmission of HIV. Latex gloves should be worn to minimize contact with infected material. They do not need to be sterile except in cases where the caregiver is changing a sterile dressing (see Chapter 10). Fingernails should be kept short to avoid puncturing gloves. **All gloves must be disposed of after one use.**

Rules for Using Disposable Latex Gloves

- There is no special technique for putting on nonsterile gloves; they should be carefully *removed,* however, to avoid hand contamination. See Chapter 10 for more information on putting on and removing sterile gloves.
- Keep boxes of gloves handy throughout the house—in the bathroom, bedroom, and kitchen. You never know when or where you might suddenly need some. They should always be within reach when administering care. It's a good idea to keep a spare, clean pair in your pocket.
- Always wear gloves when:
  — bathing, cleaning, or shaving a PWA.
  — coming in contact with the PWA's rectal or genital areas, feces, urine, vomitus, or blood (such as when emptying a bedside commode or cleaning the bathroom).
  — giving mouth care.
  — changing nonsterile dressings.
  — handling the PWA's bed linens, and towels. Do not assume that such items aren't soiled with body fluids because you can't see an obvious stain—wear gloves anyway.
- Do not walk around the house touching doorknobs and things with contaminated gloves. Always remove and dispose of them immediately after use in the receptacle you keep contaminated trash in.

Note: Proper and frequent handwashing is a must even when gloves are worn.

Handwashing

To wash your hands properly, lather with soap and hot water for at least 30 seconds. A liquid soap in a pump bottle is recommended to prevent germ transmission. Always wash your hands, wrists, and forearms, as well as any jewelry, such as rings or bracelets, that you had on while providing care. Dry your hands with disposable paper towels if available to minimize the spread of germs. (Cloth towels are a breeding ground for germs.)

Rules for Handwashing

- Wash hands before **and** after wearing gloves as well as before and after providing any direct care involving contact with a PWA's skin or mucous membranes.
- Wash hands before and after using the bathroom.
- Wash hands before cooking and before eating.
- Wash hands before and after touching your own mouth, nose, and eyes.
- Use hand cream, moisturizer, or petroleum jelly to prevent rough, dry hands.

Sharing Items with a PWA

Sharing items is perfectly fine in some cases, but not in others. Remembering the following rule should make it easy for you to decide if sharing is acceptable in a particular instance: **If sharing involves any risk of blood or body fluid exchange, then do not share the item.**

Following are some examples of what can be shared and what should not be shared. If you have any questions about items covered here, ask your doctor.

Do Share

- toilet, if properly cleaned
- dishes, cups, utensils, pots, pans, if properly washed in very hot, soapy water
- kitchen appliances, such as the stove, refrigerator, toaster oven, microwave, and dishwasher
- washer/dryer
- telephone, headphones, earphones, earplugs
- bed, if the PWA is not incontinent of urine or feces
- tables and chairs
- clean clothing

Do *Not* Share

- previously used tissues, handkerchiefs, towels, washcloths
- bar soap
- toothbrushes
- razors—electric or blade, including used disposables
- sexual toys or aids, such as dildos or vibrators
- contact lens holders
- denture cups
- eyebrow tweezers
- nail scissors or clippers, cuticle nippers, nail files, or emery boards

- enema or douching equipment
- makeup, such as eyeliner, mascara, or lipstick
- pierced earrings

Household Cleaning, Laundry, and Kitchen Activities

Maintaining the home or apartment of a PWA need not be difficult. Keep in mind that it is perfectly acceptable for PWAs to cook and clean for themselves and others as long as they follow the rules for handwashing.

General Household Cleaning

Everyone feels better in clean surroundings. A clean living space also helps decrease the presence of various viruses and bacteria that are dangerous to an immunocompromised person.

What to Do

- Keep living areas well ventilated and at a comfortable temperature.
- Keep the household neat and clean.
- Use a 10 percent chlorine bleach solution (see box, page 46) to:
  — clean up spills of blood or body fluids with paper towels while wearing gloves. Dispose of the paper towels by flushing them down the toilet (if this won't damage the plumbing) or by placing them in a sealed plastic garbage bag for disposal.
  — clean the toilet, bedpan, commode, and/or urinal weekly or as needed. Full-strength bleach can be poured down the toilet for disinfection. **Always wear gloves.**
  — clean the bathtub and shower.
  — soak all cleaning materials between uses, including the brush used to clean the bathroom bowl, sponges, and rags. Make up a fresh bleach solution to use before your next cleaning job. Keep the contaminated soaking solution out of the reach of children and confused adults.
  — mop the kitchen and bathroom floors at least once a week. Pour the dirty water from the pail down the toilet or a washtub drain, **not** down the kitchen sink where food is prepared.

What *Not* to Do

- Do not use the same sponge to clean the bathroom that you use to clean the kitchen. Keep a separate sponge for each room.
- Do not use a sponge contaminated from the cleanup of a body fluid spill to wash dishes or to clean food preparation areas. It is not necessary to store sponges in bleach solutions unless they have been used to clean contaminated surfaces. You can continue to use one sponge for contaminated cleanup and a separate one for food preparation areas.

Chlorine Bleach Solutions

Chlorine bleach solutions are used to disinfect items that have been contaminated by the PWA's blood or body fluids. **Use only chlorine bleach** (scented types are acceptable), as it is the only kind of bleach known to kill HIV. Liquid formulations are best because they disperse most easily and mix most thoroughly with water. **Do not use antiseptics** (like betadine) for this purpose, because they only slow the growth of microorganisms without killing them. **Do not use alcohol,** as it evaporates too quickly to be effective.

Making Chlorine Bleach Solutions

The recommended strength of the chlorine bleach solution is 10 percent. **To make a 10 percent (1:9) chlorine bleach solution, add 1 part chlorine bleach to 9 parts water.** Using a standard measuring cup, measure out the water first, then add the bleach to the water. (This is a safety precaution, to avoid having the bleach splash up as it might if the water were added to it.)

Caution: Be careful not to splash either the bleach or the bleach solution in your eyes. Avoid getting it on your clothes or other fabrics, as it may discolor them permanently.

Using Chlorine Bleach Solutions

- **For household cleaning jobs:** Make up a fresh batch of solution for each use **unless** you plan to store it in a spray or pump bottle and dispense a fresh application for each job. For example, you cannot make up a pail of solution, use it to mop the floor, and then use it again later to mop up another spill, because you will be mopping up the second spill with contaminated solution. However, if you have a small spill to clean up, you can spray fresh solution directly onto the affected area from a spray bottle, and clean with a sponge. This never contaminates the solution in the pump bottle. Just remember to soak and then rinse the sponge before its next use.

  Keep in mind that 10 percent solutions lose their potency after 24 hours, so **fresh batches need to be made up daily.**

- **For laundry:** You can approximate the 10 percent solution needed to disinfect a washerload of contaminated clothing by adding 1 cup of **full-strength** bleach to the water as the washer is filling. (Add your clothes after you have added in the bleach to prevent pouring undiluted bleach directly onto the fabric and discoloring it.) You can use any water temperature you would normally use to wash your clothes, as it is the bleach and *not* the hot or cold water temperature that kills the virus.

  You do not need to presoak laundry stains, although if you desire to do so, it is acceptable to do so in your customary manner. Remember, though, that the item must still be washed as indicated here. If a stained item is properly washed in the 10 percent chlorine bleach solution, it will be disinfected and usable, even if the stain is still visible.

- **For soaking contaminated items:** Common household items that become contaminated with blood or body fluids must first be thoroughly cleaned with soap and water, then fully submerged in the chlorine bleach solution for 10 minutes at room temperature, and then rinsed with hot water. Just dipping an item in, or wiping it with, the solution—or straight chlorine bleach—does not kill germs.

Laundry

What to Do

- Change linen soiled with blood or body fluids immediately and change unsoiled linen at least once a week. Place chucks on the sheets to protect the mattress from blood and body fluids. **Always wear gloves** when handling the PWA's used linen and chucks.
- Wash clothing, towels, linens, and so on, that are *not* soiled with blood or body fluids with the rest of the household's as you normally do.
- Wash contaminated laundry (items soiled with blood or body fluids) separately from other laundry. It may be washed by hand (**always wear gloves**) or in a washing machine. Use your regular laundry detergent, and add 1 cup of full-strength chlorine bleach (see box, page 46). The water can be any temperature. It is the bleach, not the water temperature, that kills the HIV virus. Dry in a dryer set on a hot setting, or air dry.

What *Not* to Do

- Do not burn or discard stained clothing, linens, or towels. Items that remain stained after proper laundering are still clean and can be used.

Kitchen Activities

What to Do

- Wash all dishes, pots, pans, utensils, and cups in hot, soapy water. Rinse thoroughly and allow them to air dry. Automatic dishwashers may also be used. There is **no need** to separate the PWA's utensils.
- Clean the inside of the refrigerator regularly according to the manufacturer's instructions to control mold.
- Dispose of all old, stale, or spoiled food.

What *Not* to Do

- Do not place a fork or spoon you've used to taste while cooking back into the pot if someone else is also to eat the food in the pot. This will help to prevent the caregiver and the PWA from infecting each other with microbes that can be a danger—especially to someone with a weakened immune system.
- Do not eat from someone else's utensil or finish someone else's partially eaten food. To taste another's food, place a sample of untouched food onto your plate using a clean utensil.
- Do not use disposable plastic or paper plates, cups, or plastic utensils for the PWA unless you do so for everyone. There is **no need** to dispose of items the PWA has eaten from.

Waste Disposal

Waste disposal need not be a problem, even when items are soiled with blood or body fluids. The exact rules for disposing of your contaminated trash vary according to where you live, so check with the proper authorities in your areas. Contact the municipal department of sanitation, private trash collectors (if used in your area), or the health department, or ask the advice of your doctor or home care nurse.

Rules for Safe Waste Disposal

- Always wear gloves when disposing of waste and remember to wash your hands after removing them.
- Dispose of all "clean" waste—waste not soiled by blood or body fluids—as you would normally.
- Flush all paper items—such as paper towels, tissues, and toilet paper—down the toilet if they are contaminated by blood or body fluids, assuming your plumbing is adequate for this purpose. Otherwise, throw them out in a sealed plastic bag.
- Dispose of all wound dressings, heavy paper products, sanitary napkins, and disposable plastic items such as chucks by placing them in heavy-duty plastic bags tied shut. Throw these out with the regular trash; they are much too thick and heavy to flush down the toilet.
- Place all sharp items (syringes, blades, lancets, and so forth) in the sealed heavy-duty plastic containers available from surgical supply stores for this purpose or make a container out of an empty coffee can or bleach or liquid laundry detergent bottle. It's a good idea to add a small amount of chlorine bleach solution (see box, page 46) to the bottoms of these containers. To avoid injury, make sure you don't force sharp items into already-full containers and that the containers are properly sealed and labeled when ready for disposal. Again, check with local authorities about pickup of these containers.
- Flush all body fluids from urinals, bedpans, and commodes down the toilet.
- Line all garbage cans in your home with plastic bags rather than paper bags. Do not reuse garbage bags. Throw them away with the trash.
- Be sure your garbage cans are sealed so that children and pets do not come in contact with infected waste, especially if you are living in a house where garbage is picked up at the curb.

CHAPTER **4**

Maintaining the PWA's Lifestyle

It is often unnecessary for the PWA to dramatically change her lifestyle. She may continue to work, travel, participate in recreational activities, and so forth. Precautions, however, may have to be taken. This chapter addresses common concerns about how to maintain a safe yet high-quality lifestyle.

Work, Sports, and Recreation

A PWA can continue working, enjoying sports, and participating in any recreational activity that she has always engaged in, with her doctor's permission. In the case of contact sports or those involving potential injury (such as skiing), proper medical facilities must be available to handle emergencies. This includes the availability of gloves and bandages on-site in case of bleeding. She must wear a Medic Alert tag so that if she is injured, the personnel on-site will know how to take proper precautions. If the PWA plans to travel alone—on a business trip, to a sporting event, or for any other purpose—she should always let someone know her itinerary.

To the PWA: Safety Tips for Work and Play

- Tell the doctor your intentions before you return to work, change your type of employment, or participate in any sport or recreational activity. Obtain permission and any advice or restrictions on your activity from the doctor.
- Know your limits. Schedule rest periods to avoid fatigue and stress. Be sure to take breaks for meals, resting, bathroom use, and taking medications.
- Do not continue in or accept employment situations that put you at risk of injury, infection, or excessive physical or mental stress.
- Participate only in activities that you are comfortable doing.

Traveling

Travel can be fun, fascinating, and very tiring. There is no reason why a PWA can't travel, but it must be done wisely. If the distance is short and the PWA is well rested prior to embarking, the trip can be wonderful, especially if her needs along the way have been anticipated. Problems arise when traveling long distances. Fatigue becomes a problem, and discomfort can occur when riding in a car, bus, or airplane for prolonged periods. The PWA must be able to take breaks to stretch stiff limbs, bathrooms must be available, and medications must be taken on time. Travel outside the country or for long distances may require advice from the doctor.

If the PWA is too ill or weak to travel by conventional means, seek the advice of a physician. Many ambulettes or ambulance companies will take someone to the desired destination for a fee.

What to Do

- Write out (or ask the doctor to write out) a health history that includes all relevant information regarding past and present health problems, current medications, allergies, persons to be notified in an emergency, and so forth. Make sure the PWA takes this information with her when she travels. She should keep it on her person (in a wallet or purse) and have a duplicate copy in her luggage where a traveling companion can find it.
- Take enough medication for the entire trip, plus an extra supply in case the PWA is late in returning. She should take extra prescriptions with her to fill on the road, if necessary. (But remember that prescriptions may not be honored in other states or foreign countries.)
- Ask the doctor to recommend a physician in the area the PWA will be visiting, if she is planning to be away for a week or longer.
- Find out where the nearest hospital emergency room is when the PWA reaches her destination.
- Anticipate the need for rest stops, if traveling by car, to stretch legs, use a bathroom, have a snack, take medication.
- Anticipate possible motion sickness in cars, buses, airplanes, and boats. Discuss with the doctor the possibility of taking medication for this problem.
- Tell the caregiver, a friend, or a family member where the PWA is going, give him or her a phone number where she can be reached, and call periodically to let them know she's okay.
- Anticipate comfort needs, such as a pillow for the PWA's back, walking shoes, and comfortable clothes to wear while traveling. The PWA should consider wearing light clothing and packing a sweater to help adapt to temperature changes while on the road.
- Try to select hotels or motels with elevators or ground floor rooms to avoid climbing stairs. This may mean making reservations in advance.
- Remember that foreign travel may require vaccinations. The PWA should see her doctor early on so that if vaccines are necessary and she has a reaction, there will be plenty of time to recover before embarking. Avoid traveling to exotic places where disease is endemic and hygiene and medical facilities are poor, such as third world countries.

- Take full advantage of special privileges allowed for people who are traveling when they are ill. These include: early boarding on planes, special meals, wheelchairs at airports and cruise ship terminals, and transportation from one airplane to another if the PWA must change planes en route. Contact the airline or cruise line in advance and discuss the PWA's needs with them.
- Consider using services that provide nurses or traveling companions for ill persons. These services, however, can be costly.

What Not to Do

- Do not allow the PWA to be pressured into traveling by well-meaning family or friends. If she is too tired, she should say so and stay at home.
- Do not be afraid to cancel a trip. Most travel industry companies will refund the money (or a portion of it) if you provide a letter from the doctor explaining that the PWA was too ill to travel.
- Do not leave special equipment or devices at home, thinking that an airline, hotel, or cruise line can provide them. When in doubt, call ahead and ask. If the answer isn't satisfactory, bring your own equipment.

Pets

Pets are an important part of many people's lives. It is generally recognized that pets can help fulfill basic human needs such as the need for companionship, love, and emotional support. They help to promote relaxation and decrease stress. **Regardless of these benefits, having a pet is NOT recommended to immunosuppressed people such as those who have AIDS.** The reason is that pets pose an increased risk of infection and opportunistic illnesses by virtue of the viruses and bacteria that they harbor in their waste products. This applies not only to cats and dogs and other mammals, but to fish, birds, and reptiles as well.

If the PWA already has a pet, it is recommended that she try to find it a new home or take it to an animal shelter that does not destroy animals. If this is not what she chooses to do, or if she has no pet but has decided to get one despite the risk, she can take care of herself while caring for her pet by using the following precautions.

Caring for a Pet

- Avoid having the PWA clean up after pets. Be especially careful of their waste products. PWAs should not clean animal spills, litter boxes, aquariums, or bird cages if someone else is available to do these chores. **A PWA who does take care of her pet herself should wear a mask and gloves when cleaning up feces or urine and when changing the pet's paper, litter, or tank water.**

- Wash your hands thoroughly after cleaning up after a pet even though you wore gloves during the task.
- Attend to the health needs of the pet promptly—especially vaccines recommended by the veterinarian.
- Keep pets indoors exclusively, if possible, so they do not pick up any opportunistic infections they can pass along to humans.
- Keep pets away from other animals—including other people's pets—even if they seem healthy, because they can carry diseases PWAs may be susceptible to.
- Do not allow a pet to sleep with the PWA. An animal may accidentally bite or scratch while it is sleeping and dreaming, and the PWA may be injured if she moves and startles it awake from a sound sleep. Furthermore, a pet may be incontinent in the bed, which is an additional source of infection for the PWA.
- Do not allow the PWA to clip or file a pet's nails or claws to avoid scratches. Animal scratches can lead to bleeding and infection. Nail or claw grooming needs to be carried out by another person on a regular basis to minimize the risk of scratches during casual contact. Consider having cats declawed.
- If the PWA is accidentally scratched or bitten by a pet, clean the wound with soap and water, bandage it, and notify the doctor no matter how minor the injury. Change the bandage at least once a day and assess the site for possible infection (redness, drainage, and swelling). If this occurs, see the doctor immediately.
- Periodically reassess the PWA's ability to care for her pet. If you decide to find the pet a new home, take pictures of the pet as keepsakes. If a friend or family member adopts the pet, be sure to have the PWA ask for regular updates and arrange for occasional visits.

PART III

Managing Symptoms

CHAPTER **5**

Checking for Signs and Symptoms of Illness

Assessing the PWA's General Condition

Many opportunistic infections are associated with AIDS (see Chapter 1). These infections manifest themselves in numerous physical, mental, and behavioral changes. When you are examining someone who has AIDS, you must use your eyes, ears, and sense of smell just as a doctor would use a stethoscope and other diagnostic tools. You know what you see, hear, and smell every day. **By noting any change from what you have come to know as normal for the infected person, you are doing a physical examination.** Any change, however minor, should be reported to the PWA's physician. Small changes, such as occasional *insomnia,* can be reported at a routine office visit. Large, dramatic, or drastic changes (such as a temperature of 104°F for two or more days) require immediate reporting. Write down the changes you observe, noting the time, circumstances, and other important details so that they are not forgotten.

What to Look For

- Unexplained fever, especially when not responsive to temperature-lowering medications
- Shaking chills
- Night sweats, especially if they happen often
- Unexplained, persistent fatigue
- Complaints of pain anywhere, especially severe headache, stiff neck, or abdominal pain
- Swollen glands (also called enlarged lymph nodes) anywhere on the body. These usually occur in the neck, armpits, and groin (see Figure 5.1).
- Changes in skin texture, color, or the appearance of a visible lesion, wart, or rash
- Unusual bruising or bleeding, when there is no known cause
- Any change in vision
- Persistent white spots or coating in the mouth or on the tongue, especially if painful
- Shortness of breath that occurs frequently or at rest

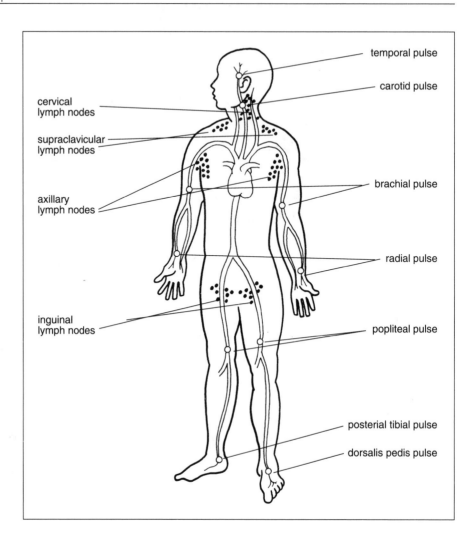

FIGURE 5.1
Locations of Pulses and Lymph Nodes

- Persistent cough, especially a cough that produces sputum
- Any abnormality of the pulse or complaint of chest pain
- Unexplained weight loss, or weight loss of ten pounds or more in one or two months
- Excessive loss of body fluid (*dehydration*) due to vomiting, diarrhea, or decreased fluid intake
- New, worsening, or persistent diarrhea, especially if it is bloody (red), tarry (black), or mixed with mucus
- Unexplained vaginal bleeding, discharge, or itching
- Unexplained penile bleeding, pain, or discharge
- Pain or bleeding with urination; difficulty starting or stopping the stream
- Mood, personality, behavior, speech, or memory changes, especially if the PWA himself notices a change

- Change in gait or mobility
- Dizziness, light-headedness, or weakness
- Seizure or suspected seizure (see Chapter 20)
- Persistent insomnia
- Signs of infection at a wound or catheter site. These include redness, swelling, pain to the touch, odor, and/or drainage of any color or amount.

Reporting Health Information to the Doctor

- Record any changes and report them to the PWA's physician as soon as possible. Do not assume a change will go away or that it is unimportant. Remember: Most opportunistic infections are treatable, especially if caught early. **Call the doctor immediately for dramatic or severe changes in mental status, temperature, pulse, and respirations or if there is a sudden onset of bleeding, diarrhea, vomiting, pain or seizures.** Severe headache, sudden and unexpected loss of vision, sensation, or movement of an arm, leg, or other part of the body may signal a stroke and is also an emergency.
- Be specific in what you report. For example, if you are reporting an elevated temperature, know the exact temperature, the method used for determining the temperature (oral or rectal thermometer; Fahrenheit or centigrade), how often the temperature was elevated, how many days it has lasted, and what the response was to temperature-lowering medications.
- Note how long the problem has existed.
- Give an objective description of the problem. For example, if you are reporting new episodes of confusion, be prepared to give an example of what you mean. But do not diagnose—that is the doctor's job. The information on the "seven parameters" (see box, page 58) will assist you in giving a succinct, accurate, and useful description of the problem to the doctor.
- Inform the PWA's physician if you believe a change is related to something specific, such as rash related to a new medication, and explain why.
- Report to the doctor what effect the change has had on the PWA and his quality of life.
- Encourage the PWA to report these problems on his own. Offer help in reporting problems when necessary. Be honest with the details in reporting changes.

Checking Temperature, Pulse, and Respiration

As part of your general assessment, it's important to know how to check temperature, pulse, and respiratory rate (breathing). You will be using these techniques to assist you in your care of the PWA—in particular, to quickly and accurately identify and report problems.

The Seven Parameters

In medicine, a maxim called the "seven parameters" is used to outline and clarify the nature of a pain or problem. The doctor will probably want you to describe the PWA's symptoms in terms of these parameters, which are:

1. location
2. quality
3. quantity
4. timing
5. setting
6. relieving or exacerbating factors
7. associated symptoms

This means, if you are reporting a pain, it is important to describe to the doctor:

where the pain is located;
what it feels like (e.g., sharp like a knife or dull like a toothache);
how severe it is;
when and **where** it began;
what makes the pain better or makes it worse; and
what other manifestations (e.g., nausea and vomiting with abdominal pain) were
      present.

Taking a Temperature

Normal body temperature is 98.6°F (37°C) when taken orally. A rectal temperature may be slightly higher; a temperature taken under the arm may be slightly lower.

To take a temperature, choose a method: oral, rectal, or *axillary* (under the armpit). Before beginning, remember to shake down the thermometer or reset it (if it's a digital model) to a reading below 96°F.

To take an oral temperature, make sure that the person has not had anything hot or cold to eat or drink for 30 minutes beforehand. (Bathing and smoking will also affect the accuracy of temperature readings.) Insert the thermometer (bulb end) under the tongue and make sure the person closes his mouth and doesn't bite down on the thermometer. Keep the thermometer in place for 9 to 10 minutes. Read the thermometer by holding it up to the light and manipulating it until the numbers are clearly visible. The temperature is that number at which the horizontal marking (usually red or silver fluid) stops. (Digital thermometers, like digital clocks, give you a direct numerical reading that appears on a small screen.) **Do not attempt to take oral temperatures on confused or comatose persons.**

To take a rectal temperature, lubricate the bulb end of the thermometer with petroleum jelly and gently insert 1 to 1½ inches into the rectum. Hold in place for 2 to 5 minutes, then remove, wipe the tip and read in the same manner as for an oral temperature. **Do not attempt to take a rectal temperature on**

PWAs with diarrhea, rectal bleeding, or any rectal infection or lesion (such as a hemorrhoid) unless advised to do so by a doctor. Never leave someone alone with a rectal thermometer in place.

To take an axillary temperature, place the thermometer under the arm (deep into the armpit) and position the person's arm against his side to hold the thermometer in place. Wait 11 to 15 minutes and read as you would for rectal and oral temperatures. **This is the least accurate method and should be reserved for uncooperative people.**

Taking a Pulse

A normal pulse is what's normal for the individual, although the usual range is 60 to 100 beats per minute (bpm). When counting a pulse, the PWA should be sitting quietly.

To find pulse locations, refer to Figure 5.1. The easiest place to feel a pulse is at the wrist. To find the pulse in the wrist, run your index and middle fingers down the side of the thumb to the wrist and continue on for about one-half inch until you feel the throbbing sensation. If you cannot feel the pulse and seem to be in the correct location, try a lighter touch (it's a common mistake to exert too much pressure). Count each throbbing sensation as one beat; count for 60 seconds, using the second hand on your watch or clock as a timer. (Example: 78 throbbing sensations in 60 seconds = 78 beats per minute). **Do not use your thumb to feel another's pulse.**

Measuring Respiratory Rate (Breathing)

Normal respiratory rates vary from 12 to 18 breaths per minute. The PWA should be sitting or lying quietly and not speaking. Ideally, you should attempt to count a respiratory rate when the PWA is unaware that you are doing so, because it is natural to alter your breathing when you are being observed.

To count the respiratory rate, watch the rise and fall of the chest for 60 seconds. The number of times the chest rises and falls equals the rate of respiration, reported as "breaths per minute."

CHAPTER **6**

Fever

Defining Fever

Deciding what is and isn't a fever can be difficult. A temperature of 98.6°F or 37°C when taken orally is considered by most people to be a "normal" temperature. Many individuals, however, have a normal body temperature that is slightly higher or lower. Therefore, the normal range is considered to be within two degrees of 98.6°F in either direction (96.6°F–100.6°F). For this reason, it is suggested that you consider an elevated temperature to be one over 101°F, no matter how it was measured (orally, rectally, or under the arm). (See the information in Chapter 5 on how to take a temperature.)

Causes of Fever

Temperature elevations can occur for a variety of reasons, not all of which are due to illness. Fevers may be noted in people who have just finished a vigorous exercise workout or who have just come from a very hot environment, such as the beach. Fever may also be a reaction to a medication (called a "drug fever") or to dehydration, inflammation, or infection.

Treatment of Fever

What to Look For

- Increased skin temperature (skin feels warm or hot to touch)
- Unusual inactivity or *lethargy* in a previously active person
- Headache
- Flushed look to the face, especially the cheeks
- A complaint of feeling very hot or cold
- Shaking chills or sweating
- Body aches, especially joint pains
- Hot, dry skin
- Lack of appetite

- Accompanying symptoms, such as: nausea, vomiting, constipation, diarrhea, chattering teeth, and a glassy or watery look to the eyes
- Rapid heartbeat (more than 100 bpm), especially with fever of 103°F or greater
- Shortness of breath; again, especially with excessive temperature elevations
- **Convulsions, delirium, or confusion may occur in the presence of a very high body temperature (104°F or more) but can occur with lesser fevers in sensitive individuals. These situations require emergency assistance with ambulance transport to the hospital.**

What to Do

- Follow any directions given to you on a previous occasions by a doctor regarding the use of temperature-lowering medications such as Tylenol (acetaminophen), aspirin (salicylic acid), or Advil (ibuprofen).
- Give lots of fluids to anyone with an elevated temperature. Any fluid that does not contain caffeine will do: water, juice—even ice pops. An increased fluid intake helps to prevent dehydration and cools the system.
- Encourage the PWA to rest or sleep as needed.
- Cover the person with only a sheet, except if she is feeling cold or experiencing chills. Then extra blankets are fine.
- Administer a tepid water bath or sponge bath (especially if the fever is 103°F or more) to help bring down the elevated temperature more rapidly.
- Apply ice packs or cold, damp towels under the arms and/or in the groin for fevers of a least 103°F. Place them in these areas for 15 to 20 minutes, then remove them for 15 to 20 minutes, repeating the cycle as often as necessary until the fever breaks. Stop immediately if chills begin or if the PWA feels discomfort.
- Take the temperature every two to four hours and keep a written record. Note the time, the temperature, how the measurement was taken (e.g., orally), and any associated symptoms (such as chills, body aches, vomiting). Also record what interventions you used to lower the fever, such as baths or medications. Note when a temperature-lowering medication was taken, whether it was effective and, if so, by how many degrees the fever was reduced. Report these findings to the doctor.

What *Not* to Do

- Never give any medications unless so instructed by a doctor.
- **Never give fluids to a sleepy or lethargic person, because he may choke.**
- Never use an alcohol bath to bring a fever down; it can cause the fever to drop too quickly, resulting in chills and exhaustion.

When to Consult Your Doctor

- **If the feverish person has a convulsion, or becomes delirious, combative, or confused, CALL AN AMBULANCE. This requires an emergency room visit and immediate medical attention.** Call your doctor to report **mild** confusion or *delirium;* follow instructions accordingly.
- If the PWA feels a "bounding heartbeat" (*palpitations*) or any shortness of breath.
- If a fever has been over 101°F or greater for 24 hours or more, or if the fever is accompanied by any cough, nausea, vomiting, or diarrhea.

CHAPTER 7
Fatigue

Defining Fatigue

Fatigue is also known as tiredness or weariness and is characterized by decreased energy, strength, or endurance. A person who is fatigued will seem lethargic, disinterested in her surroundings, or just sleepy.

Causes of Fatigue

Fatigue may be caused by excessive exercise or physical activity, malnutrition, circulatory disturbances (such as anemia or decreased oxygen supply as sometimes happens in individuals with respiratory problems). Fatigue may also have a psychological component. It is common in people who are bored, anxious, depressed, or suffering from severe emotional stress.

Anyone, at any time, can suffer from fatigue—be they well or ill, PWA, or caregiver—at any age and for a host of reasons. But do not ignore fatigue in the PWA, or assume it is unimportant. It may be a sign of a more severe underlying problem, such as a new opportunistic infection or cancer.

Treatment of Fatigue

What to Look For

- A lack of energy or complaint of feeling excessively tired, coupled with an increased need for sleep at night or in the form of daytime naps
- A complaint of feeling sad or "blue"
- Decreased desire to even try to do usual activities
- Less attention to personal hygiene and appearance
- Slower movements and/or the inability to rise from a sitting or lying position as quickly and easily as before
- Forgetfulness or a shortened attention span
- Poor appetite

- Shortness of breath
- Tearful or fearful behavior

What to Do

- Attempt to provide a restful and quiet environment.
- Incorporate naps and rest periods into the daily routine.
- Encourage the PWA to conserve energy to do the tasks she considers to be most important.
- Limit phone calls and vists, if necessary.
- Provide assistance with personal hygiene or household chores.
- Serve six small meals a day instead of three large ones, or consider having the PWA snack on favorite foods to maintain nutritional intake.
- Try relaxation tapes, meditation, reading, and listening to music to enhance relaxation.
- Consider consulting a psychiatrist, psychologist, social worker, or nurse therapist for professional guidance.
- Reassure the person and offer emotional support if she feels guilty about feeling fatigued or about not completing tasks.

What *Not* to Do

- Do not administer over-the-counter medications to "pep up" the PWA or help her to sleep.

When to Consult Your Doctor

- If the PWA is too lethargic to do anything for herself, even if she should be physically able to do so.

What to Discuss with Your Doctor

- Any physiological or psychological change in the PWA's life that might explain fatigue.
- The feasibility of using mood elevators and/or sleep aids.
- A referral to a therapist for help in dealing with *anxiety,* depression, or other emotional issues.
- The possibility of having a homemaker, home health aide, or visiting nurse help in the home with tasks that the caregiver is unable to perform because of fatigue or time constraints.

CHAPTER 8

Pain

Defining Pain

Pain is a subjective phenomenon—one that has been the subject of countless books, songs, sonnets, works of art, and medical articles. Yet even today, with all of our high-level technology, its exact description eludes us. We do know that our brains manufacture chemicals, known as *endorphins,* that function as natural and internal painkillers to induce a state of lessened pain and heightened amnesia. For example, a woman who has experienced severe pain while giving birth will, by the next day, only remember in very general terms what the pain felt like. If asked to call it to mind again, she won't be able to remember the exact nature of the feeling. Try this exercise yourself: Try to recall the exact feeling you experienced the last time you were in pain. You will find this is difficult, if not impossible, to do. You may only recall that it was sharp, dull, or throbbing, but generally you cannot relive the sensation.

Pain, in general, is a sensation in which individuals experience discomfort, distress, or suffering to varying degrees according to their own tolerance or threshold for pain. This is why no two people will feel a toothache in quite the same manner and why to some a toothache may be unbearably excruciating while to others it is merely an annoyance.

Causes of Pain

Physiologically, pain occurs as a result of stimulation of sensory nerves and varies from mild to severe, thus provoking an appropriate protective reaction from the body. A toddler feeling the heat of a flame on the stove doesn't have to consciously reason, but instead reflexively pulls her hand out of the way. Pain perceived as mild by the mind is fairly well adapted to, whereas chronic or severe pain is not.

Treatment of Pain

Mild pain is often treated without medications, by use of ice packs, massage, warm baths, special breathing techniques, *biofeedback,* meditation, or guided imagery, to name a few nonpharmacological approaches to pain management (see Appendix C). When pain medications (*analgesics*) are used, they are usually nonnarcotic prescription or over-the-counter drugs, such as Tylenol (acetaminophen), aspirin (salicylic acid), or Motrin (ibuprofen).

Severe pain is usually helped somewhat by these same nondrug treatments, but it generally requires supplemental medications to lessen the pain to tolerable levels or to alleviate it altogether. **Although some of the narcotic pain relievers can be either physically or psychologically addicting, it is crucial to remember that addiction is a secondary concern when someone is either terminally ill or in excruciating pain. Withholding narcotics (morphine, Percocet (oxycodone and acetaminophen), Dilaudid (hydromorphone), Tylenol with codeine, etc.) because of fear that the person is or will become addicted, or because the caregiver believes that the pain is not as severe as the person states it to be, is inappropriate and cruel.** If, on the other hand, the caregiver feels that the PWA is experiencing side effects or is requiring dosages in excess of what is safe and recommended to manage his pain, then this must be discussed with the doctor so that an alternative medicine or schedule may be instituted.

What to Look For

- Pale skin, most commonly with sudden, sharp pain
- Goose bumps
- A tendency to touch, hold, or protect and favor the area that hurts
- Widened (dilated) pupils, especially with sudden, sharp pain
- Increased pulse
- Increased respirations—often rapid, shallow breathing
- Increased muscle tension, as when someone braces himself or stiffens to endure the pain
- Change in the tone of voice, usually to a higher pitch when in pain, although, in some individuals, the voice may lower to a whisper.
- Change in the rate of speech, either to a very rapid pace or to a very slow and halting pattern
- Moans, groans, crying, or tearful behavior
- Rocking—this is frequently exhibited with abdominal pain. The person may hold his abdomen and rock.
- Vomiting
- Cold sweats
- Insomnia

What to Do

- Assess the pain according to the Seven Parameters—location, duration, nature, etc.—as described in the box on page 58.
- Administer pain relievers as prescribed by the doctor. Record any side effects.

- Try nonpharmacologic measures if the pain is mild, such as watching television, listening to music, or other such distractions. Or, consider the use of biofeedback, relaxation exercises, meditation, or guided imagery (creative visualization). See Appendix C on holistic and adjunct therapies.

What Not to Do

- Never ignore any complaint of pain.
- **Never permit the PWA to drink alcohol of any type while taking pain relievers.** This can cause nausea, vomiting, disorientation, confusion, *convulsions,* and even death.
- **Never allow the PWA to drive or operate machinery while under the influence of pain relievers.** Pain medications can impair judgment and reflexes. They may also sedate the person and cause him to fall asleep while driving or while using a dangerous tool.
- Do not withhold, or attempt to prolong intervals between doses, of properly prescribed pain medications because you fear that the PWA is or may become addicted. **In cases of excruciating pain or terminal illness, addiction is a secondary concern.**
- Do not assume someone is lying about or exaggerating his symptoms simply because he appears comfortable or isn't behaving as you think someone in pain should. Everyone handles pain differently. No one can feel someone else's pain.
- Do not "double up" on pain medicines. Giving more than the prescribed dose may alleviate pain at the cost of serious side effects, including nausea, vomiting, confusion, and memory loss.
- Do not administer any pain reliever unless it is prescribed by a doctor. You may mask pain that is a symptom of something more serious.
- Do not use a pain-relieving medication that was prescribed for another purpose. First, seek the advice of a doctor.
- Do not use medication prescribed for someone else. The drug may interact with one of the PWA's medications and/or cause potentially life-threatening side effects.

When to Consult Your Doctor

- **For any pain that is sharp, severe, and/or accompanied by vomiting, unconsciousness, seizures, changes in vision, or problems with breathing, GO DIRECTLY TO THE EMERGENCY ROOM OR CALL AN AMBULANCE.**
- To report any new pain the PWA experiences, or the return of pain he has experienced in the past.
- To report any side effects of pain medication, such as sedation, confusion, abdominal pain, or nausea.

What to Discuss with Your Doctor

- The efficacy of pain medications.
- The PWA's objective in taking pain relievers. For example, if given the choice between being alert and oriented but a little uncomfortable, and being totally pain-free but lethargic, what is the PWA's preference? Together, he and his doctor can work toward maximizing quality of life while minimizing the pain.
- The proper use of the pain relievers that he or she has prescribed, such as when the medicine should be taken and what side effects to expect.

CHAPTER 9

Swollen Glands

The medical term for the glands referred to in "swollen glands" is "lymph nodes." Lymph nodes act as filters, keeping bacteria and viruses from entering the bloodstream. They wall off infection and prevent it from spreading throughout the body and, in particular, to vulnerable areas such as the heart.

Causes of Swollen Glands

Lymphadenopathy and enlarged lymph nodes are medical terms for swollen glands. The most common form of lymphadenopathy occurs with sore throat, when there is swelling of the glands in the neck or beneath the jaw. Lymph nodes, however, are located throughout the body (see Figure 5.1), and any lymph node can be swollen in any area of the body when an infection is present.

Lymphadenopathy can be caused by several types of cancer, bacterial infections, or inflammatory conditions. In AIDS, lymphadenopathy is often seen in people with Hodgkin's lymphoma, Kaposi's sarcoma, tuberculosis, mycobacterium avium intracellulare (MAI), cytomegalovirus (CMV), Epstein-Barr virus (EBV), herpes simplex I (cold sores), herpes simplex II (genital herpes), and herpes zoster ("shingles").

Characteristics of Swollen Glands

Inflammation of a lymph node, known as *lymphadenitis,* causes the gland to become swollen, red, painful, hard, and/or warm to the touch.

A lymph node will often remain swollen for several weeks, even after the infection is gone. During this time the redness, tenderness, and warm feeling will gradually subside. However, a condition called *persistent lymphadenopathy* can exist in chronically ill people, especially people with AIDS. Persistent lymphadenopathy is said to occur when lymph nodes are swollen for more than six months in two or more locations not including the groin; for example, a gland under the arm and one in the neck.

Treatment of Swollen Glands

Treatment of *lymphadenitis* may include an incision and drainage of infected fluid at the site, a biopsy (removal of a sample of the tissue for diagnosis), antibiotic therapy, and/or warm, moist dressings or soaks to increase comfort and decrease the amount of swelling.

What to Look For

- Discomfort in any area where a lymph node is located (the neck, armpit, and groin are the most commonly affected areas)
- Swelling, heat, redness, or a hard, marblelike ball in any lymph node area
- Elevated temperature (see Chapter 5 on how to take a temperature)
- Recent illness, such as a sore throat, flu, stomach virus, or injury

What to Do

- Note where the swollen gland is, especially if there is more than one in more than one location.
- Note any signs or symptoms of lymphadenitis, such as redness, a warm sensation, pain, or hardness, suggesting that the lymph node has become filled with infected material.
- Note any associated symptoms, such as fever, fatigue, nausea, vomiting, diarrhea, constipation, sore throat, or cough.
- Note any and all changes in the PWA's body, especially in areas nearest to where the lymphadenopathy is present. For example, if there is a cut on the arm, there might be a swollen gland in the armpit.
- Note anything that makes the area feel better or worse.

What *Not* to Do

- Never try to cure the PWA yourself. Administering medications prescribed on a previous occasion or for another condition might decrease the present inflammation and reduce painful swelling, but this can be dangerous as it may also mask a more serious problem that needs to be diagnosed.

When to Consult Your Doctor

- If a swollen gland is found or suspected. The doctor will need to know the PWA's general state of health, how long the swollen node has been there, and whether there has been any heat, pain, or redness. Be prepared for the possibility that blood tests may need to be done or other diagnostic tests (e.g., a lymph node biopsy) ordered to determine the underlying cause of the lymphadenopathy.

CHAPTER 10

Skin Care

Functions and Characteristics of the Skin

The skin is actually an organ of the body—in fact, it is the *largest* organ in terms of surface area. As such, it serves many vital purposes: it provides a barrier to infection; it shields us from harmful chemicals and from harsh sunlight; and it safeguards us against dehydration from excess water loss. We experience hot and cold, pressure and pain, itching, wetness, and a variety of other sensations through our skin. If it were not for our skin, we would not synthesize vitamin D, a chemical essential to our metabolism. In addition, our body eliminates wastes through its pores. Close off enough skin pores and you will suffocate. In addition to performing these functions, the skin is also the body's insulator, regulating heat loss and conservation.

One of the most significant characteristics of skin is its color. "Normal" skin color means what's normal for you. If you are normally fair-skinned with a blotchy complexion, a change would be noted if you were to develop a darker tone to your skin. Likewise, a dark-skinned person who develops white patches is said to have developed a change in skin color.

Many factors affect skin color. Overexposure to the sun's ultraviolet rays will cause darkening (tanning) or redness (burning) of the tissue. Some medications, such as Lamprene (clofazimine), will cause a darkening or discoloration of the skin that in some people resembles a suntan but in others causes the skin to assume a grayish-blue or purplish hue. Allergies to certain medications, laundry detergents, soaps, cosmetics, or creams often cause skin redness or rash. A bluish look to the skin means that the body is not getting enough oxygen (*hypoxia*) and is called *cyanosis*. A red hue is seen in people with elevated temperatures or with a localized inflammation. Individuals are yellow or *jaundiced* when the liver isn't doing its job properly. Pale patches on the skin (most notable in black people) may be from a harmless fungal infection called *tinea versicola*. And of course, we are all familiar with black-and-blue marks from bruises.

Skin is unique because it's an organ we can see and as such can be an indicator of health. It's important to take note of normal skin color and texture in the PWA. Changes in color as well as other skin characteristics (e.g., bumps, bruises, rashes, lesions, or sores) may be the first sign of illness or disease and should be reported promptly to your doctor.

This chapter gives you some tips about how to keep skin healthy as well as how to identify and treat some of the common skin problems encountered in AIDS.

Keeping Skin Healthy

The key to keeping skin healthy is knowing how to strike a balance between keeping it clean and germ-free with careful washing while not overdoing. Too frequent or rigorous washing with harsh chemicals can dry skin excessively and even damage it. Breaches in the skin can then serve as portals of infection.

What to Do

- Wash with warm water and a mild (nondrying, nondetergent, and nonperfumed) soap once daily—more often only if a specific area becomes soiled.
- Apply fragrance-free lotion or oil after washing to areas prone to dryness.
- Avoid applying alcohol, perfume, or cosmetics; they can promote drying or provoke an allergic reaction.
- Protect the skin from sunburn by applying sunscreen with a sun protection factor (SPF) of at least 15 for prolonged sunlight exposure.
- Protect delicate tissues (especially ears, fingers, and toes) from extreme cold by providing appropriate outerwear in cold weather.
- **Examine the PWA's skin thoroughly at least once a day**—a good time is while bathing—checking for evidence of dryness or skin lesions. **Skin changes can be the first sign of a problem.**
- Pay particular attention to the skin of the weak, immobile, or nearly immobile PWA. **People who are malnourished, dehydrated, and/or those who cannot move are extremely vulnerable to severe skin problems—bedsores in particular. These are much easier to prevent than to cure.**
- Encourage the intake of healthy foods and adequate fluids where possible.
- Follow the advice in Appendix E concerning moving people who cannot move themselves.
- Provide adequate padding on beds and chairs. "Egg crates" (foam pads with bumpy surfaces that resemble the cartons that eggs are sold in), sheepskins, and air mattresses may be purchased from surgical supply stores for this purpose.

How AIDS Affects the Skin

Kaposi's sarcoma, an opportunistic cancer seen in AIDS, looks like a dark purple or brown freckle or patch on the skin. *Candida* (yeast) infections look like white or red, scaly eruptions. Sometimes a fungal infection may be mistaken for *eczema* or *psoriasis*—both of which are chronic forms of dermatitis (inflammation of the skin) causing dry, flaky, and reddish areas.

Skin changes are also common in PWAs who are confined to bed and unable to move. Lying in bed or sitting in a chair day after day in the same position can break down the skin. These changes are called *pressure sores,* bedsores, or *decubitus ulcers* (see page 77). In sensitive persons, merely sliding down or inching up in bed can cause sheet burns.

Many other changes in the skin are seen in people with AIDS. These may include hives from an allergy or the classic fluid-filled pimples associated with herpes simplex or chickenpox. (See also "Skin Lesions," page 76.)

Dry Skin and Itching

Dry skin lacks moisture or oil. It can result from bathing too frequently, over-using alcohol-based products such as perfumes, which cause excessive dryness, or taking certain medications that cause dry skin as a side effect.

Itching of the scalp or skin may be caused by a variety of factors including: dry skin, insect bites, allergic reactions to foods or medications, illnesses such as chickenpox, or infections like the fungus that causes athlete's foot. The itch in itself, although annoying, is not a problem. However, scratching the itch can be. Scratching can cause damage to the skin, which must be intact to serve as a natural barrier against infection. Scratching to the point of causing burrows and/or bleeding must be avoided. Therefore, it's important to discover the cause of the itch so that it can be corrected.

What to Look For

- Skin that feels and looks dry; there may be a pattern of fine lines.
- Flaking, scaling, or patchy areas
- Itching or scratching
- Redness, dryness, rashes, insect bites, evidence of scratching (burrows, nail marks, tiny areas of bleeding that may have been caused by scratching too intensely)

What to Do

- Assess the PWA's skin **daily** for areas of dryness, most often seen on the face, arms (especially at the elbows), or lower legs.
- Try to ascertain the cause of any itching. If ignored or unnoticed for even as much as a day, scratching can cause serious skin breakdown. Furthermore, the underlying cause of the itch can grow more serious.
- Urge the PWA to drink lots of water to help prevent dry skin.
- Use a humidifier or vaporizer at night to moisten the air. Be sure to clean it properly and change the water daily.

- Bathe only once daily in warm (not hot) water and for less than ten minutes (except for cleansing after vomiting or incontinence).
- Use a bath oil that does not contain alcohol or perfumes.
- Pat the skin dry after washing rather than rubbing it, which reddens the skin and removes its natural oils.
- Use a moisturizer on damp skin after bathing. Choose one without alcohol or perfume.
- Trim the PWA's nails neatly to minimize the chance of injury to the skin from scratching.
- Discourage the PWA from scratching; however, if he must, advise him to use the pads of his fingers instead of the nails. Recommend massaging the area in lieu of scratching it.
- Put cotton gloves or mittens on the PWA's hands to prevent skin damage if he is confused or tends to scratch in his sleep.

When to Consult Your Doctor

- If itching becomes a problem, scratching has damaged the skin, and/or an area is not healing.
- If you suspect that a medication, an infection, or an allergic reaction is causing the dry skin and/or itching; until you discuss this with the doctor, **continue to give any prescribed medication.**
- To discuss the use of oatmeal baths, calamine lotion, and/or *antihistamine* tablets to help relieve the itching.

Skin Lesions

A skin lesion is any visible abnormality of skin tissue, such as a rash, a boil, a blister, a wound, an injury, a tumor, a pimple, or a cyst. A lesion may have a crust, pus, or other discharge. It may cause a change in skin color or pigmentation. Lesions may be benign (noncancerous); malignant (cancerous); diffuse (covering large areas), or focal (small areas).

What to Look For

- Any change in the skin, including a change in color, texture, or temperature or the appearance of something not noted before, such as a pimple, mole, or discolored area
- Any pain, itching, tingling, burning, odor, or drainage. If there is a draining sore, note the color, odor, consistency, and approximate amount of fluid present.
- Any growth of hairs or appearance of crusting, dryness, scaling, or itch, in the abnormal area

What to Do

- Check daily to see if the abnormality is going away or changing in any manner.
- Use only the medication prescribed for the condition.

What *Not* to Do

- Do not allow the PWA to scratch! This can spread an infection, cause a secondary infection, or damage the skin so that it's cut or scraped and more vulnerable to becoming infected. (See also page 75 on scratching.)

When to Consult Your Doctor

- If the PWA has itching or pain; call immediately.
- If a skin lesion seems to be changing or persists for three or more days. Skin problems are hard to diagnose over the phone, so it is likely that the physician will want to see the person. In some cases, a biopsy—a scraping or sampling of the tissue—may be taken for further analysis.

Pressure Sores

A pressure sore, also known as a bedsore or decubitus ulcer, is any area of skin breakdown, redness, or discomfort. Anyone with decreased mobility, from inability to walk to inability to shift positions while sitting in a chair to inability to turn in bed unassisted, is vulnerable to bedsores.

Pressure sores occur most often when there are prolonged, unrelieved periods of sitting or lying in the same position. However, they may also be caused when a person slides down in bed against the sheets or tries to pull herself up by bracing herself against her elbows or heels. This friction against the sheets creates rough, raw skin vulnerable to breakdown. Pressure sores can occur in as little as one or two hours in a sedentary person and can eventually lead to irreversible tissue death if ignored. To prevent the problem, knowledgeable skin assessment, good skin care, and correct positioning, turning, and body alignment are absolutely essential (see Appendix E).

Bedsores are also caused by poor nutritional intake and poor hydration. Weight loss from poor nutrition means less fat to cover bony prominences. Less commonly, excess weight against the mattress will exert more pressure and thus cause more skin breakdown.

Loss of bladder and/or bowel control also leads to skin irritation and increased breakdown. A warm, moist area of skin provides a breeding ground for bacteria and fungi that cause infection.

What to Look For

- Areas of swelling, particularly in gravity-dependent areas like the ankles. Swelling is a sign of poor circulation; that is, blood flow is poor, tissues are not being constantly replenished with vital oxygen, and their waste products are not being efficiently eliminated. Tissues become toxic and can even die, leaving a telltale skin lesion.
- The early signs of skin breakdown: swollen, pink or red areas most commonly seen over bony prominences such as the hips, shoulder blades, sacrum, elbows, or knees (see Figure 10.1). Be alert to the fact, however, that sores can start anywhere—even in fatty areas such as the buttocks.
- Later signs of breakdown, which include active breaks or ulcers in the skin, bleeding openings, and even blackened areas. The latter are sores in the advanced stages of disease, when there is actual tissue death (*necrosis*).

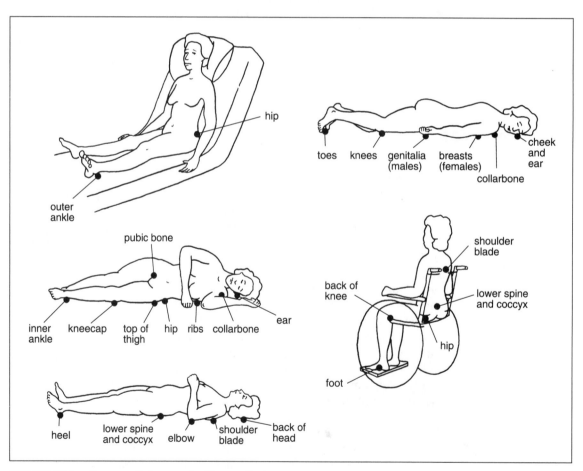

FIGURE 10.1   *Pressure Points on the Human Body*

What to Do

- Follow the general rules set forth in the preceding section on maintaining healthy skin.
- Provide a well-balanced diet (assist the PWA with feedings if she is unable to feed herself) and assess nutritional intake (see Chapter 15). This is crucial to the prevention and healing of pressure sores. Wasted individuals have bony areas over their bodies that are prone to skin breakdown. And once sores form, they utilize a large number of calories and proteins to repair themselves, diverting this needed energy from performing other vital body functions, such as staving off infection.
- Encourage and assist with exercise, activity, and movement. **Change the position of a bed-bound individual every one to two hours.** Assist the less-debilitated PWA out of bed and into a chair several times a day, even if it is only for 15-minute periods (see Appendix E).
- Use pads to protect elbows, knees, ankles and heels, as these are high-risk areas for pressure sores for the immobile person. Pads must be removed every few hours so skin can be checked. They are available at pharmacies and surgical supply stores. A good homemade version of these pads is a tube sock or sweatsock with the foot part cut off and a piece of sheepskin sewn inside. Pull the sock over the area, but be sure it's not too tight, as you don't want to restrict the circulation.
- Use egg crates, sheepskins, and foam or air mattresses on beds and as seat covers in addition to pillows for immobile people. These are available at most pharmacies and surgical supply stores.
- Request that air or foam mattresses as well as elbow, ankle, and knee pads be sent home with the PWA after hospitalization.
- Consider the use of a bed cradle (see the section on equipment in Chapter 2).
- Use diapers, bedpans, Texas catheters, or urinals if the PWA is incontinent. Change soiled sheets and bathe the PWA as soon as possible after an episode of soiling to maintain clean, dry, undamaged skin.

What Not to Do

- Do not allow an immobile PWA to remain in the same position for more than two hours, even if she is asleep or insists she is comfortable. Explain why a position change is so important and encourage the PWA to tell you how she'd like to be repositioned.

When to Consult Your Doctor

- Whenever a pressure sore develops; these usually require the application of topical medications, special dressings, and possibly even oral antibiotics.

Wound Dressings

People with AIDS require dressings of a variety of types for many reasons. Reddened areas, for example, may require protection with little more than a thin layer of padding backed by an adhesive strip to hold it in place. An example of these simple dressings is *Duoderm dressings.*

Pressure sores require anything from a *dry gauze dressing* to a more complicated covering involving the sterile application of medications ordered by a physician. These more complicated sterile dressings are frequently called *wet-to-dry dressings* because the layer of gauze placed onto the wound or against the skin is moistened with betadine or another medication ordered by the doctor and then covered with a layer of dry gauze.

Dressings over reddened areas of skin are usually done at the PWA's or caregiver's discretion, to prevent an at-risk area from breaking down. Other, more complicated dressings are usually ordered by the physician and are implemented, at least initially, by a visiting nurse or home care nurse, who can then teach the PWA or caregiver the proper technique for changing the dressing.

The following sections will help the caregiver to decide when and how to apply various types of dressings, as well as how to select an appropriate one for a particular type of wound. **The information provided here is in no way intended to replace face-to-face, hands-on teaching by a doctor or nurse.**

Note: Other treatments are sometimes used along with dressings when your doctor decides that they would be beneficial. They may include: exposure of the damaged area to air; heat lamps; and powders, foams, and jellies that are applied directly to the wound. The belief in the benefit of these various treatments is highly individual. Consult your doctor for further information regarding what might be appropriate for you.

Applying a Duoderm/ Padding-Type Dressing

Duoderm is a soft, padded-type of bandage with an overlying layer of adhesive that anchors to the skin. It is useful for protecting areas of skin at risk for breakdown: those that are reddened or have minor skin trauma. It allows the skin to breathe, as it disperses drainage within the pad rather than through it. It should not be applied to a heavily draining wound or bleeding area of skin breakdown because it doesn't permit proper assessment of the wound or necessary drainage to occur. It also won't adhere to the wound properly.

What to Do

- Wash your hands and wear gloves.
- Wash and dry the area thoroughly.
- Select the correct size dressing to cover the entire reddened area.
- After the area is dry, place the dressing against the area to be covered. Peel off the paper backing and apply the adhesive side against the skin, covering

the desired area. (A Duoderm dressing placed over moist or wet skin will not adhere properly.)

- Keep the dressing in place until it begins to roll up at the edges or comes off by itself—usually in three to five days.
- Change the dressing if it becomes soiled and dispose of it. (See Chapter 3 for information on proper waste disposal.)

Applying a Dry Gauze Dressing

You may choose to use a plain dry gauze as a dressing in cases of protecting a scab, a surgical site, and in areas not practical for fitting a Duoderm, which come only in standard sizes and shapes.

What to Do

- Choose the size of gauze you will need to cover the identified at-risk area, for example, $2'' \times 2''$ or $4'' \times 4''$.
- Gather all needed equipment, such as scissors and tape, beforehand. (Paper tape is preferred, because it doesn't cause a great deal of pain or difficulty in removal.)
- Cut strips of paper tape before beginning and place them within reach.
- Wash your hands and wear gloves.
- Wash and dry the area to be dressed gently and thoroughly.
- Place dry gauze over the area. Use a sufficient amount to cover but not to be cumbersome or uncomfortably bulky for the PWA. Usually two pieces of gauze placed one on top of the other are enough.
- Tape the gauze in place using the paper tape. Again, use only enough to hold the dressing in place. Too much tape is uncomfortable and also can damage the skin as it is removed.
- Change the dressing at least twice daily—more often if necessary—and immediately, if it becomes soiled with urine or feces. (See Chapter 3 for information on proper waste disposal.)

Applying a Wet-to-Dry Dressing

Wet-to-dry dressings are usually ordered by the doctor for more serious wounds, such as deep bedsores, that require the application of medications directly to the skin lesion or onto a wet gauze, which is then covered by a layer of dry gauze and secured with tape.

What to Do

- Have all the necessary equipment within easy reach before beginning. This means **sterile** gloves, drapes, gauze pads, tape, and any liquid agents (such as saline, betadine, or hydrogen peroxide) and medicinal ointments or creams. Often your doctor or nurse will recommend using a sterile dressing kit, which contains everything you will need. **Remember gloves!**
- Avoid improvising. Follow your doctor or nurse's instructions carefully and completely for all dressing changes.

- Wash your hands carefully with soap and warm water.
- Open a sterile drape onto a smooth, flat, dry surface that is comfortable for you to maneuver from. You'll do the sterile wet-to-dry dressing change from this sterile surface.
- Carefully open the packets containing the sterile gauze bandages by peeling them down and let them fall onto the sterile field so as not to let your unsterile hands or packaging come into contact with the sterile gauze or field.
- Unscrew the cap or break the seal on the moistening agent or medication ordered by your physician or recommended by your registered nurse. This is usually betadine, hydrogen peroxide, or normal saline. (*Normal* in this context means that the pH [relative acidity/alkalinity] of this salt water solution has been adjusted to match what is normally found in the fluids and tissues of our bodies.) **Take care not to touch the rim of the bottle to the wound or with nonsterile hands.** If the bottle is not brand new, pour off the first few drops of liquid into a basin or sink. Next, pour the approximate amount you'll need to wet the gauze into a sterile container.
- Put on sterile gloves, following the technique described in the box below.
- After you have your sterile gloves on, you can touch the sterile gauze freely. Dip the gauze into the moistening agent in the sterile container and squeeze out any excess liquid from it. The gauze should be moist, not wet. Oversaturating the gauze with moistening agents will be of no benefit to the PWA and will only wet his clothes, sheets, and furniture. It also makes it difficult for tape to stick.
- Use the moistened gauze to cleanse the wound, by moving the pad in concentric circles, always working outward from the most central portion of the wound. Make one circular sweep of the area—from the inside to the outside—and discard the gauze. Do this with clean gauzes moistened with the agent the doctor prescribes for three or more repetitions.
- Leave a moistened gauze in place, or apply a medicinal ointment to a fresh sterile gauze pad and place the pad over the wound, according to what the doctor or nurse has advised.
- Cover the moist gauze with a dry piece of gauze.

How to Put On Sterile Gloves

1. Tear open the outer wrapper and drop the inner wrapper containing the gloves onto your disposable sterile field.
2. Pick up the first glove by its cuff and place it on your dominant hand. In other words, if you are right-handed, lift up the right glove with the left hand and put it on. **Do not touch the finger portions of the glove.**
3. Then, with the glove now firmly on your dominant hand, reach that hand into the bent-up cuff portion of the remaining glove and open it sufficiently to allow you to slide in your other hand.

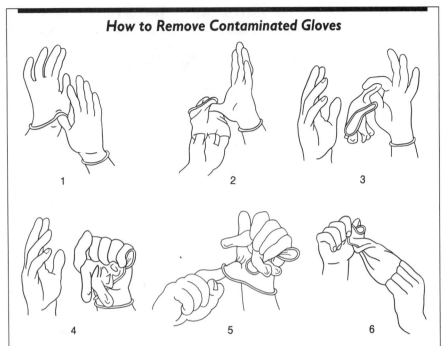

How to Remove Contaminated Gloves

1   2   3

4   5   6

Grasp the edge of the cuff of your nondominant hand and pull the glove off so that as you do, you turn it inside out (steps 1 to 3). Hold that glove in the palm of your other hand (still wearing a glove) (step 4). Now grasp that cuff and pull off the other glove, turning it inside out, and enclosing the contaminated glove from the other hand as you do so (steps 5 and 6).

- Remove your sterile gloves, following the technique described in the box above. Dispose of them as you would any contaminated trash (see Chapter 3).
- Tape the gauze in place. Remember to use the smallest amount of tape needed to hold the dressing in place.
- Change the dressing as often as is recommended by your doctor. Always perform dressing changes on schedule.
- Assess the wound site at every dressing change for potential complications, such as odor, drainage, swelling, bleeding, or increased redness or pain. Check to see if the area feels warm or hot and/or if the PWA is running a fever.
- Take your time when doing a dressing change. Rushing through it will be uncomfortable for the PWA and make it more difficult for you to assess the wound.

What Not to Do

- **Never do dressings on deep, bleeding, or draining wounds without *gloves*, for your own protection. Furthermore, sterile dressings re-**

quire *sterile* **gloves.** Your health care provider will decide if a dressing must be done using sterile technique and will teach you how to do so.

When to Consult Your Doctor

- To get advice if you are unsure about whether to use a dressing or what type to use.
- To ask any questions regarding dressing changes even if they seem foolish or obvious. Never take chances.
- To inform your physician of any changes in the skin, including odor, drainage, bleeding, swelling, or heat at a site already undergoing dressing changes. A more complicated dressing may be needed if drainage or bleeding has increased or developed.

CHAPTER II

Hair Care

Caring for your appearance and looking your best helps you to feel better about yourself and promotes self-esteem. It is especially important for a person who is ill, because this is when she tends to feel the least good about herself.

Hair Washing

The method of shampooing used for a PWA depends entirely on the PWA's general condition. Safety is always the primary consideration.

What to Do

In All Cases

- Assemble all the necessary equipment before starting: shampoo, conditioner, basin, cups, shampoo tray, towels, combs, and brushes.
- Use a mild shampoo and conditioner, one containing the least perfume and alcohol (such as baby shampoo).
- Be careful not to scratch the scalp with fingernails when shampooing, applying conditioner, or massaging.
- Avoid excessive washing, as it will dry out the scalp.
- Rinse hair thoroughly, making sure all the shampoo and conditioner has been washed out.
- Squeeze excess water from the hair and towel dry or blow dry.
- Forget the mousse, spray, or styling gels. These contain alcohol and perfumes that will dry the scalp and hair.
- Avoid hot curlers, curling irons, and excessive blow drying.

If the PWA Is Up and Around

- The PWA can wash her hair in the shower or over a sink. She should not attempt this, however, if she is dizzy, tremulous, or generally tired.

If the PWA Can Sit Up

- Have the PWA either sit in the bathtub, on a chair at the sink, or on a chair or up in bed with a basin of water on a table in front of him.

- Follow the preceding shampooing directions, making sure that the PWA closes her eyes when you rinse out the soap. If the PWA is in the tub or at the sink, a hand-held shower nozzle is very helpful.
- Protect the PWA's clothing with towels and protect yourself from falls by taking care not to slip on spilled water and soap on the floor.

If the PWA Is Unable to Sit Up

- Place the PWA so that her head and upper torso are either up at the head of the bed or to one side of the bed without the head hanging over. Be sure her head and neck are supported.
- Remove any pillows from under the PWA's head.
- Place a chuck, towel, or other protective pad under the PWA's head and shoulders.
- Gently free the hair trapped under the person, being especially careful with long hair so as not to cause pain by pulling it.
- Use a shampoo tray (see Figure 11.1). This plastic or inflatable device with raised sides acts as a trough to collect and drain off water into a basin on the floor beside the bed. These trays may be purchased at pharmacies or surgical supply stores and are reusable.
- Shampoo and condition as you normally would with mild products, and be careful not to get shampoo or conditioner in the PWA's eyes or mouth.
- Empty the water container as often as necessary, but do so quickly so that the PWA doesn't lie with wet hair for long.
- Remove the shampoo tray, slip a towel under the PWA's head, and wrap the towel around the hair to remove excess moisture.

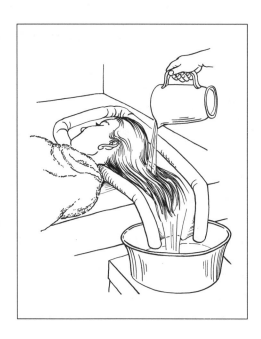

FIGURE 11.1
Shampoo Tray (From *Basic Nursing: A Psychophysiologic Approach* by Karen Creason Sorensen and Joan Luckman. W. B. Saunders, 1979. Reprinted with permission.)

What Not to Do

- Do not leave a bedridden PWA to empty or fill the water container without someone watching the PWA or without safety rails in place if she is confused, lethargic, or unconscious.

Hair Loss

Most people think of hair loss (or *alopecia*) as a loss of part or all of the hair on one's head. This is frequently true; it's important to remember, however, that hair loss may also be from the arms, legs, trunk, pubic areas, face, eyebrows, and eyelashes.

Causes and Characteristics of Hair Loss

Hair may be lost as part of the normal aging process, but it may also be lost due to certain endocrine disorders, serious illnesses, skin disorders, medications, and radiation therapy. There are distinct patterns of hair loss: hair may fall out completely, or in patches, or it may simply become thinner overall. How hair is lost depends somewhat on the underlying cause. For example, someone undergoing chemotherapy may have patchy hair loss all over the body, whereas someone else with a skin disorder localized to one area may only have alopecia in the one affected site.

Hair loss is generally not physically painful (except in the case of some skin disorders). It can, however, be emotionally traumatic. The PWA who has lost his hair has to readjust to his new body image and to the reactions of others who are seeing his new appearance for the first time. In some cases, dealing with hair loss may be as difficult as coping with the diagnosis of HIV or AIDS itself.

What to Look For

- Large amounts of hair (more than what is normal for the person) in the brush or comb, on the pillow or sheets upon waking, in the sink or shower drain after washing, or in your hand after running your fingers through the hair
- A thinning of hairy areas anywhere on the body
- Bald patches anywhere on the body

What to Do

- Take note of thinning hair or bald patches. This may be a sign of illness or a medication side effect that the doctor should be made aware of.
- Support the PWA and try to minimize his distress, because, in many cases, the hair grows back.
- Seek professional counseling or support groups as needed.

- Talk honestly and openly about how you both feel.
- Help the person to decide if he'll use wigs, hairpieces, scarves, hats, or nothing at all. He should wear them if that is what he wants to do and feels comfortable with.
- Avoid the use of over-the-counter medications, "cures," or cosmetics for baldness. They may be expensive, ineffective, and damaging to the skin and scalp.
- Look at and treat the person with hair loss the same as before. Be sensitive, however, to his insecurity and change in self-image.

To the PWA: Look at yourself in the mirror. You will get used to your new appearance more quickly the sooner you confront it. Learn to accept and appreciate yourself. You are still the same person you always were. Don't hide in your house. Face the world. Behave normally. Don't be afraid to use humor to help you and others to deal with your condition. Laughter is often the best medicine and will certainly help to put others at ease.

What to Discuss with Your Doctor

- The possibility of hair loss as a side effect of medications; it is better to know what to expect than to be surprised by this unwelcome occurrence.
- What, if anything, can be done to delay the onset of hair loss.
- Ways the PWA can best be helped to deal with hair loss and body image changes. Obtain information about therapists and support groups in your area.

Shaving

Shaving (most frequently men's facial hair or women's leg and underarm hair) is permitted for people with AIDS except in the case of a low platelet count or a bleeding disorder (see the section on laboratory tests in Appendix A). The doctor may also prohibit shaving (or advise it very cautiously) when the PWA is on an *anticoagulant* medication such as Coumadin (crystalline warfarin sodium) or heparin. These substances slow the body's ability to clot blood; thus, severe bleeding might occur in the event of a shaving accident. In any case, use extreme care when shaving so as not to cut the skin and thus interfere with its natural barrier against infection.

Shaving with an electric shaver is most often recommended for the PWA, because it is less damaging to the skin and less likely to cause accidental scrapes, cuts, or nicks. It's also easier for the caregiver to use an electric razor, because she won't fear hurting the PWA and it's not necessary to apply soap or shaving cream. Long hair, however, can be difficult to shave with an electric razor. In the case of longer hair or when no electric shaver is available, a disposable razor, which can be used once and thrown away, is recommended.

You can also use clippers to trim longer hair down to a length that can be negotiated with an electric razor. Reusable blades are not recommended because of the tendency to reuse them too often without changing the blade, thus causing cuts and skin damage.

What to Do

- Assemble all the equipment you'll need (your razor [electric or disposable], water, shaving cream, soap, towels, and mirror) before beginning.
- Wear gloves.
- Take your time when shaving someone. Rushing leads to cuts and skin irritations.
- Begin by softening the area to be shaved (if using a blade) before shaving either with a nondeodorant soap or shaving cream and water. The skin needs no preparation when using an electric razor.
- Avoid the use of deodorant soaps and aftershave lotions containing perfume or alcohol. They not only dry the skin by removing its natural oils but also can sting freshly shaved areas. Avoid using underarm deodorants and antiperspirants immediately after shaving the underarms, as they too can sting.
- When shaving, it is usually recommended that you pull taut with one hand the area to be shaved and use short, firm, but gentle strokes in the direction in which the hair grows. This decreases skin irritation and prevents ingrown hairs.
- Apply a warm towel to the face after shaving to cut down on skin irritation.
- Discard disposable razors after use in the manner in which you throw away other sharp objects that have come in contact with the PWA (such as needles). (See the section on waste disposal in Chapter 3.)

What *Not* to Do

- **Never share razors. Make sure the PWA has his own razor and that no one else uses it.**
- Do not use depilatories; they tend to be made from harsh chemicals that can cause drying or other skin damage, or provoke an allergic reaction.

When to Consult Your Doctor

- If the PWA is taking anticoagulant medications or suffers from low platelets or other bleeding disorders; your doctor can recommend a shaving method for him.
- If the PWA has a rash or skin lesion in the area you would like to shave.
- If you are unable to stop a cut, nick, or irritation from bleeding after shaving.

CHAPTER 12

The Eyes

Some eye problems or vision changes cannot be avoided. It is always wise, however, to avoid potential problems. This chapter explains how proper eye care and protection can help maintain the best vision possible. It focuses also not on specific eye conditions but on what a change in vision will look or feel like and what the proper response to a detected change should be.

Proper Eye Care

What to Do

- Visit the ophthalmologist at least once per year. **PWAs should consult ophthalmologists, not optometrists, for eye care.** An optometrist is qualified to perform eye exams, and to prescribe and make glasses and contact lenses. However, he or she is not a physician. An *ophthalmologist* is a medical doctor who can diagnose and treat illnesses of the eye as well as perform surgery.
- Keep eyeglass and contact lens prescriptions current.
- Keep glasses clean, in good repair, and adjusted for comfort.
- Wear glasses as prescribed.
- Keep contact lenses clean using recommended techniques and solutions. Remove lenses to allow the eyes to "breathe" according to the schedule the doctor prescribes. Replace them as needed. **Make sure that your eye doctor knows that you have AIDS, since contact lenses may be ill-advised or contraindicated with some HIV-associated conditions.**
- Always read and do close work in well-lighted areas.
- Wear sunglasses outdoors in the daytime all year round to protect the eyes from glare, ultraviolet light, wind, and foreign bodies.
- Avoid smoke-filled areas, aerosol sprays (such as hairspray and room air fresheners), and other chemicals that produce fumes.
- Use only your own eye makeup; it is a breeding ground for bacteria! This includes: eye shadow, eye liner, mascara, false eyelashes, and eyelash glue. Replace makeup that is more than three months old or that has developed an odor or changed its color or consistency.
- Rest tired eyes by closing them gently, not tightly.

- Apply cool compresses or an ice cube wrapped in a towel—**lightly**—if a slight puffiness develops around the eyes; never apply heavy pressure.
- Avoid eyestrain by reading large-print books or using a magnifying glass. Books on audiotape are available through the local library and in major book chains for those who have impaired sight.
- Report any problems to your physician or ophthalmologist as soon as they develop.
- Wash your hands before and after touching *each* eye or its surrounding tissue. (Caregivers should also wash their hands before and after they touch the PWA's eyes.) This decreases the likelihood that an infection will be spread from one eye to the other.

Vision Changes

Certain vision changes (such as nearsightedness, farsightedness, and astigmatism) are quite common among the general population and may, of course, affect persons afflicted with AIDS as well. Very often, however, a change in vision or in the appearance or comfort of the eye may be the first warning sign of an infection or other AIDS-related problem. Only the physician or ophthalmologist can tell whether a particular symptom is a relatively minor problem or an indication of a severe underlying condition.

What to Look For

- A complaint of blurry or fuzzy images—not being able to see things clearly, either nearby or far away
- Squinting
- A complaint of visual field loss. For example, when reading a book, one side of a page will seem to be missing as though one side of the eye is blind. This is usually temporary and can come and go.
- Double vision with or without dizziness
- Difficulty adapting to darkness or light
- The appearance of a halo or rainbow around lights
- A sensation that a curtain is coming down over the eyes
- Spots or floaters before the eyes. These look like black dots or debris wandering across the field of vision.
- Pain in one or both eyes, or a portion of one eye
- A discharge from the eyes. This is particularly evident upon awakening in the morning. Frequently, it will seem as though the eyelid is glued closed by a crusty or sticky material.
- Increased tearing of one or both eyes
- Dryness of the eyes, causing a scratchy sensation, like sandpaper
- A sensation that there is a foreign body in one or both eyes

- An obvious growth on the lid, around the eye, or on the lash lines
- Swelling of the eyelids or around the eyes
- Itching of the eyelid or lash line, or around the eyes

What to Do

- Remain calm. Not all changes in vision, eye appearance, or comfort are serious, permanent, or life-threatening. Reassure the PWA and offer emotional support.
- Note the symptoms, such as: redness, swelling, pain, discharge, tearing, dryness, sensitivity to light, vision changes, or any growths on or around the eye. Also note how long the symptom lasts.
- Note problems that occur together with the eye symptoms, such as dizziness, headache, nausea, or vomiting, since many eye problems are related to other medical conditions.
- Always use clean items, such as tissues, washcloths, and towels, on or near the eyes. Dispose of tissues after one use.
- Remember the importance of household safety for someone with vision problems. Be sure that the floor is kept free of obstacles that the PWA could fall over, and ensure adequate lighting. Keep frequently used and essential items within reach or close by. (See Chapter 2 for more information on keeping the home safe.)
- Remove contact lenses immediately upon identifying an eye problem, discomfort, or pain. If you are unfamiliar with contact lenses and have to do this for the PWA, speak to the ophthalmologist first. (See page 94 for instructions on how to do this.)

What Not to Do

- Never permit PWAs to wear contacts overnight, because PWAs are prone to eye infections.
- Do not attempt to treat an eye problem yourself with someone else's medication or a medicine you have from a previous condition, even if the symptoms appear to be the same.
- Do not use over-the-counter medications, as this may delay proper treatment and diagnosis, mask symptoms, or otherwise compound the problem.
- Do not apply pressure to the eye via the application of a tight dressing or compress.
- Do not patch the eye unless directed to do so by a doctor.
- Do not attempt to remove a foreign body from the eye yourself. (Contact lenses are an exception, if you have been instructed to remove them by the PWA's physician or nurse.)

When to Consult Your Doctor

- **For any loss of vision, double vision, or severe pain or swelling of the eye, the eyelid, or any surrounding tissues, GO TO THE EMERGENCY ROOM.**

- To schedule yearly checkups (or as recommended by your ophthalmologist).
- For any eye complaint, call the ophthalmologist immediately. If, after you have explained the problem, you cannot be seen on the same day, call your regular doctor.
- For information on moistening agents and the use of patches for PWAs who cannot completely close their eyelids (as when in a coma) (see the sections at the end of the chapter for administering drops and patching eyes.)

What to Expect at the Doctor's Office

- Medications may be prescribed to treat the condition. These might include: anesthetic drops, antibiotic drops or ointments, lubricating drops or ointments, and/or oral medications. Be sure you understand the proper route and schedule by which to use these medications.
- If the doctor has ordered eye drops or a patch, be sure that you understand exactly how to apply them; if possible, practice before you leave the office.

Removing Someone Else's Contact Lenses

These techniques can be used only if the person is able to cooperate with you. If the person is unable to cooperate, **do not** attempt to remove the lenses without first talking to an eye care professional.

First and foremost, wash your hands and put on gloves.

For Soft Contact Lenses

Have the person look up while you gently pull down her lower lid with one hand while sliding the contact lens off the iris (the colored part of the eye) with the other hand.

Once the lens is situated on the sclera (the white part of the eye), use your thumb and forefinger to gently pinch up the lens and remove it from the surface of the eye. Remember to do this **gently,** as pinching or pressing too hard may damage the eye, the lens, or both.

For Hard Contact Lenses

Use your forefinger to apply firm pressure as you pull the skin at the outer corner of the person's eye in an outward direction toward the ear. While maintaining the pressure, have the person blink. This will cause the lens to pop out of the eye. Make sure either you or she has a hand ready to catch the falling lens. Place the lens (soft or hard) in its case in a fresh solution of sterile saline.

Putting In Eye Drops

Wash your hands thoroughly prior to handling the eye, and don gloves. Remove the cap of the bottle, taking care not to allow it or the open lip of the container to touch your fingers or the countertop. (You want to keep the medication sterile.)

Have the person look up, and use your index finger to gently pull down the lower eyelid. (Use the finger of the hand on the same side as the eye to which you are applying the medicine.)

Squeeze the prescribed number of drops directly into the pocket of the lower eyelid. The person will naturally blink, which will spread the medicine over the surface of the eye.

Replace the cap and return the bottle to its storage area. (Many eye drops must be kept in the refrigerator. Check with the pharmacist about proper storage of this and all medications.) Wash your hands again.

Follow the same basic procedure for eye ointments, except place a thin ribbon of the medicine along the lower lid sufficient to coat the surface area. Be careful not to touch the tip of the medicinal container to the eyelid.

Patching an Eye

You'll need two eye patches to perform this task correctly. These can be purchased anywhere that first aid supplies are sold, such as drugstores and supermarkets.

Remove any eye makeup and administer any eye medication before patching the eye. Then, have the person close both eyes. Fold one eye patch in half the long way and place it gently in the hollow of the socket. Next, apply the second patch directly on top of the first.

Have the PWA hold the patches in place while you secure them with paper tape, applied diagonally from the center of the forehead across the patch to the side of the face in front of the ear. Make the tape secure enough so that the PWA is unable to open his eye or raise his eyebrow, but he should feel no more than *gentle* pressure.

Change patches daily, or whenever medications need to be instilled.

CHAPTER 13

Mouth Care

Dental Care and Oral Hygiene

The oral hygiene and dental care needs of the PWA aren't really very different from those of a healthy individual. Special care must be taken, of course, when a PWA has a low platelet count or anemia, because of the possibility of bleeding. It cannot be emphasized enough, however, how vital it is to take good care of the mouth to maintain and increase comfort, body weight, and self-esteem while decreasing the potential for dental and/or medical problems centered in the mouth.

What to Look For

- The presence of food particles, plaque, or discoloration of the teeth, which may indicate poor brushing technique or the omission of brushing or flossing
- Receding, swollen, or bleeding gums
- Loose, chipped, or jagged teeth, or broken dentures and other appliances, such as caps, crowns, and braces
- Complaints of mouth pain, sore or bleeding gums, toothaches, or the inability to chew and/or swallow
- Mouth odor that develops during the time elapsed between brushing and rinsing sessions
- Sensitivity of the mouth or teeth to hot or cold foods

What to Do

- Brush the teeth and tongue after each meal with a soft-bristled toothbrush or toothette (see Chapter 2 for information on toothettes).
- Change the PWA's toothbrush every three months or sooner if the bristles become frayed or uneven.
- Use a minimal amount of toothpaste or baking soda solution (see box, page 98) to clean the teeth.
- Floss at least once daily unless advised not to by your doctor or dentist due to bleeding problems.

Mouth-Care Solutions

The doctor or dentist will recommend the correct solution to use, but in general, avoid using a baking soda or salt solution when there are open sores in the mouth, as these solutions may cause stinging. **Do not swallow** any of the following solutions.

Baking Soda Solution
Mix 1 teaspoon of baking soda to 2 cups of warm (not hot) water. Rinse your mouth with the solution and then gargle with it and spit it out.

Baking Soda and Salt Solution
Mix ½ teaspoon of salt with 1 teaspoon of baking soda and 1 quart of warm water. Rinse your mouth with the solution and then spit it out.

Hydrogen Peroxide Solution
Mix 1 part (e.g., 1 oz) hydrogen peroxide (available over the counter in pharmacies) to 3 parts (e.g., 3 oz) warm water (not hot) water. Mix just prior to use. Hold the solution in your mouth for 1 to 1½ minutes and then spit it out. **Do not gargle;** this substance foams in your mouth and might cause gagging if you attempt to gargle with it.

Note: These mixtures are meant to be used as a comfort measure only and in no way replace medical care from your doctor or dentist. If the PWA is unable to rinse, the caregiver can apply these solutions to the mouth using a soft toothbrush or toothette.

- Clean dentures as directed and keep them in a denture cup. Remove them once a day to examine the mouth and gums. Use a small flashlight to observe for redness; irritation; white, red, or purple patches; and ulcers.
- Rinse the PWA's mouth at least every two hours with a mouth-care solution (see box above) if she is unable to brush.
- Keep the PWA's lips moist with lip balm or petroleum jelly.
- Schedule dental visits every six months, or more frequently if necessary.
- Follow the instructions in the box on page 99 to provide mouth care to a weak or comatose PWA.

What Not to Do

- Never insert your fingers into the PWA's mouth for any reason. You might be accidentally bitten.
- Do not floss the PWA's teeth unless an appliance for flossing is used. It is too difficult and can cause choking for the PWA as well as pose a danger of being bitten to the caregiver.
- Do not floss the teeth if
  — the hemoglobin, hematocrit, or platelet count is low,
  — there is a disorder in the body's blood-clotting mechanism, or
  — the PWA is on an anticoagulant medication.

Assisting a Weak or Comatose Person with Mouth Care

Help a weak or unconscious person with oral hygiene in the following manner. First, if she is able to sit up or be turned to the side, use a soft toothbrush or toothette with baking soda solution (see box, page 98). This is preferable to toothpaste because it cleans and freshens the mouth but does not require rinsing. Be gentle in brushing, using minimal pressure in a back-and-forth, up-and-down motion. Allow the baking soda mixture to drain from the mouth into a receptacle.

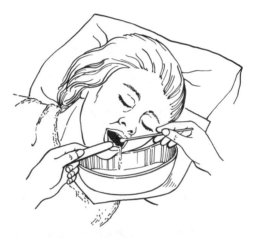

   Do this only if the PWA is cooperative. Never attempt to pry open her jaws. If the PWA bites the toothette or brush, don't pull it out of her mouth, because you may break teeth or cause other injuries. Wait for her to open her mouth.

(Drawing from *Basic Nursing: A Psychophysiologic Approach* by Karen Creason Sorensen and Joan Luckman. W. B. Saunders, 1979. Reprinted with permission.)

When to Consult Your Dentist or Doctor

- To report any abnormal findings associated with the mouth—for example, redness, pain, irritation, or ulcers in the mouth; gum problems; inability to chew or swallow, and so on.
- For all accidents resulting in chipped, cracked, or loosened teeth.
- For deep gum or lip lacerations; they may need sutures and require an emergency room visit if bleeding does not stop with the application of ice and direct pressure.

To the PWA: When seeing your dentist for regular checkups (at least every six months), be prepared to tell her about any medications you are taking. Certain medicines can affect the teeth and condition of your mouth. Inform the dentist of all allergies and your current health problems. It is a good idea to make your dentist aware that you are HIV positive or have AIDS. **Some medical conditions associated with AIDS may complicate some types of dental work (e.g., tooth extractions). Therefore, it is recommended that you obtain your physician's permission and take special precautions, which often include taking antibiotics before and after dental work.**

Mouth Sores

Mouth sores, or any inflammation of the mouth, are often referred to as *stomatitis*. Stomatitis may be caused by infections of a bacterial, viral, or fungal origin or by exposure to radiation treatment, drugs, or chemotherapy. Mouth sores may also be a symptom of a vitamin deficiency or trauma such as that caused by jagged teeth rubbing against the lining of the mouth.

PWAs are most frequently at risk of stomatitis from thrush (oral candidiasis), herpes simplex, poor dentition, and/or as a side effect of chemotherapy or radiation therapy for Kaposi's sarcoma.

What to Look For

- A sensation that the tongue is sore or has been burned
- Generalized mouth pain
- A white patch with a defined border on the tongue but not in the oral cavity, which is often associated with *oral hairy leukoplakia*
- White patches that are thick and curdlike, resembling cottage cheese, which frequently occur with thrush or candidiasis
- Generalized redness, punctuated by brownish or whitish patches, which may be seen along with bacterial infections
- Red or purple patches or nodules, which are often a sign of Kaposi's sarcoma
- Foul breath or mouth odor even after rinsing the mouth and brushing the teeth
- Increased salivation or drooling
- Decreased appetite and food intake
- Sensitivity to spicy foods, acidic foods, or beverages (things that are too hot or too cold)
- A change in the PWA's eating habits, such as his changeover to soft or pureed foods
- Poor condition of the teeth and gums
- A feeling of dryness in the mouth or tongue
- Swelling of the gums and tongue
- Bleeding gums, especially after brushing or eating
- Swollen and/or tender lymph nodes under the chin or along the throat and neck

What to Do

- See the previous section on oral hygiene and dental care for general instructions, including how to brush and rinse.
- Use any topical analgesic prescribed by your physician or dentist according to the directions given to you.
- Constantly survey the PWA's weight, appetite, and nutritional status.
- Use straws or small spoons if it is easier for the PWA to consume food and fluid in this manner.

What *Not* to Do

- Do not use commercial mouthwashes and breath sprays that contain alcohol, phenol, or other harsh chemicals that might burn the mouth.
- Do not use lemon glycerin swabs. They dry out one's lips, tongue, and mouth.
- Do not allow the PWA to wear dentures that are loose or in ill repair. Do not insert any dentures at all if mouth sores are very severe or painful.
- Do not serve excessively spicy, hot, or cold foods. Lukewarm or room temperature preparation is best.
- Do not provide citrus fruits or juices if they burn the mouth.
- Do not permit the PWA to smoke or drink alcohol.
- Do not try home remedies unless you discuss them first with the doctor. They sometimes do more harm than good.

When to Consult Your Dentist or Doctor

To inform the doctor or dentist of any mouth sores, bleeding gums, and associated fevers or swollen glands. Be prepared to describe the problem as outlined in Chapter 5 and specifically in terms of how it interferes with eating, drinking, and oral hygiene.

The PWA may need an examination (including blood work and X rays) and medication. Frequently, these prescriptions include the following: oral antibiotics, topical ointments, pain relievers, lozenges, mouth rinses, or a mixture of several types of remedies. More severe conditions may require a hospital stay for intravenous antibiotics, chemotherapy, and/or radiation treatments.

Bleeding in the Mouth

Bleeding in the mouth is not an illness in itself, but rather a sympton of something else that is occurring in the body. Mouth bleeding can simply stem from poor oral hygiene showing itself in the early stages of *periodontal disease.* It may be a result of a vitamin deficiency (usually vitamin C), which frequently occurs in PWAs experiencing difficulties with eating and digesting. In some

PWAs, mouth bleeding may be due to trauma to the gums in association with a low platelet count during and after chemotherapy or radiation.

What to Look For

- Bright red blood in the mouth or sink after rinsing or brushing
- Brown (old, dried) blood on the teeth, or in the sink after rinsing, especially upon awakening in the morning when bleeding has occurred while sleeping and has dried in the mouth overnight
- Bad breath or mouth odor that recurs after rinsing or brushing
- Swelling or recession of gums
- Loose teeth
- Mouth pain or discomfort (may or may not be present)
- A change in appetite, sense of smell, and/or taste perception
- Nausea from the taste of dried blood in the mouth or from bad breath

What to Do

- Note the exact location of any actual bleeding observed; for example, lower gums.
- Ascertain any change in appetite and eating and drinking habits. Maintain good nutrition and hydration.
- Follow the instructions given in the section on oral hygiene and dental care concerning how to brush, rinse, and floss.
- Eat softer, lukewarm foods cut into small pieces and chewed carefully, if necessary.

When to Consult Your Dentist or Doctor

- For any bleeding and associated problems in the mouth. Expect an exam, possibly including blood tests and X rays. For additional information, see the previous section on mouth sores.

Dry Mouth

A dry mouth is a common and annoying condition for people who have AIDS. The causes vary and may include everything from excess smoking, drinking, or caffeine to the side effects of chemotherapy or radiation of the head and neck. Certain medications may also cause a dry mouth, as can dehydration from poor eating or frequent vomiting and diarrhea. In addition, people with certain metabolic disorders and those who snore, mouth breathe, or have a dysfunction of their salivary glands may suffer from this affliction.

Dry mouth can be uncomfortable as it may interrupt speech and cause cracking of the lips, a sore tongue, and bad breath.

What to Look For

- Constant licking of the teeth and lips by the PWA
- Dry, cracked lips and/or tongue
- Dry or painful mouth, tongue, and/or lips
- Mouth odor that returns quickly, even after frequent brushing and rinsing
- Decreased or nonexistent saliva
- Additional signs of dehydration, such as dry skin, sunken eyes, and decreased urine output.

What to Do

- Encourage the PWA to sip nonalcoholic beverages throughout the day to keep the oral cavity moist. In addition to fluids, try offering ices, ice cream, jello, hard candies, and lollipops.
- Maintain good dental hygiene (see information provided earlier in this chapter).
- Use lip balm or petroleum jelly on cracked lips and in a thin line along the teeth as needed.
- Keep a glass of water by the bedside in case of awakening with a dry mouth sensation.
- Use a humidifier or vaporizer, especially when the person is sleeping or if the person is a mouth breather.

What *Not* to Do

- Do not use mouthwashes or breath sprays containing alcohol or phenol.
- Do not permit the PWA to drink caffeinated or alcoholic beverages if at all possible.
- Do not allow the PWA to smoke or remain in a smoke-filled room, if he can avoid it.
- Do not have the PWA remain in a room with dry heat.

When to Consult Your Doctor

- If you suspect the dry mouth is caused by dehydration.
- If you suspect the condition is caused by a medication (**continue giving the medication** until you discuss it with the doctor).

CHAPTER 14

The Heart and Lungs

Keeping the Heart and Lungs Healthy

Following are a few simple rules to help prevent the development of cardio-vascular and respiratory problems.

What to Do

- Discourage the PWA from smoking and don't permit others to smoke around him.
- Avoid pollutants, toxic fumes, and chemicals.
- Prevent the PWA from being exposed to others with respiratory infections.
- Recommend that the PWA be vaccinated against influenza and pneumovax. Flu shots need to be updated each season (between October and February), according to the particular strain that is expected to be prevalent. Pneumovax is generally good for five years.
- Use a humidifier to thin secretions and keep respiratory passages moist.
- Provide fluids—ideally eight 8-ounce glasses per day.
- Encourage a balanced diet of heart-healthy foods whenever possible. Keep in mind, however, that fat, salt, and cholesterol concerns are generally secondary for PWAs, who should be permitted to eat whenever and whatever they want.
- Provide fresh air and exercise, for example, by taking the PWA on walks in the park.

Chest Pain

Chest pain can have its origin in the heart, lungs, upper abdominal muscles, bones, and other supporting structures (i.e., tendons, ligaments, and nerves) of the neck, shoulders, or chest. A detailed accounting of the nature of the pain and associated symptoms is needed to help determine the cause and origin of the pain.

Causes of Chest Pain

Much of the chest pain experienced by PWAs is respiratory in origin and is due to shortness of breath and cough. Together, shortness of breath and cough may comprise the symptoms of pneumonia, tuberculosis, pneumothorax (collapsed lung due to a collection of air or gas in the chest), or pulmonary embolism (blood clot formation in the lungs). Some chest pain may be cardiac, since PWAs may suffer heart attacks and heart infections (bacterial endocarditis) or inflammations (pericarditis; myocarditis). In addition, heartburn, gallbladder disease, pancreatitis, and even ulcers may have chest pain as their principal symptom. There may also be chest pain associated with acute anxiety states and, of course, direct injury to the chest wall.

Treatment of Chest Pain

Evaluating Chest Pain

- Is the pain mild, moderate, or severe?
- Is the pain sharp, dull, burning, or like a weight pressing on the chest?
- Does it come and go or is it steady?
- When did the pain start?
- How long does it last?
- Where exactly is it located? (Have the person point with one finger to the spot where the pain is most intense.)
- Does the pain travel to the jaw, back, abdomen, or down one or both arms? **Note: The sensation may be described as a tingling or a numbness rather than a pain.**
- Does the person clutch his chest with one or both hands?
- Does the person cushion his chest with a pillow or rock back and forth?
- Are there any associated symptoms such as: nausea; vomiting; poor appetite; belching; sweating; cold, clammy skin; dizziness; increased or irregular heartbeat; fainting; cough; shortness of breath; wheezing; anxiety; or restlessness?
- Is there pallor or cyanosis (a bluish-gray skin tone associated with insufficient oxygen uptake in the tissues)?
- Does the pain worsen with exertion (e.g., climbing steps), with certain movements, with coughing, sneezing, breathing deeply, or eating specific foods, or on an empty stomach?
- What, if anything, relieves the pain (e.g., belching may relieve a gas pain)?
- Is there known cardiac disease, abdominal problems, recent respiratory illness, bodily injury (as from falls or car accidents), or exposure to sick individuals?

What to Do

- Remain calm. Reassure the PWA. Excitement may only worsen the symptoms.
- Take the PWA's pulse, respiratory rate, and temperature (see Chapter 5). Write them down.
- Encourage rest in a comfortable position.

Giving Nitroglycerin

Nitroglycerin tablets are usually good for up to three months once the bottle is opened. (When you open a new bottle, write the date it was opened on the label.) Keep nitroglycerin tablets in their original brown bottle to minimize the weakening effect of exposure to light.

The recommended dosage is one tablet to be placed under the tongue. Wait 3 to 5 minutes and administer another if the pain persists. Do this until there is relief of the chest discomfort, or until a maximum of three to five tablets have been used. **If there is no relief after three to five nitroglycerin tablets or the pain persists for 20 to 25 minutes, call an ambulance and go to the emergency room.**

Do not go anywhere without the nitroglycerin, and never allow the prescription to run out or expire.

- **Administer nitroglycerin tablets if there is a known history of cardiac disease and the PWA has a prescription for them (see box above).**

  Note: It's a good idea for caregivers to take a CPR course familiarizing themselves with proper rescue procedures. These courses are offered by various community organizations, including the American Red Cross and the American Heart Association (see Appendix G).

When to Consult Your Doctor

- When three doses of nitroglycerin have been taken to no avail by a PWA with known coronary artery disease, **CALL AN AMBULANCE.**
- In PWAs without known cardiac disease, call the doctor as soon as possible anytime a PWA experiences a new onset of chest pain or a worsening of existing pain. Be prepared to provide a complete description of the pain. It's helpful for the physician to know the person's pulse, temperature, and respiratory rate. It's important to let the doctor know if the PWA has been around others who are ill. Inform the doctor of any injury to the chest. Also let her know if nitroglycerin was given and/or if there has been a lapse in antibiotic therapy in a PWA who is on antibiotics for PCP *prophylaxis*.

What to Expect at the Doctor's Office

The evaluation of chest pain, which is usually done at the hospital, may include the following: blood tests (e.g., cardiac enzymes to see if a heart attack has occurred), chest X ray, *electrocardiogram (EKG)*, lung scans, *gallium scans,* bronchoscopy (see Appendix A). A picture of the heart done with sound waves called an *echocardiogram* may also be ordered. If there is a possibility that the chest pain is intestinal in origin, the PWA may be asked to swallow a chalky liquid called *barium* after which X rays will be taken of the esophagus and stomach. This is called an **upper GI series.**

Depending on what is determined to be the underlying cause of the chest pain, the PWA may be placed on a variety of medications to manage pain or anxiety and/or to open up the blood vessels. When the blood vessels that carry oxygen to the heart—the coronary arteries—are too narrow to carry sufficient oxygen to meet our needs, we experience chest pain as a warning sign to stop our activity. Heart medications like nitroglycerin widen blood vessels so that they may carry more oxygen-rich blood. In addition, when medications cause blood vessels in the extremities to widen, this pools more blood there, diverting it away from the heart. If less blood reaches the heart, it doesn't have to work as hard to pump blood through the body. Reducing the workload on the heart reduces the likelihood of a heart attack occurring. Hospitalization may be necessary for prolonged, recurrent, severe, or undiagnosed chest pain.

Shortness of Breath

Causes of Shortness of Breath

We all know how it feels to be short of breath. It may have happened to us while we were out jogging or during the course of being very upset or anxious. Illness-related shortness of breath, however, (*dyspnea*) may stem from high fevers and can accompany a variety of lung diseases including asthma, emphysema, pneumonia, tuberculosis, bronchitis, and allergies. Any partial collapse or blockage of the lung will also cause difficulty in breathing. Certain heart conditions—including those that cause fluid to accumulate in the lungs, such as congestive heart failure, *arrhythmias,* or subacute bacterial endocarditis—can also manifest themselves in shortness of breath.

Shortness of breath can occur at any time: while sleeping, while at rest, during minor activity, or, of course, during exertion. It may be accompanied by other symptoms, including cough, chest pain, chest tightness or heaviness, and wheezing.

Treatment of Shortness of Breath

What to Look For

- Rapid breathing, which may be shallow or deep. The average person breathes 18 to 20 times per minute. Shortness of breath usually increases the respiratory rate to at least 30 breaths per minute. (See Chapter 5 for information on how to check a respiratory rate.)
- A sudden onset and/or rapid progression of difficulty breathing; increasing shortness of breath with less and less exertion
- The need to pause while speaking to catch a breath
- Audible or labored breathing
- Wheezing. A wheeze is a high-pitched noise that may sound like a whistle when the person attempts to inhale or exhale.
- Cough. A cough may or may not be present with shortness of breath. Furthermore, the character of the cough may vary. For example, with irritation

of the respiratory passages from exposure to cigarette smoke, there may be a dry, hacking cough. When pulmonary infection or postnasal drip is present, the cough may yield sputum. It's important to note the color and consistency of the mucus and whether there is blood present. It's also important to note the approximate amount of sputum produced (e.g., a teaspoon, tablespoon, etc.) and how often it is present.

- Temperature of 101°F or more
- Flared nostrils
- Use of so-called accessory muscles, muscles not normally used for breathing. These include the abdominal muscles.
- Heaving chest
- Chest pain
- Sweating or cold and clammy skin
- Increased heart rate or a sensation that the heart is beating faster or skipping beats (called palpitations). *Note:* The normal heart rate is from 60 to 100 beats per minute. Any pulse greater than 100 is rapid and may be an indication of respiratory as well as cardiac distress. (See Chapter 5 for information on how to take a pulse.)
- Anxious facial expression
- Fear of choking or not being able to catch a breath
- Loss of appetite or inability to eat because of poor breathing
- Fatigue, malaise, or exhaustion
- Restlessness or confusion
- **Cyanosis—a bluish, grayish, or ashen look to the lips, face, and/or nailbeds. Again, this is a sign of low oxygen and constitutes a medical emergency.**

What to Do

- Reassure the person. Remain calm; a distressed demeanor on your part may increase his anxiety and worsen his shortness of breath.
- Check the PWA's pulse and respiratory rate (see Chapter 5) and record them.
- Take the PWA's temperature rectally (*not* orally—this method would doubtlessly be inaccurate and increase breathing difficulties). See Chapter 5 for instructions on how to take a rectal temperature.
- Follow any instructions given to you by your doctor on similar occasions, if an emergency room visit or doctor's visit does not seem indicated.
- Elevate the PWA's head and upper body, if he is in bed, to at least a 45° angle, and to 90°, if possible. Prop him with pillows under his head and behind his back. He may feel more comfortable slightly bent over with his shoulders hunched.
- Instruct the PWA to try to breathe through pursed lips as follows: Inhale through the nose and exhale as if blowing out a candle. This should be repeated, slowly and deeply, at an approximate rate of 18 times per minute.
- Use a vaporizer or humidifier to moisten the air.

- Administer oxygen, if home use has been prescribed.
- Have the PWA drink fluids if he is able. This thins secretions, keeps the mouth moist, and prevents dehydration. Using a straw might help the PWA to drink fluids more easily.
- Encourage rest and decreased movement.

What *Not* to Do

- Do not allow the PWA to lie flat.
- Do not force the PWA to eat or drink if he seems unable.
- Do not administer other people's medications (e.g., asthma inhalers) to the PWA.

When to Consult Your Doctor

- **CALL AN AMBULANCE**
  - For cyanosis
  - For severe agitation
  - For airway obstruction. If someone's air passages are blocked (either from a foreign body or from the person's own tongue, which can occur when a person becomes unconscious), he cannot speak, breathe, or cough. He will look distressed and may be clutching at his throat. **This is a medical emergency that can rapidly lead to respiratory and cardiac arrest and death. You must perform immediate rescue measures (CPR) to prevent brain damage and death.**
  - For chest pain, accompanied by nausea; vomiting; pain or numbness in the left arm, jaw, or neck; or any chest pain experienced by a PWA with a cardiac condition
- **GO TO THE EMERGENCY ROOM**
  - For a respiratory rate of 36 breaths per minute or more (unless this is usual for the PWA and his doctor is aware of this)
  - For new-onset confusion
  - For shortness of breath that doesn't resolve after resting, sitting upright, and doing breathing through pursed lips
  - If the PWA is restless (this may progress to severe agitation)
- If the shortness of breath does not seem serious. Be prepared to tell the doctor the PWA's respiratory rate, pulse rate, and temperature. Inform him of the presence of other symptoms, such as sputum production, chest pain, cough, or wheezing. It will also be important to relate the circumstances surrounding the shortness of breath. For example, was the PWA awakened from sleep? Did it occur during activity? How long did it last? You should also inform the physician of the PWA's recent medical history, including any known allergies or exposure to persons with respiratory illnesses.

What to Expect at the Doctor's Office

The PWA will probably need a chest X ray and blood tests. The latter might include a sample of arterial blood taken from the wrist to check the amount of oxygen present. If the PWA is coughing up sputum, samples might be obtained for analysis to check for tuberculosis or other infections common among PWAs. Other more advanced diagnostic testing might include: pulmonary function tests, a gallium scan or a bronchoscopy, an electrocardiogram (EKG), a cardiac stress test, and/or an echocardiogram.

Pulmonary function tests are conducted by having the individual breathe into a machine that records various measurements of his lung capacity. These tests are generally not painful, although they may be tiring. In addition, arterial blood samples are sometimes performed in conjunction with the test; this procedure does cause some moderate but very temporary discomfort. Gallium scans and bronchoscopies are discussed at length in Appendix A.

Among the treatments used to manage shortness of breath (depending on its underlying cause) are antibiotics, *bronchodilators* (oral and inhalant types), cough medications, intravenous drugs, and oxygen.

Cough

The cough reflex serves a vital purpose: to remove foreign substances and to clear mucus that might be obstructing the respiratory passages.

Causes and Characteristics of Cough

The nature of the cough (e.g., dry and hacking versus sputum-producing) can tell a great deal about the nature of the underlying illness. Coughs may be chronic, as in cigarette smokers, or they may come on suddenly and be short-lived. The latter type usually occurs with colds, allergies, and asthma attacks. The sputum produced may be thick or thin, clear or colored. A brown sputum is frequently seen among cigarette smokers. Green signals certain infections. Blood may indicate the presence of trauma, a tumor, pneumonia, or asthma.

Blood-tinged sputum is often frothy. It is important to observe whether it is **coughed or vomited**. Someone with low platelets may cause bleeding to occur when he coughs. Coughing up significant amounts of blood may lead to anemia.

Severe coughs sometimes cause throat irritation and/or chest pain that resolve once the cough is quelled.

Treatment of Cough

What to Look For

- A lingering cough, or a change in a chronic cough; for example, a dry hacking cough that is now producing secretions
- Thick or colored sputum

- Coughing up blood
- Chest pain during or just after the cough
- Throat pain or irritation during or after the cough
- Wheezing or shortness of breath
- Associated fever, or increased pulse or respiratory rate (see Chapter 5)
- Associated swollen glands, fatigue, or abdominal pain

What to Do

- Administer any medications or treatments prescribed by the doctor.
- Use a humidifier or a vaporizer to moisten the air. If none is available, and the PWA is strong enough, turn on the hot water in the shower and have him sit in the bathroom and inhale the steam for as long as he can tolerate it, up to about 10 to 15 minutes.
- Encourage good hydration. Have the PWA drink water or clear, noncaffeinated fluids frequently to thin secretions.
- Offer candies or lozenges to moisten the throat and mouth.
- Encourage rest whenever possible.
- Turn the immobile PWA from side to side every one to two hours to keep secretions from thickening. If the PWA is able, get him out of bed and into a chair several times a day (see Appendix E to learn how to move people safely). Mobility is important to keep secretions thin and to prevent pooling of infected material in the lungs. Otherwise, the PWA may develop pneumonia.
- Encourage deep breathing to decrease the pooling of secretions in small airways (see the following section on keeping the lungs clear).
- Help the PWA to cough up any mucus (see the next section).
- Prohibit smoking.
- Eliminate exposure to respiratory irritants, such as wet paint, smoke or fumes, dust, ragweed, and pollen.
- Minimize exposure to others infected with respiratory illnesses.

What Not to Do

- Never diagnose the PWA yourself. What you may think is pneumonia may simply be a cold or allergy. Conversely, it's dangerous to assume symptoms are from a minor virus when in fact they may be from pneumonia.
- Do not ignore a cough that persists for more than a few days. It may be a sign of a serious medical problem such as tuberculosis or pneumonia. This is especially true if there is sputum production. Large amounts of mucus and/or sputum that is yellow, green, or blood-tinged signal the need for antibiotics.
- **Do not give hard candies or lozenges to a confused or semiconscious person, as this can cause choking.**
- **Do not confine a person with AIDS to bed** if he is able to be up and around.

When to Consult Your Doctor

- If the PWA is coughing up large amounts of blood (greater than a teaspoon) or blood clots or is vomiting blood (especially in a PWA known to have a low platelet count or bleeding disorder), **GO TO THE EMERGENCY ROOM.**
- If the cough is a chronic problem and is unchanged, then discuss its management with your physician at your next office visit.
- If the cough is chronic but is now different in some way (e.g., it is usually dry and now it is sputum-producing or it is usually productive of clear sputum and now the sputum is blood-tinged), call your doctor as soon as possible.
- If the cough is a new symptom or is *acute* in your judgment. Be prepared to tell the doctor when it started, whether there is sputum present, and what it looks like. Inform him of any fever as well as what the PWA's respiratory rate and pulse rate are. Tell him if there are any associated symptoms, such as nasal congestion or mucus, earache, sore throat, chest pain, shortness of breath, or abdominal discomfort. Be sure to tell him of any recent exposure to persons with respiratory illnesses, allergens, fumes, or other irritants (including cigarette smoking).
- If the PWA is unable to cough and deep-breathe effectively enough to clear his airway and lungs of dangerous secretions

What to Expect at the Doctor's Office

The PWA should be prepared to have blood and/or sputum obtained for analysis. He may also need a chest X ray, allergy or tuberculosis testing (see Appendix A), a bronchoscopy, a gallium scan, a urinalysis, and/or an electrocardiogram (EKG).

Medications may be prescribed to suppress the cough at night and to help thin secretions.

Keeping the Lungs Clear: Deep Breathing and Postural Drainage

When to Use Deep Breathing and Postural Drainage

Deep-breathing exercises and *postural drainage* (positioning the person to let gravity assist in draining secretions) are performed only on the recommendation of a physician or other health care professional. They are techniques used to help lung expansion and to clear mucus from the lungs and airways. These techniques are most often recommended after surgery, pneumonia, bronchitis, lung abscess, or other respiratory problems. Deep breathing is generally performed when a PWA has a weak cough that is ineffective at bringing up secretions, complains of feeling congested, and is unable to take a deep breath.

Deep breathing and postural drainage can be successful only if the PWA is able to cough effectively enough to clear his own airway or if the caregiver is trained to suction the fluids. Suctioning requires special equipment to be set up in the home and instruction by a trained health care professional until the caregiver is proficient and able to remove the secretions without supervision. The need for suctioning at home is determined by the PWA's doctor.

Performing Deep Breathing and Postural Drainage

What to Do

Deep Breathing

- Use an *incentive spirometer* or blow bottle. These are plastic disposable devices that can be obtained from the hospital if a person is admitted or from a surgical supply store. Have the PWA inhale deeply with the mouthpiece in place to raise a series of tiny, marblelike plastic balls in the bottle. This causes the person to breathe deeply and expand his lungs. This is best accomplished by having the PWA sit upright with his back supported.
- Use the pursed-lips method of breathing. Again, in a sitting position, the PWA inhales deeply through the nose and exhales slowly through pursed lips (as if blowing out a candle).

Postural Drainage

- Begin the procedure by assisting the PWA into a position whereby gravity will help secretions to drain (see Figure 14.1 for some common positions for postural drainage). (Remember to provide tissues or a small basin to catch the secretions.) The PWA can also lean over the side of the bed with his elbows or hands resting on a pillow placed on the floor. The caregiver gently pounds on his back with cupped hands while the PWA coughs (see

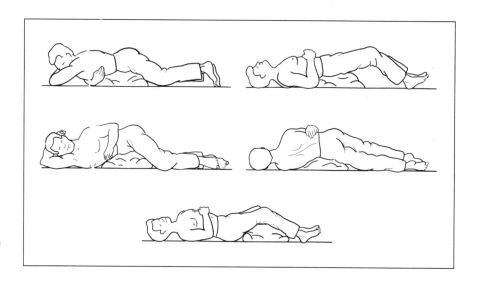

FIGURE 14.1
Positions for Postural Drainage

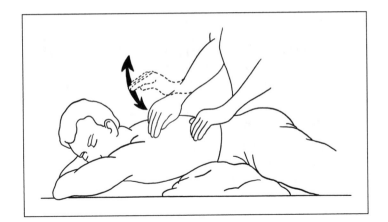

FIGURE 14.2
Correct Hand Positioning for Pulmonary Toileting ("Cupping and Clapping")

Figure 14.2). The vibrations help to loosen and dislodge retained secretions. This should take place for about **five minutes, or less** if the PWA is unable to tolerate the position or the procedure for that long.

Other positions for postural drainage include: lying on one side without a pillow under one's head, with the lower body elevated on pillows so that the head is lower than the rest of the body; or bending at the waist while sitting.

- Do postural drainage prior to meals or wait at least two hours after eating. Otherwise, you may cause nausea and vomiting. It is recommended that postural drainage be performed before bedtime as well, to help the PWA sleep more soundly and comfortably. **Caution: Observe the PWA's position carefully throughout the procedure to ensure that he does not fall.**
- Stop postural drainage when the PWA can't tolerate the position any longer; when no more secretions are heard, felt, or drained; if the PWA's cough is dry; if he becomes tired or short of breath; or if his skin color is bluish.
- For people who are too weak to tolerate postural drainage, the caregiver can use his fingertips to tap the PWA's chest in an attempt to loosen secretions.

What Not to Do

- Never initiate deep breathing and postural drainage without a doctor's order and instructions.
- Never force a PWA to do postural drainage if he is cyanotic or unable to effectively clear his airway on his own by coughing.
- Never slap or hit the PWA during postural drainage. Cup your hands and use a rhythmic motion. This procedure properly performed should never cause pain.
- Do not attempt to perform deep breathing on a PWA who is too tired, too short of breath, in pain, appears cyanotic, or is nauseous or vomiting.

- Do not perform this procedure on PWAs prone to seizures or fractures; those who have low platelet counts; or those who are extremely obese, comatose, or experiencing bronchospasm (an asthma attack).
- Do not leave a person alone during postural drainage in case he becomes exhausted, nauseated, dizzy, or unable to clear his airway.

When to Consult Your Doctor

- If the PWA becomes cyanotic (bluish-gray skin, nails, and lips) or you cannot clear his airway and he appears not to be breathing or is choking, **CALL AN AMBULANCE. Perform rescue breathing if you have been trained to do so.**
- To determine the need for suctioning. *Note:* If suctioning of the PWA is necessary, he may need to be hospitalized until arrangements are made for a nurse to come into the home to perform this procedure or for the caregiver to be trained and all equipment acquired.

Hiccups

Hiccups tend to be more common in men than in women. They appear to serve no useful purpose and in most cases are merely annoying. They are usually temporary, self-limiting, and respond well to home remedies. Given time, they often will stop as unpredictably as they started. In some cases, however, hiccups start and seem to have no end, becoming exhausting and disabling.

Causes of Hiccups

Most often, the cause of prolonged hiccuping is never discovered. A few cases, however, have been found to be associated with imbalances in the body's metabolism (body chemistry), as with diabetes or uremia. Hiccups can also be related to a problem with the *diaphragm* (breathing apparatus) or nervous system, including psychological causes (e.g., anorexia nervosa). Hiccups seem to be more common with alcohol consumption, in association with certain medical conditions (e.g., heart attack, pancreatitis, hiatal hernia), and after surgery, particularly if it was performed under general anesthesia.

Treatment of Hiccups

What to Do

- Allow time for the hiccups to resolve themselves (about 15 to 30 minutes), if the PWA is not uncomfortable.
- Try a home remedy if the hiccups continue. These include:
  — holding one's breath for as long as possible.
  — breathing into a brown paper bag that is held around the mouth so as to rebreathe the air contained within the bag.

—taking a spoonful of sugar followed by drinking a glass of water (only if not contraindicated such as in a diabetic person).

—drinking at least one full glass of water while holding one's breath.

What *Not* to Do

- Never feel foolish about contacting the doctor about such a "trivial" matter.
- Do not assume that hiccups aren't serious. They may be exhausting.

When to Consult Your Doctor

- When hiccups have been unrelenting for a half hour or more or if they stop and then start again within 30 minutes.
- **Any time** hiccups have exhausted the PWA and/or if he has been unable to eat or sleep because of them. Inform the doctor of any and all home remedies you have tried. Describe any recent surgery, abdominal pain, kidney disease, alcohol consumption, cough, or emotional problems.

What to Expect at the Doctor's Office

Although most workups for hiccups prove unproductive, the doctor may call the PWA in for diagnostic tests.

Though there are no medications that get rid of hiccups, sometimes drugs are used to sedate the sufferer. Sedation frequently causes the hiccuping to stop. Medications used to treat hiccups include antianxiety drugs, sleeping pills, and medicines usually used to overcome nausea. In particularly severe cases, surgery has been performed to sever the nerves thought to be responsible for producing hiccups.

CHAPTER 15

*Nutrition for People with AIDS**

Good nutrition is the cornerstone of good health. To preserve one's health, strength, and quality of life, maintaining good nutrition is essential. But there is more than one way to eat right. Everyone has different likes and dislikes, different ways of cooking, different amounts of time and money to invest—even different allergies. Some medications prescribed for PWAs have interactions with foods, a situation that needs to be addressed by a doctor or a registered *dietitian*. It's important to know how to make the right food choices. Caregivers have to know which foods are good for the PWA; which foods will help maintain his weight; what to include in a balanced diet along with what he likes to eat; what you and he are able to prepare; and what you can afford. Simply put, good nutrition means choosing and eating foods everyday that will provide the necessary calories, vitamins, minerals, proteins, carbohydrates, and fats needed to keep the PWA at his ideal body weight and peak of health.

The Four Food Groups

Good nutrition requires eating meals and snacks selected from the basic four food groups. A registered dietitian can provide guidance in food choices and help in deciding how many portions from each food group are needed to maintain weight or promote weight gain for the PWA. The sample menu shown in the box on page 120 can help you get started.

Group I: Fruits and Vegetables

Although they tend to be low in calories (except for dried fruits and avocados), fruits and vegetables supply many of the vitamins and minerals the body needs each day. This group includes fruit and vegetable juices, salads, and cooked and raw fruits and vegetables. Examples of one portion or serving from this group are: one medium apple, half a cup of cooked vegetables, or a small to medium glass of juice. A minimum of **four or more servings per day** is required for a balanced diet.

---

*If the PWA is diabetic, refer to the dietary information in Chapter 17; diabetics have specific nutritional needs that may not be accounted for in the information provided here.

A Sample Menu

This menu provides the minimum daily recommendations of: four servings of fruits or vegetables; three servings of protein; four servings of grains, and two servings of dairy products. It represents a moderate amount of food and allows for eating lunch at a fast-food restaurant. Notice that snacks and beverages are not included but could easily be incorporated.

Breakfast
1 scrambled egg (protein)
1 slice buttered toast (grain)
½ grapefruit sprinkled with sugar (fruit)
1 container flavored yogurt (dairy)

Lunch
1 hamburger on a bun (protein and grain)
lettuce and tomato salad with dressing (vegetable)
french fries (vegetable)
ice cream (dairy)

Dinner
1 chicken breast (protein)
rice with sauce or gravy (grain)
broccoli with butter sauce (vegetable)
1 slice chocolate cake (grain)

Group II: Protein Foods

Once called the "meat group," this is an excellent source of vitamins, minerals, and building blocks for healthy tissue. Protein is found in meat, poultry, fish, cheese, eggs, nuts, and beans. An example of a serving might be: two eggs; two slices of cheese; or two ounces of chicken, turkey, duck, beef, pork, or fish. **Three or more servings per day** from this group is usually recommended as a minimum requirement.

Group III: Grain Group

This group of foods used to be known as the "bread and cereal group." Grains contain vitamins, minerals, and some protein and are an important source of fiber. Examples of foods in this category are cereals (hot and cold), rice, pasta, breads, and crackers. A typical serving might be one slice of bread, or half a cup of noodles, rice, or hot cereal. It is recommended that **four servings or more** be eaten from this group daily. *Suggestion:* To help decrease diarrhea, try eating more of the "white" or refined grains. To help stop constipation, eat more of the "dark" or high-fiber grains.

Group IV: Dairy Group

This group provides protein, vitamins, some minerals, and a lot of calcium. Included in this group are milk, cheese, ice cream, yogurt, puddings, and custards. **Two or more servings per day** are advised. This might include an 8-

ounce glass of milk, a cup (8 ounces) of yogurt, two slices of cheese, or one and a half scoops of ice cream. *Suggestion:* Remember to use whole milk to gain the maximum amount of fat and calories.

For those who are lactose intolerant, milk products may not be easily digested because such individuals lack an enzyme in their bodies responsible for breaking down the sugar or *lactose* found in milk. Low-lactose products can often be substituted (see page 137).

Fats and Oils   Although fats and oils are not members of one of the basic four food groups, they are very important to a person who is trying to maintain or gain weight. Included in this group are butter, margarine, gravies, cream cheese, cooking oils, salad dressings, mayonnaise, sour cream, whipped cream, and sauces. Partake of these as much as you like.

Snack Suggestions

When the usual chips, cola, or fruit get boring, try some of the following healthy suggestions. They provide the protein, vitamins, minerals, and calories that you need with the taste that you may crave:

pizza
fish sticks
tacos
peanut butter and jelly sandwich
canned pasta
cheese and crackers
graham crackers
baby food fruits and desserts
rice, tapioca, or flavored pudding
Jell-O gelatin desserts
ice cream or ice cream soda

yogurt
nuts (peanuts, cashews, almonds, etc.)
dried fruits
cereal and milk
cookies, cake, or pie and milk
cheesecake
caramel popcorn
granola bars
peanut brittle
trail mix

Ten Nutrition Rules for PWAs to Break

1. *Junk food is bad.* All of our lives we have heard that junk food is bad for us. It isn't nutritious. Our parents told us not to eat it. Bunk! Junk food like pizza, tacos, hamburgers, french fries, ice cream, and malteds are basically made up of items from each of the food groups. Though it is true that they tend to be high in calories and vary in quality, the PWA need not concern himself with these issues. The goal for most PWAs is to gain weight. Aside from the high caloric content, junk foods have the added advantages that they require no

cooking, are often delivered to your door, clean up quickly and easily, and generally taste great.

Some junk foods, however, like chips, candy, and soft drinks, are composed mostly of fats, oils, and sugar; they provide little protein, vitamins, and minerals. But they do contain calories. So enjoy these junk foods along with those from the basic four food groups. It's perfectly all right as long as they do not constitute the entire diet.

2. *Megadoses of vitamins and minerals are good.* Even as children, we were aware of the virtues of taking vitamins. Many of us were given chewable vitamins every day. The truth is that if a nutritious and well-balanced diet is eaten every single day, a vitamin or mineral supplement is not needed. However, most of us do not eat a well-balanced diet every day. It's therefore a good idea to take a multiple vitamin and mineral supplement daily if your physician deems it necessary. *Megadoses* **of vitamins (i.e., doses in excess of the Recommended Daily Allowance [RDA] for adults) are** *not* **recommended because of the potential toxic side effects of some nutrients and because of the adverse reactions that may occur, such as nausea, vomiting, and diarrhea.**

Give **one** multivitamin and mineral supplement rather than several pills containing different vitamins and minerals. Shop around for these over-the-counter formulations, because prices vary greatly and most expensive does not necessarily mean best.

3. *Watch your cholesterol.* Although this is important for most people, PWAs should not be concerned with cholesterol warnings unless specifically directed otherwise by their doctors. Serve eggs, cheese, meat, and fried foods and don't worry: The PWA needs the protein, fat, and calories.

4. *Lose weight.* This is not an issue for most PWAs. Weight loss is common in PWAs, and they find it easier to lose weight than to gain or even maintain body weight. While the rest of us may be on weight reduction diets, a PWA should eat anything and everything he desires. No low-calorie, cholesterol-free, sugar-free, dietetic foods for him!

5. *Drink eight glasses of water a day.* Maintaining good hydration is important, but for the PWA this is best done by substituting the word "liquid" for water. Water has no calories, vitamins, or minerals. Better choices for the PWA are milk, shakes, sodas, fruit juices, cocoa, and fruit punch.

6. *Sugar is bad.* As far as PWAs are concerned, this is a lie. Sugar not only helps the PWA to maintain and gain weight because it is chock-full of calories, but it also makes food taste good. The PWA can eat all the sugar, jelly, syrup, honey, and candy he wants. Just be sure to maintain good dental care. Brush and floss the teeth daily and see the dentist regularly.

Special Note: PWAs with diabetes or other glucose abnormalities should consult their doctors regarding sugar intake and diet.

7. *Don't eat between meals.* Often five or six small meals per day or three regular meals with lots of high-calorie snacks in between work best for PWAs.

8. *Canned, frozen, and packaged foods are inferior.* It is nonsense to think that prepared foods are not as good as homemade. Nowadays many are nutri-

tious, delicious, and easy. Items like canned fish, frozen vegetables, canned pork and beans, chili, beef stew, frozen pizza, and boxed macaroni, potatoes, or cereal are all okay.

9. *Raw eggs will give you strength.* Have you heard about the weight lifters who put raw eggs in milk shakes to increase their protein intake? The punchline is that they all are sick from salmonella food poisoning. *Raw eggs are not recommended for PWAs or anyone else!* Provide protein through well-cooked eggs (no runny yolks or partially done scrambled eggs), meat, and cheese. Avoid *all* raw foods, including meat and sushi as well as eggs. If serving eggnog, used prepared eggnog from a carton. Don't make your own if raw eggs are in the recipe.

10. *Macrobiotic and vegetarian diets are best.* Though these diets are eaten by many PWAs, they are not recommended. The macrobiotic diet has its origins in ancient Zen temples. Its principal foods are brown rice, whole grains, and miso soup. Absolutely no sugar, red meat, or refined or processed foods are allowed. Western variations of the macrobiotic diet now allow some foods not on the stricter version.

Vegetarian diets also exclude meat, fish, poultry, and food products derived from these sources. Variations of vegetarian diets permit some leniency. For example, eating eggs might be allowed. These diets require a lot of effort to plan meals, and they are often low in calories, protein, calcium, iron, and some vitamins.

PWAs should reconsider following diets such as these. A PWA who is on such a diet or considering starting one should seek the advice of his physician and a registered dietitian.

Tips for Gaining Weight

Here are some ways for PWAs to add calories to their diets.

- Drink juices, milk, chocolate milk, cocoa, or milk shakes instead of soda, punch, tea, or coffee.
- Make hot cereals or soups with milk instead of water. Even better, use cream or half and half.
- Add powdered milk (2 tablespoons) to every cup (8 ounces) of regular milk you drink.
- Mix cheese into egg dishes such as omelettes or scrambled eggs.
- Add cooked chopped meat to soups and salads.
- Use honey on toast and in tea or hot cereals.
- Put peanut butter on everything—bread, crackers, fruit, cookies—and mix it into milkshakes or cake batter.
- Mix butter or margarine into soups and melt onto popcorn, vegetables, rice and cooked cereals. Add it to casseroles, and spread it on bread and crackers.

- Use salad dressing and/or mayonnaise liberally on salads, sandwiches, vegetables, and even potatoes.
- Try sour cream on potatoes (with butter), vegetables, chili (with some cheese), salads, and in soups.
- Put whipped cream on top of cake, pie, ice cream, hot chocolate, puddings, and other desserts.
- Fry foods rather than roasting, broiling, or baking them.
- Fry vegetables instead of steaming or boiling them.
- Prepare foods with sauces, creams, and gravies.

Liquid Nutritional Supplements

The caregiver can also use liquid nutritional supplements to add calories, especially if the PWA's appetite is poor or he is too weak to eat regular foods. Not all supplements require a doctor's prescription. For example, Carnation Instant Breakfast is delicious and can be added to milkshakes or used as a snack on its own. We recommend adding ice cream to it for a treat. "Polycose" is a powder that has no taste of its own. When added to foods and beverages, it makes them higher in calories.

Canned supplements (e.g., Sustacal and Ensure) are convenient, but they can be expensive. Your dietitian or doctor can guide you in choosing what would be appropriate to meet the PWA's nutritional requirements. Supplements vary in cost, so shop around. When prescribed by a doctor, the cost is often covered by medical insurance.

You may need to try a few canned supplements until you discover one that the PWA likes. Serve them at room temperature, cold, or over ice. Consider adding regular milk, ice cream, chocolate syrup, fruit juice, sugar, or fresh fruit to improve the taste. Most supplements are made with soy milk and therefore are lactose-free, a boon for PWAs who cannot digest dairy products.

Food Safety

Follow these guidelines when purchasing, storing, and preparing food:

- Purchase only pasteurized milk and cheese products.
- Use all food items before the expiration date on the package.
- When purchasing meat, poultry, or fish, put the package into a plastic bag in your shopping cart so that the drippings don't leak onto other foods.
- Don't buy damaged packages, such as: dented cans, swollen cans, or things that have been opened.
- Refrigerate or freeze foods as soon as possible after purchase.

- Keep shelves, countertops, refrigerators, freezers, utensils, cutting boards, sponges, and towels as clean as possible.
- Use a separate cutting board (preferably acrylic, not wood) for meats.
- Wash utensils, cutting boards, countertops, and your hands with soap and hot water after handling one food and before preparing another.
- Wash fruits and vegetables thoroughly before cooking or eating.
- Maintain the temperature of your refrigerator at 40°F.
- Use a meat thermometer when cooking. A minimum of 140°F is needed to kill bacteria. When reheating leftovers, the minimum temperature should be increased to 165°F.
- Cook eggs until the yolks are firm, not runny.
- In restaurants, always order your food to be cooked "well done" as opposed to "medium" or "rare." Fish should be flaky, not rubbery, when cut.
- Due to the risk of food poisoning, raw seafood should not be eaten. The PWA should *not* eat: sushi, sashimi, clams, oysters on the half shell, or even lightly steamed foods like mussels and snails.
- When traveling abroad, boil all water before the PWA drinks it. He should drink only liquids made with boiled water. Don't forget that one can also get ill from ice cubes, brushing one's teeth and rinsing one's mouth with tap water, or swallowing water while showering. Avoid uncooked vegetables and salads. Peel all fruit.

CHAPTER 16

Managing Digestive Problems

PWAs sometimes suffer from digestive disorders or nutritional deficiencies requiring specially designed therapeutic diets. Physicians and registered dietitians can work together to help you if you have these problems or if you need a diabetic diet, a renal diet, a low-fat diet, or a gluten-free diet.

Altered Sense of Taste

The most common cause of altered taste perception in PWAs is medication. Many drugs (intravenous and oral) used to treat the various opportunistic infections have been known to affect the taste of foods. However, the most notorious culprit is pentamidine, which is used in the treatment of *pneumocystis carinii* pneumonia. Most often, the change in taste is described as being metallic, but bitter and overly sweet are also commonly described tastes. Foods containing protein seem to be especially vulnerable to this effect.

Someone with an altered sense of taste may have no interest in eating, even favorite foods. He may complain about food tasting bad or different despite others' perception that the food tastes normal. The PWA may refuse to eat certain foods and may lose weight as a result.

What to Do

- Encourage the PWA to eat as much as he can of the foods that do not have an offensive flavor.
- Serve small, frequent meals and/or snacks between meals.
- Try to maintain a high-calorie diet if the PWA can tolerate one.
- Provide hard candies, especially mints, for the PWA to suck on.
- Serve foods at room temperature rather than when they are very hot or very cold.
- Dine with the PWA whenever possible. Eating with someone will make a meal more pleasant and may keep his mind off the change in taste perception.

What Not to Do

- Do not force the PWA to eat foods that taste bad to him. It may discourage him from eating anything.

- Do not serve spicy foods.
- Do not stop a medication you suspect of changing the person's sense of taste.

When to Consult Your Doctor

- To inform her of the change in taste. Describe the type of change (e.g., bitter, metallic, sweet, or salty); the time of day it occurs or appears to worsen; and which foods are most affected. Determine if a medication may be the cause and whether an alternate therapy may be used. If this is not appropriate, ask for suggestions about how to deal with the problem.
- For a referral to see a registered dietitian for assistance with altered taste perception, which is sometimes helpful.

Poor Appetite and Weight Loss

People with AIDS may have many reasons for having a poor appetite: emotional upset, anxiety, medications, fever, radiation therapy, infectious processes, and pain. For PWAs, weight loss, however minor, is a serious problem. Good nutrition is a vital part of helping the immune system to work.

The goal for all PWAs is to promote weight gain or prevent weight loss. This may sound simple, but for most PWAs, maintaining body weight is a complex and difficult matter. Some may be too weak to eat while others just don't feel like eating.

Causes of Poor Appetite and Weight Loss

- Pain
- Tiredness
- Nausea and/or vomiting
- Diarrhea and/or constipation
- Anxiety and/or depression
- Inability to prepare meals
- Lack of groceries in the house
- No money to purchase food
- New medication *regimen*
- Uncomfortable eating environment; for example, the PWA may have a very hot apartment in the summer or no table to eat on.
- Dental problems
- Altered taste perception
- Lack of variety in the diet
- Need for a special diet

What to Look For

- Clothing seems big
- Actual weight loss is noted on the scale
- Lack of interest in favorite foods
- Sleeping through mealtime

What to Do

- Serve several small meals a day instead of three large ones. For example, the PWA should try eating crackers and juice, a container of yogurt, or half of a sandwich.
- Remind the PWA to eat every two or three hours if he can.
- Try to serve high-calorie, high-protein foods and snacks (see pages 123–124).
- Serve juice, milk, soda, or cocoa with meals to add needed calories.
- Serve high-calorie beverages—ice cream sodas, milk shakes, hot cocoa—and creamed soups, if the PWA is unable to eat solid foods.
- Allow friends and family to help with shopping, cooking, and bringing snacks to the person.
- Make use of take-out or delivered foods, such as pizza, Chinese food, and hamburgers.
- Use canned, frozen, and microwaveable foods.
- Forget the warnings about sugar, salt, and cholesterol unless otherwise directed by the doctor. Serve ice cream, peanut butter, mayonnaise, gravies, sauces, sugar, jelly, honey, candy, fried foods, eggs, chips.
- Eat slowly in a pleasant atmosphere.
- Arrange an attractive plate to make foods more appealing. Use foods of different colors and textures to add interest.
- Allow the PWA to rest between meals if he is tired, but remember that a little exercise stimulates the appetite.
- Administer any antinausea medicine that has been prescribed as directed or about 30 minutes before eating.
- Unless you are told not to by your doctor, you should feed the PWA even if he has diarrhea. Often, if he is lactose intolerant, a lactose-free diet will help decrease the diarrhea (see page 135).
- Maintain good dental health (see Chapter 13).
- Instruct home health aides and homemakers in the preparation of the PWA's favorite foods. Have them prepare extra meals and freeze them to help take some of the load off of you, the caregiver.
- Consider services such as Meals on Wheels, which deliver at least one hot, prepared meal to the door per day.
- Use liquid nutritional supplements as they become necessary (see page 124).

What *Not* to Do

- Do not permit the PWA to eat raw protein foods like uncooked or under-cooked eggs (e.g. "sunny side up"; soft-boiled), Caesar salad, raw meat (steak tartare) or sushi. These can cause food poisoning, a particularly serious threat to PWAs.

When to Consult Your Doctor

- For any change in appetite or weight loss, however insignificant it may seem.
- To discuss the use of pain medication as well as drugs to combat nausea, diarrhea, or constipation if needed.
- To inquire about appetite-stimulating medications.
- To consult a registered dietitian.
- To find out how to sign up for Meals on Wheels, a homemaker, and/or other services.

Difficulty Swallowing

Difficulty in swallowing *(dysphagia)* can stem from a physical blockage or a *neurological* problem that affects the esophagus and prohibits the act of swallowing. It may first be identified as a problem swallowing liquids, solids, or both. Furthermore, it may be described as inability or difficulty in performing the act of swallowing, pain or hesitancy during the course of swallowing, or a sensation that something is remaining in the throat after swallowing has taken place.

Some of the conditions PWAs are at risk for that lead to problems with swallowing include brain damage (e.g., after a stroke); muscular or nerve disorders; and strictures (narrowing), tumors, inflammatory disorders or trauma (e.g., from *chemotherapy* or *radiation*) of the esophagus. These are some of the more serious conditions causing dysphagia; most problems, however, are temporary and easily solved.

What to Look For

- Holding food in the mouth longer than is usually necessary, especially when accompanied by excessive chewing
- Drinking large amounts of fluid to "push down" solid foods
- Vomiting, gagging, or coughing while or soon after swallowing
- Feeling that something is stuck in the throat after eating a meal or snack
- Pain in the mouth or throat while eating and/or drinking
- Requests for soft or pureed foods (or the observation that more solid fruits, vegetables, or meats are left on the plate)
- Drooling and the inability to swallow saliva

What to Do

- Encourage the PWA to eat *any* food and drink *any* liquid that can be comfortably consumed.
- Watch for gagging, choking, or coughing. Be prepared to perform the Heimlich maneuver, as needed.
- Monitor PWA for signs of malnutrition by weighing her every two or three days and noting any weight loss. Do not judge the person's nutritional status by sight. When you're with someone day after day, it is difficult to notice weight changes of one or two pounds.
- Determine whether the PWA is becoming dehydrated by checking for dry skin, dry mouth, a dry or sunken look to the eyes, and little or no urinary output. A dehydrated person might also have a very dark, concentrated urine. (Don't be confused by medications that can also alter the color of the urine.)
- Serve foods and beverages at the temperature and consistency the PWA can best tolerate.
- Feed the PWA at the time of day that she is most able to eat and drink.
- Remember that some of the conditions that cause dysphagia can cause difficulty in breathing as well. **Observe the PWA carefully for any signs of labored breathing, which can be life-threatening and merits immediate attention.**

What *Not* to Do

- Never leave the PWA alone during a meal if gagging is a problem, as there is always the danger of choking.
- Do not try to force or coerce the PWA into eating things she can't swallow. She may choke.
- Do not assume that just because small amounts of food and liquid are consumed the person cannot become dehydrated or malnourished.

When to Consult Your Doctor

- For persistent vomiting during or after meals for two or more days.
- For any fever of 101°F or higher for two or more days, pain, weight loss, gagging, drooling, or sensations that there is something stuck in the throat. Be prepared with a complete history of the problem as outlined in Chapter 5.

What to Expect at the Doctor's Office

Be prepared for a physical examination that might include a throat culture and blood tests initially, possibly followed by more sophisticated tests and/or a referral to an ear, nose, and throat specialist *(otolaryngologist or ENT doctor)*.

Nausea and Vomiting

Nausea is a queasy feeling when a person has the urge to vomit. Vomiting is the actual expulsion of partially digested food and fluids from the stomach. Although it is more common to have nausea without vomiting, you also can vomit without first feeling nauseated.

Nausea and vomiting in people who have AIDS can be caused by a variety of things: medications, opportunistic infections, radiation therapy, chemotherapy, pregnancy, psychological factors, headaches, overeating, or eating spoiled food.

What to Look For

- The onset of the nausea and vomiting, how long it lasts, and what might have caused it
- Projectile vomiting (vomiting that shoots out in a forceful stream that may or may not be preceded by nausea). **This type of vomiting is very rare and is usually a medical emergency**.
- The color of the vomitus (red, brown, yellow, like coffee grounds, etc.) and whether there is a fecal odor to it
- The approximate amount of fluid expelled
- Any accompanying symptoms, such as heartburn, abdominal pain, dizziness, headache, diarrhea, constipation, fever, or jaundice
- Nausea and vomiting episodes that occur after taking certain drugs or medical treatments

What to Do

- If the PWA is nauseated but not vomiting, he should
  - try to eat small, frequent meals.
  - eat dry, bland foods, like crackers, dry toast, or dry cereals.
  - stick to plain, simple foods that require little or no preparation and cooking, such as: broths, puddings, ice cream, rice, pasta, yogurt, cereals, fruit, cheese, and eggs.
  - eat cold foods instead of hot because hot foods tend to have odors that can aggravate nausea.
  - avoid drinking liquids with his meals. It's better to have them either before or after the food.
  - take any *antiemetic* (antinausea) medication prescribed by the doctor.
  - stay out of the room where cooking is being done to minimize exposure to food odors.
- Help the PWA into a sitting position if he complains of nausea or is actually vomiting. If he is unable to sit, turn him onto his side so that the stomach contents can be expelled without causing choking.

- If the PWA has vomited into a bucket or other receptacle, don gloves before emptying it into the toilet.
- Monitor the PWA for signs and symptoms of dehydration (sunken eyes, decreased urine output, dry mouth, and dry skin).
- Maintain good hydration. Have the PWA sip on flat sodas, noncitrus juices, water, weak tea, jello, or lukewarm broths. He can also suck on ice chips or ice pops.
- Help the PWA to brush his teeth and rinse his mouth often.
- Assist the PWA to take slow, deep breaths and try to consciously relax the abdominal muscles to ease nausea and retching.
- Have the PWA rest quietly in an upright position.

What *Not* to Do

- Never leave a nauseated or vomiting person lying on his back or stomach. This increases the chances that he may inhale vomit into his lungs or choke on it.
- Never force a weak, frail, or immobile person to go to the bathroom if he feels the urge to vomit. Provide a receptacle and stay with him.
- Do not allow the PWA to lie down flat for at least two hours after eating. If he must rest, he should sit or recline with his head and upper body at least four inches higher than his head.
- Do not assume nausea or vomiting is from a medication. Consult the doctor to assure a proper diagnosis.
- Do not force the PWA to eat or drink if he has been vomiting. On the other hand, when nauseated, it sometimes helps to eat something.
- Do not try to get the PWA to eat his favorite foods when he feels queasy, because this may turn him off to them later.
- Do not serve greasy, fried, and/or spicy foods when the PWA is nauseous; these foods may worsen the sensation.
- Do not cook foods that have strong odors (e.g., avoid frying fish or brewing coffee).

When to Consult Your Doctor

- **If the PWA has projectile vomiting or if he vomits bloody fluid, black fluid, or material that has a fecal odor or looks as if it has coffee grounds mixed with it, GO TO THE EMERGENCY ROOM.**
- If nausea and/or vomiting persists for more than a day. The doctor will want to know how often the episodes occur; the amount, color, and odor of the material expelled; what started the symptoms (if known); and what, if anything, makes it better or worse.
- If you suspect dehydration. Convey whether the PWA is able to eat and drink.

- If antinausea medication is needed; the present medications are not working to combat vomiting; or to discuss hospitalization for intravenous replacement of fluids lost from vomiting.

Diarrhea

Diarrhea is the passage of several loose or watery *bowel* movements within one day. The stool must be both frequent and fluidlike to truly be diarrhea. Two or three formed stools in a day when you usually only have one, or one watery stool, does not mean that you have diarrhea.

Diarrhea may only last a day or two, as with a minor stomach virus, or it may be chronic and debilitating. Unfortunately, PWAs often suffer from the latter situation. One common cause of daily diarrhea among PWAs is *Cytomegalovirus (CMV) colitis.* Other causes of diarrhea include other opportunistic infections, chronic abdominal conditions (e.g., colitis, Crohn's disease, irritable bowel syndrome), food intolerances, laxative use, and emotional stress. Recent travel, particularly to a foreign country or a rustic area (e.g., while on a camping trip), where diarrhea -causing parasites may be acquired, is another possible cause of loose stools.

What to Look For

- Abdominal pain or cramping
- The feeling of needing to *defecate* urgently and immediately; inability to make it to the bathroom in time
- Many watery stools, with or without blood and/or mucus mixed into the feces
- Associated symptoms, such as fever, nausea, vomiting, decreased appetite, hemorrhoids
- Signs of dehydration (see page 137)

What to Do

- Assist the PWA to the bathroom frequently if he is mobile and check on him.
- Provide the PWA with a way to communicate with you should he need to use the bathroom.
- Provide a bedside commode or bedpan, if the PWA cannot be assured of reaching the bathroom in time. Use adult diapers or chucks as well.
- Maintain good skin care. Use baby wipes or cotton moistened with warm water to clean the rectal area if bathroom tissue is too abrasive to the skin.
- Remove dried feces by first applying baby oil or petroleum jelly to the skin.

Dietary Guidelines for Managing Diarrhea

Specific alterations may be made to this diet for individual situations. Always check with your doctor and/or registered dietitian for advice.

Foods to Eat

Provide foods from the following list:

bananas	plain crackers
plain white rice	cooked cream of rice, cream of wheat,
applesauce	or farina cereal
plain pasta	mashed potatoes (no gravy or butter)
dry white toast	

Provide plenty of clear fluids (tea, apple juice, water, jello, broth, flat ginger ale, or flat lemon-lime soda).

Replace lost potassium by serving bananas, fish, lean meat, and potatoes.

Do not serve *any* dairy products, or spicy, fatty, or greasy foods, until the person has been free of the diarrhea for at least 48 hours and has been able to tolerate foods from the preceding list as well as lean meats, fruits, and vegetables.

Foods to Avoid

Spicy Foods

pizza	East Indian cuisine
chili	Asian cuisine (e.g., Thai, Szechuan)
tacos	

Fatty, Greasy, or Fried Foods

potato chips	gravies
french fries	fried chicken or fish
bacon	stews
sausage	hamburgers or hot dogs

Gas-producing Foods

dried beans	carbonated sodas
cabbage	chewing gum

High-Fiber Foods

raw vegetables	whole wheat breads
raw fruits	nuts and seeds
corn	

- Protect the intact skin in the rectal area and buttocks by applying vitamin A&D ointment or a similar emollient after each bowel movement.
- Offer fluids to prevent dehydration.
- Modify the PWA's diet (see box above).

What *Not* to Do

- Do not stop giving a medication, even if you suspect it of causing diarrhea. Speak to the doctor first.
- Do not clean up fecal material without gloves.
- Do not give alcoholic beverages, as this will worsen dehydration.
- Do not serve foods that stimulate diarrhea (e.g., coffee, tea, prunes).

When to Consult Your Doctor

- If diarrhea persists beyond 24 hours; if it is weakening the PWA; if it is causing dehydration; if it is accompanied by fever, nausea, vomiting, abdominal pain; or if the stool is mixed with blood or mucus.

What to Expect at the Doctor's Office

Diagnostic tests may include intestinal X rays performed after barium is introduced as a contrast medium; stool tests for bacteria and parasites; lactose tolerance tests; and/or *sigmoidoscopy* or *colonoscopy*. If asked to bring in a stool specimen, collect one in a bedpan or by first covering the commode with plastic wrap to catch the specimen. Use a tongue depressor, dixie cup spoon, or popsicle stick to transfer it to a clean, covered container. **Always wear gloves.**

Sigmoidoscopy and colonoscopy involve the insertion of a rigid or flexible fiber-optic scope into the rectum to directly view the intestines to look for signs of infection, inflammation, cancer, or any other growths.

The doctor may prescribe medicines to combat the diarrhea and calm the intestines. It may also be necessary to alter the present medication regimen if a drug is causing diarrhea as a side effect. Referral to a registered dietitian can also help in many cases.

Lactose Intolerance

Many people blame diarrhea and other digestive problems on *lactose intolerance*. Only a physician can diagnose true lactose intolerance, which is an inability to digest the sugar (called lactose) found in milk and dairy products because the person is lacking the enzyme that breaks down lactose.

If the PWA has been diagnosed as lactose intolerant, or you suspect that she has this condition, you should know that it is fairly common. For some PWAs, lactose intolerance is a temporary problem. The principal symptoms include bloating, swelling of the abdomen, gas, and diarrhea brought on by eating foods containing lactose.

The main foods to avoid are regular milk, yogurt, cheese, ice cream, and ice milk. Often, however, these items are well tolerated in small amounts, as, for example, milk in coffee. You can also substitute products specially processed to prevent the symptoms, such as Lactaid, which is a special brand of

---

Dietary Guidelines for Lactose-Intolerant PWAs

Avoid
> regular (whole) milk, skim, low-fat, evaporated, and powdered milk
>
> most cheese
>
> cocoa, chocolate, and chocolate beverages
>
> whipped cream
>
> sour cream
>
> puddings and custards
>
> pancake mix
>
> ice cream and ice milk
>
> gravies, sauces, and soups made with milk or cream

Substitute
> sweet acidophilus milk
>
> lactose-reduced milk
>
> buttermilk
>
> soybean milk
>
> natural cheeses that have aged 90 days or more (such as many cheddar and swiss cheeses)
>
> ices
>
> certain yogurts
>
> powdered coffee creamers
>
> kosher foods marked "pareve"—they are milk-free

---

milk, and eat non-dairy foods, such as Tofutti, in place of ice cream or frozen yogurt. Ask the doctor about Lactaid or Dairy-Ease tablets, which can be purchased in drugstores. They may be taken in pill form before eating or added to milk to help digest the lactose. See the box above for lists of foods to avoid and food substitutions.

Dehydration

Excessive loss of body fluid can occur when someone sweats profusely or has severe diarrhea or vomiting. It can also happen when the intake of fluid is insufficient. This condition is known as dehydration. The consequences of dehydration can be extremely serious; therefore, fluid must be replaced—by drinking, or intravenously if the PWA is incapable of meeting his fluid needs on his own.

What to Look For

- Excessive thirst
- Dry mouth, gums, teeth, and throat

- Decreased skin elasticity. Normally skin is very moist, plump, and supple from the fluids that are present. If the skin appears very dry and, when it is pinched, it remains in "tents," this is an indication of severe dehydration.
- Dry, possibly cracked, skin
- Dry and sunken eyes
- Lack of tears
- Elevated temperature
- Restlessness, agitation, and confusion
- Dark, concentrated urine (brownish or tea-colored)
- Urinating in smaller amounts and less frequently

What to Do

- **Act quickly if you suspect dehydration!** Early intervention can prevent serious complications such as shock and kidney failure.
- Note how often the PWA urinates, what color the urine is, and how much is produced (use a bedpan or urinal to collect the urine for measurement). Remember that certain medications alter the color of urine, so it may be hard to judge urine color in some cases.
- Administer antinausea and antidiarrhea medicines as directed.
- Maintain good hydration by encouraging the PWA to drink as much of any fluid as he can tolerate. If possible, have the person drink the special fluid mixtures described in the box on page 139 to help replace necessary body chemicals (*glucose* and *electrolytes*).
- Encourage the PWA to sip, not gulp, beverages.
- Provide a straw or teaspoon if it helps the PWA to drink.
- Experiment with hot and cold beverages to determine which is better tolerated.
- Try ice chips, popsicles, jello, and sherbet as alternatives to plain drinks. Freeze favorite beverages in ice cube trays to suck on.
- Monitor the amounts of fluids consumed and eliminated.
- Make sure the skin is kept moisturized to prevent breakdown (see Chapter 10).
- Protect a confused or agitated PWA from harm by providing a safe environment and staying with him.

What *Not* to Do

- Do not force fluids, but encourage the PWA to drink.
- Do not allow alcohol or caffeine-containing liquids. They can increase fluid loss.

When to Consult Your Doctor

- Whenever there is severe vomiting, diarrhea, or perspiration that you suspect may lead to dehydration. Be prepared to relate the signs and symptoms

---

Fluid Mixtures for Treatment of Dehydration

Mix up these "cocktails" to help regain the normal glucose and electrolyte balance that may be upset by severe vomiting or diarrhea.

Mixture A

½ teaspoon salt
1 to 2 ounces white Karo syrup
8 ounces apple juice

Add water to make 1 quart and sip throughout the day if able. Try to drink one 8-ounce glass after each bowel movement.

Mixture B

8 ounces apple, orange, or other fruit juice
½ teaspoon honey or corn syrup
1 pinch salt

Mixture C

8 ounces water
¼ teaspoon baking soda

Drink 4 ounces of mixture B alternating with 4 ounces of mixture C after each loose bowel movement or sip from the glass containing mixture B throughout the day.

Mixture D

Gatorade (any flavor)

Drink 8 ounces of Gatorade after each bowel movement.

---

you have noticed, such as: dry skin, dry mouth, dry eyes, decreased or dark urine, new confusion, restlessness, agitation, or fever. You should be able to give the doctor an estimate of fluid intake and loss. Based on the severity of the situation, a hospital visit may be warranted. There, blood tests can identify chemical imbalances indicative of dehydration that may not be readily apparent. In addition, intravenous fluid replacement may be carried out.

Constipation

Constipation is the passage of infrequent or very hard, dry stools. This frequently causes discomfort because the person must strain to eliminate the stool from his body. Constipation results when something interferes with the normal frequency of bowel movements so that they slow down from daily or several times per day to maybe only a couple of times per week or less. As the stool sits in the intestines and is not eliminated from the body in a timely fashion, water contained within the feces is continually absorbed into the intestines, making the stool progressively drier, harder, and more difficult to pass.

Causes of Constipation

Common causes of constipation include the use of narcotics for pain relief, dehydration, immobility, ingestion of barium (as part of medical testing), an underactive thyroid gland, bowel disorders, malfunctioning of the nerves regulating the intestines, emotional problems, and poor bowel habits. Constipation may be a short-lived problem (as, for example, when a PWA is taking a drug that causes this as a side effect) or it may be chronic with some illnesses.

The diagnosis of constipation is relative to the individual. If it is normal for the PWA to have only two bowel movements a week and he continues to have two formed, soft bowel movements a week, he is not suffering from constipation. But a PWA who slows down from three stools a day to only one may indeed be constipated, even though he is having a daily bowel movement.

Treatment of Constipation

What to Look For

- Increased hardness of stools, difficulty in moving the bowels, and/or decreased frequency of bowel movements
- A swollen or bloated abdomen
- Leakage of stool in tiny amounts from the anus. This may mean that there is a solid mass of feces lodged in the rectum that can't be eliminated, thus blocking the normal passage of waste materials.

What to Do

- Increase fluid intake as much as possible.
- Add more fruits, vegetables, cereals, and grains to increase the fiber in the PWA's diet. Fiber adds bulk to the stool and helps it to absorb water; this produces a wetter, softer stool that is easier to pass.
- Ensure quiet, uninterrupted periods of time in the bathroom.
- Increase activity. If able, the person should walk and exercise lightly.
- With the doctor's permission, perform a fecal disimpaction by inserting a lubricated, **gloved** finger into the anus and manually removing the stool.

What Not to Do

- Do not give over-the-counter anticonstipation medications without first checking with the doctor.
- Do not overuse laxatives, which can cause the bowels to rely on chemical signals to trigger a bowel movement. If you try to stop the laxatives, the body has to relearn what to do on its own.

- Do not automatically assume that the person is constipated if his pattern changes from daily or every-other-day bowel movements to a less-frequent pattern just as long as feces remain soft and formed.
- Do not stop giving pain medication if it's still necessary.

When to Consult Your Doctor

- When stools are hard, dry, and difficult or uncomfortable to pass.
- To discuss the continued use of constipating narcotics for pain relief (the doctor may be able to change the painkiller or add a stool softener).
- To ask if you can try over-the-counter or prescription medications such as bulking agents (Metamucil), milk of magnesia, mineral oil, stool softeners (Colace), enemas, or *suppositories.*
- To discuss dietary changes to decrease constipation. Ask for a consultation with a registered dietitian.
- If you think the PWA is developing hemorrhoids or if preexisting ones are becoming inflamed. *Hemorrhoids* are swollen and bulging veins that develop in the rectum, much like varicose veins occur in the legs. When a person strains to move his bowels, hemorrhoids may become painful or itchy. Relieving constipation as well as giving sitz baths, topical anesthetics, hydrocortisone creams, and suppositories will alleviate most hemorrhoidal tissue. (However, the PWA should see his doctor for an exam before trying these medicines.) Occasionally surgery is necessary to remove hemorrhoids.

Rectal Bleeding

When dealing with rectal bleeding, it is important to differentiate between minor bleeding that is easily identified by seeing small drops of bright red blood on the toilet tissue after use and what is improperly referred to as major rectal bleeding. In truth, when the stool appears to be black and tarry or when there is copious bright red blood often accompanied by the passage of clots, the bleeding is not actually from the rectum. In the case of black tarry stools, the blood is actually originating high up in the intestinal tract and is transformed in appearance because it is old or partially digested. **Black stools (*melena*) or the passage of large amounts of blood indicate bleeding from a site above the rectum and can be a medical emergency because of the large volume of blood lost.**

Minor rectal bleeding is not a medical emergency because only minute amounts of blood are lost, even though it may look like a lot due to the absorbency of the toilet tissue. Most minor rectal bleeding is due to hemorrhoids (some are internal; that is, they don't protrude through the rectum and therefore can't be seen though the bleeding is there), constipation (dry, hard stool scratches the delicate tissue lining the wall of the rectum, causing bleeding as stool is forcibly pushed out), or other trauma (such as that caused by anal intercourse).

What to Do

- Use soft toilet paper and wipe gently.
- Use moistened cotton, Tucks, or baby wipes in lieu of toilet tissue.
- Keep this area clean and dry. If there is rectal pain with the bleeding, use a squirt bottle filled with warm soapy water or sitz baths for cleansing rather than rubbing the area with your hands or a washcloth. Pat dry. Do not rub the rectal area with toilet tissue. You may cause further pain and bleeding.
- Look for any visible hemorrhoids, trauma (lacerations, abrasions), or growths.
- Avoid further trauma (as from anal sex).
- Maintain a diet that includes adequate fiber and fluids to avoid constipation.
- Keep the person mobile if able.
- Ensure quiet, relaxing, uninterrupted time in the bathroom.

When to Consult Your Doctor

- At the first sign of rectal bleeding, whether it is minor bright red blood or significant amounts present as red, black, or tarry stools. As with other gastrointestinal symptoms, the doctor may prescribe diagnostic tests and possibly hospitalization for observation and treatment. Follow the instructions given and report back to him.

CHAPTER **17**

Diabetes

Diabetes is such a common consequence of some of the medications (e.g., pentamadine) and therapies (such as total parenteral nutrition) used to treat AIDS, and it is such a complex condition, that it merits a chapter to itself.

What Is Diabetes?

Let's say that you have lasagna and salad for dinner. A complex digestive process transforms that food into simple proteins, sugars, starches, fats, vitamins, and minerals capable of being absorbed from the bloodstream into the tissues of the body. Large, complex sugars and starches are changed into a simpler sugar molecule called glucose. Glucose differs from ordinary table sugar (called *sucrose*) in that it is smaller and therefore travels into the cells more readily.

Glucose remains in the circulation unless a hormone called *insulin* is present and functioning properly. Insulin links up to sugar molecules and carries them across the cell membranes from the blood to the individual cells that rely on glucose to carry out their day-to-day operations. Glucose is to humans what gasoline is to cars. If there's not enough present, the car or the body just won't run.

Without insulin, sugar continues to break down through digestion, but it builds up in greater and greater amounts in the blood and is not able to reach the body tissues where it is so urgently needed. Hence, a diabetic will have a high content of sugar in his blood while he literally starves to death in his cells.

Insulin is produced and stored in an organ of the body that lies near the stomach, the *pancreas*. Normally, the pancreas releases insulin in proportion to the amount (and type) of food that needs to be processed. Thus, a small amount of insulin release follows a small meal and so on. In diabetes, there is either a complete lack of insulin production, or the insulin produced is defective and/or inadequate to meet the needs of the body.

Diabetics who do not produce any insulin have *Type I*, or *insulin-dependent diabetes*, or, since it generally shows itself early on in life, *juvenile onset diabetes*. The latter term is not completely accurate, however, because many adults, including many PWAs, develop insulin-dependent diabetes later in life because of other diseases and/or medications.

More than 90 percent of diabetics fall into the category of *Type II, non–insulin dependent diabetes* or *adult onset diabetes*. These individuals produce at least some insulin in the pancreas; however, this insulin is inadequate in some way: either there is too little of it or it is defective. People with Type II diabetes sometimes take insulin shots short term to get their disease under control, but they do not need to inject themselves with insulin to survive. Generally, their disease is less serious and can be managed with diet, exercise, and one of a group of oral medications called *sulfonylureas*. These medications, in pill form, enhance the action of what insulin Type II diabetics possess, while the diet attempts to reduce the body's demand for insulin by lowering caloric intake. The doctor will provide instruction on the types and side effects of these medications as well as the diet therapy required. The information in this chapter is otherwise equally applicable to Type II diabetics.

Although diabetes poses an even greater challenge to people with AIDS, it can be managed successfully with proper care and commitment. The PWA, the caregiver, and the doctor will need to work together toward achieving specific goals to manage diabetes. They include:

- Learning about the disease and how to monitor it
- Designing and implementing a plan of diet, insulin, and/or oral medications to successfully keep blood sugar levels within a normal range
- Preventing the long-term complications of the disease, which may include: heart attack, stroke, kidney disease, blindness, and circulatory and nerve damage to the limbs resulting in severe infections and/or pain

What to Look For

Especially with non–insulin dependent diabetes, the onset may be insidious, with few or no symptoms. Here are the classic symptoms to watch for:

- Frequent urination and excessive thirst; the kidneys work overtime to filter more sugar from the blood, thus diabetics urinate more often. As they eliminate more water from their bodies, they feel very thirsty and attempt to compensate for the loss and prevent dehydration. You may not notice increased thirst and urination during the day, but the red flag is often raised at night, with diabetic PWAs needing to get up out of bed to use the bathroom or have a glass of water.
- Sudden, severe weight loss and intense hunger; if no glucose is reaching the cells because insulin is inadequate, the body starts to use its own fat and protein tissues as energy sources. Thus, the body wastes away and doesn't gain back the lost fat and muscle mass despite feelings of hunger and increased food intake.

    Note: PWAs are less likely to suffer from non–insulin dependent diabetes as a consequence of their immunodeficiency. However, in this case, the typical picture is of an *overweight*, not wasted, individual. These diabetics must follow a special calorie-restricted diet to try to match their food intake to their insulin production.

- Weakness and fatigue
- Aches and pains, especially abdominal pain
- Nausea and vomiting
- Numbness, tingling, or burning sensations in the fingers or toes
- Blurred vision
- Cuts that don't heal
- Itching and skin rashes
- Worsening yeast infections
- Infections of the gums or bladder that seem persistent

What to Do

- Follow the regimens in the following sections concerning the testing of urine and blood; diet; exercise; foot care; and administration of insulin.
- Get the PWA a Medic Alert tag or bracelet to wear signifying that he is a diabetic.
- Practice good hygiene and skin care to prevent the infections that PWAs and diabetics are extremely vulnerable to (see Chapter 10).
- Ensure that the PWA sees the podiatrist and ophthalmologist regularly, because diabetes can cause major limb problems and blindness.
- Monitor for signs and symptoms of a high or low blood sugar as described in the next section and report them to your doctor.

What *Not* to Do

- Do not change an insulin regimen or stop administering diabetic pills without first talking to the doctor.
- Do not allow the PWA to cheat on his diet or skip meals—especially if on insulin.
- Do not go anywhere without emergency insulin and candy.
- Do not stop giving pentamadine or other medications suspected of causing diabetes without consulting your physician.
- Do not permit the person to smoke cigarettes or drink alcohol.

Hypoglycemia (Low Blood Sugar)

In PWAs on insulin, watch for the signs and symptoms of *hypoglycemia*. This is a **low blood sugar reaction** from too much insulin and not enough glucose. **Hypoglycemia, also called *insulin shock* or an *insulin reaction*, is a medical emergency and requires immediate intervention.**

What to Look For

- Excessive sweating
- Trembling with cold, clammy skin

- Pallor
- Faintness progressing to seizures or loss of consciousness if not caught early
- Headache
- Hunger
- Heart palpitations
- Blurred vision
- Nervousness, irritability, or personality change

What to Do

- Give the PWA a glass of milk if hypoglycemia is suspected. If none is available, give the PWA sugar or food with a high sugar content, such as honey, candy, fruit, or orange juice into which you have mixed 2 to 3 tablespoons of sugar.
- Check the PWA's blood sugar using a home monitoring device (refer to page 150 and Fig. 17.1) to see if it is within normal range (ideally, 70–120 mg/dl) after 20 minutes. If it is still low, give another snack and call the doctor for further advice.
- Give the PWA an injection of *glucagon* (see box below, or follow the instructions of your doctor or nurse), **if he is unconscious**.

    Once the glucagon elicits a response, it should be followed by giving the person juice, candy, or another sugar source. If the person remains

---

Emergency Injection of Glucagon for Hypoglycemic Attacks

Glucagon is available in vials containing 1 milligram of powder accompanied by a diluting solution that is then mixed and injected using an insulin syringe. Glucagon is stable without refrigeration for four to five years and up to three months once it has been premixed and stored in the refrigerator.

You inject it into the individual either under the skin, into a muscle, or into a vein if he becomes unconscious and unable to eat or drink something to raise his blood sugar. A nurse or doctor should instruct you in injection techniques if you are the caregiver and may need to perform this procedure.

To inject glucagon
1. Rub the tops of the two vials with an alcohol swab.
2. Insert a sterile needle attached to a syringe into the rubber stopper on top of the bottle containing the fluid.
3. Withdraw all of the fluid and inject it into the second vial containing the powder.
4. Mix the powder and liquid without withdrawing the syringe.
5. Invert the vial and draw up the entire contents.
6. Put on gloves; then inject.

(See Appendix B for further instructions on injection techniques.)

unconscious for more than 20 minutes, he needs an intravenous infusion of glucose. In any case, **the doctor or ambulance should be summoned once glucagon has been administered**. Don't be surprised if the person experiences nausea and vomiting following a glucagon injection—these are common side effects.

Do not hesitate to give a diabetic person who appears to be hypoglycemic some sugar. If you are wrong, the worst thing that may happen is that it will raise his blood sugar slightly. On the other hand, withholding sugar may be a fatal mistake.

- Try to determine the reasons for the hypoglycemia: too much insulin; too little food; skipped or delayed meals; vomiting; or an unusual amount of exercise.

Hyperglycemia (Elevated Blood Sugar)

Unlike hypoglycemia, which occurs rapidly, **high blood sugar** (also called *hyperglycemia*) is slower and more subtle. It can result from too little insulin, failure to comply with the diabetic diet, infection, fever, or emotional stress.

What to Look For

- Increased hunger
- Thirst
- Excessive urination
- Weakness
- Achiness
- Abdominal pain
- Nausea, vomiting, poor appetite
- Heavy and labored breathing

What to Do

- Test the PWA's urine or preferably his blood sugar and report the results to the doctor, if you suspect hyperglycemia (see pages 148–151).
- Give the PWA non-sugar-containing fluids.

Diabetic Ketoacidosis

Although the signals of too much glucose tend to come on gradually, there are cases when the situation worsens to the point that a metabolic imbalance occurs: a tremendous elevation of blood sugar, which spills out of the kidneys into the urine, accompanied by a wasting of body fat and muscle mass. This condition is called diabetic *ketoacidosis*.

What to Look For

- Nausea, vomiting, lack of appetite, and abdominal pain as if the person had a stomach virus
- Extreme thirst with a dry mouth and dry, flushed skin from dehydration
- Deep, rapid, and labored breathing
- Fruity or acetonelike odor to the breath (acetone smells like nail polish remover)
- Disorientation that can progress to coma if left unrecognized

What to Do

- **GO TO THE EMERGENCY ROOM for insulin and intravenous fluid replacement at once.**

When to Consult Your Doctor

- For coma, seizures, or hypoglycemic attacks that recur within two hours of treatment, **CALL AN AMBULANCE.**
- If blood sugar measurements are greater than or equal to 240 and/or if the PWA is experiencing hyperglycemic or diabetic ketoacidosis symptoms, **GO TO THE EMERGENCY ROOM.**
- If the PWA develops symptoms that suggest diabetes, hypoglycemia, hyperglycemia, or diabetic ketoacidosis.
- If the PWA's hypoglycemia is not responsive to a sugar source within 20 minutes.

What to Expect at the Doctor's Office

Serial blood tests will be taken before and after eating or before and after drinking a special liquid containing glucose in order to diagnose or monitor diabetes. *A blood sugar of 140 mg/dl or greater after a 12-hour fast is diagnostic of diabetes.*

Monitoring Diabetic Control: Blood Sugar and Urine Testing

There are two ways of checking diabetic control. One is by testing the urine for the presence of sugar and *ketones*. The second is by using a small meter or reagent strip to directly measure the sugar content of a drop of blood.

The preferred method of testing is with home blood glucose reagent strips or meters. Refer to Figure 17.1 for tips on the use of these reagent strips. In

How to Test

Obtaining Blood
1. Wash hands to warm them.
2. Hang hand low.
3. Puncture side of tip of finger.
LARGE HANGING DROP.

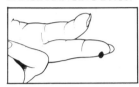

Blood on Strip
1. Cover pads completely.
2. ONE application.
3. DO NOT SMEAR.
4. Start timing IMMEDIATELY.

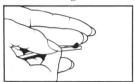

Wipe at 60 Seconds
1. Dry cotton ball.
2. Moderate pressure.
3. Remove ALL traces of blood.
4. DO NOT BLOT.

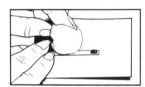

Compare Colors
1. Match pads with both colors on vial label.
2. Estimate if in-between color blocks, e.g., between 80 and 120 equals 100 mg/dl.

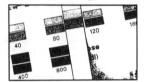

FIGURE 17.1
Use of Blood Sugar Testing Reagent Strips (©Copyright 1986, Boeringer Mannheim Corporation. Used by permission.)

addition, your doctor or nurse should instruct you in the specific operation of a particular glucose monitoring device. Following are some general guidelines.

Urine Tests

Urine testing was the first method taught to diabetics before the invention of compact, fast, accurate, and nearly painless blood monitoring devices. But it is not the monitoring method of choice any longer, because it is an indirect, not a direct, measure. Because different people's kidneys have different capacities for retaining glucose, the amount lost in the urine varies widely and is not a very accurate assessment of how much is contained within the blood. **In fact, blood levels may be twice normal before the abnormality shows itself in the urine.**

If urine testing is to be performed, dipsticks are available. These are specially treated pieces of paper coated with plastic that are dipped into the urine; a color change is read to interpret the presence of sugar and ketones. When testing, the second specimen of the day is the most accurate. For example, if you use the urine that has been in the bladder overnight as the first specimen of the day, you may get an inaccurately high sugar content reading because this urine has been stagnating in the bladder all night. The **best method** is to have the PWA urinate upon awakening, and then check a *second* specimen approximately a half hour later.

When there is poor diabetic control, the body becomes starved for energy sources and begins to break down its own protein (muscle mass) and fat. By-products of this breakdown process are ketones, which then show up in the urine during a bout of diabetic ketoacidosis.

Although urine glucose testing is rapidly becoming obsolete, **urine testing for ketones is still important.** Check the urine for ketones in the presence of very high blood sugar readings (240 mg/dl or higher), or when ill or stressed, or if there is abdominal pain, a fever, and/or signs and symptoms of hyperglycemia.

Blood Tests

Blood tests provide the most accurate measurement of glucose levels. Use special devices designed to quickly and almost painlessly prick the finger rather than attempting to do this with a blade or lancet. This will minimize the chance of injury to you or the PWA. The results may be read either by a machine (styles and costs of machines for this purpose vary) or visually, as is illustrated in Figure 17.1.

Blood sugar generally ranges for diabetics between 70 and 180 mg/dl depending on the specific circumstances of the test (see Table 17.1). The doctor will design a testing schedule tailored to the PWA's needs.

Do's and Don'ts for Accurate Diabetic Monitoring at Home

- **Do remember to always wear gloves when handling blood or urine.**
- Do keep a log of test results along with the time of day, relation to meals, insulin intake, and any special circumstances such as stress or severe infection. Report the information to the doctor.
- Don't store reagent (test) strips in direct sunlight, humid places (like the bathroom), or hot environments. Keeping them anywhere else is fine.
- Don't place your fingertips directly on the treated paper, because moisture and oils from your hands might react with the chemicals and affect the results.

TABLE 17.1   *Normal Blood Sugar Ranges in Relation to Time of Day*

Testing Time	Blood Sugar (mg/dl)
Before breakfast	70–105
Before lunch and dinner	70–130
One hour after eating	Less than 180
Two hours after eating	Less than 150
Overnight (2 A.M. to 4 A.M.)	70 or more*

*Too much insulin in the evening can cause hypoglycemia in the middle of the night. To prevent this, give a bedtime snack.

- Don't use expired or obviously spoiled reagent strips or test chemicals.
- Don't alter the insulin dose or schedule based on monitoring results without first consulting the doctor.
- Don't forget or neglect to check glucose levels as scheduled to avoid the detrimental effects of fluctuations, which, left unnoticed, can lead to hypo- or hyperglycemia.

When to Consult Your Doctor

- Any time blood sugar levels fall below 70 or climb above 120 mg/dl (unless your physician has given you other parameters).
- To report ketones in the urine.
- To ask questions about how to use monitoring equipment and the timing of testing.
- For "official" blood sugar tests conducted by the doctor's laboratory as well as for *glycosolated hemoglobin* checks. This test examines overall blood sugar control during a period of a couple of months as opposed to looking at one random sample.

Insulin and Injection Techniques

People with AIDS generally become diabetic as an adverse effect of a medication they must take to manage an aspect of their disease. At least initially, most PWAs have to be on insulin. Taken by mouth, insulin gets broken down during digestion. Therefore, it must be injected directly into the body, bypassing the digestive tract.

If too much insulin is given or if too little sugar is available for it to work on, hypoglycemia may ensue. But not giving enough insulin or noncompliance with the diabetic diet can put a person at risk for hyperglycemia and diabetic ketoacidosis. Both can lead to irreversible coma and are medical emergencies. (See the beginning of the chapter for more information on how to recognize and treat deficits and excesses of insulin and blood sugar.)

Insulin Types, Dosages, and Schedules

A doctor will prescribe the type, dose, and schedule of insulin that is necessary. Some formulations are derived from other animals (pork and beef), and there is now a type that is exactly like human insulin but is totally synthetic and is made through a process called genetic engineering. The latter type is more expensive but won't cause the allergic reactions or resistance that animal insulins may.

Some insulin formulations start to work quickly and wear off quickly, and other types have a more gradual onset and a longer duration of action. Depending on his needs, the PWA may be placed on one or more than one type of insulin.

A diabetic PWA may need one or more injections each day. After you overcome the psychological barriers, you will find that giving an injection is not that difficult. Follow the diagrams included in Appendix B for proper technique. Always have a nurse teach you in person first, and practice with her; then use the information in this book as a supplement and a refresher. **Note: Some people require a mixed injection of two kinds of insulin into the same syringe. The illustrations and instructions provided in Appendix B do not account for mixed insulin injections. Ask your nurse or diabetic educator how to prepare and inject this type.**

Managing Insulin Use

What to Do

- Keep insulin refrigerated or in a cool, dry place. Do not freeze it or expose it to sunlight. Don't keep open vials for longer than a month at room temperature or three months in the refrigerator.
- **Always wear gloves when injecting insulin.**
- Follow blood and body fluid precautions as you would normally, taking special care with needle and syringe disposal (see Chapter 3).
- Make necessary adjustments once a particular type, dose, and schedule of insulin has been begun to better balance with food intake, activity, stress level, and sick days. To do that, it's essential to keep track of and report the following information:
  — how the person feels between insulin injections.
  — how different levels of activity influence how he feels and what the blood sugar measurements are.
  — how eating, not eating, and vomiting or diarrhea change the way the PWA feels and what his blood sugar reading is.
  — whether the PWA is experiencing any of the signs and symptoms of either hypo- or hyperglycemia and under what circumstances (time of day, relation to meals and activity) these symptoms are appearing.
- Find out from the doctor how to adjust insulin if the PWA wants to exercise or if he is ill with an active opportunistic infection.
- Remember to rotate the sites you are injecting (see Figure 17.2).
- Tell any doctors the PWA consults that he is taking insulin, because some medicines actually impair glucose tolerance and others do not work when the person is on insulin. They may also interfere with insulin's proper functioning.

What Not to Do

- **Never stop insulin unless the doctor has told you otherwise, even if the PWA can't eat.** Test the blood sugar and call the doctor for specific instructions.

- Never use outdated insulin or insulin that looks different than usual. Insulin is normally cloudy, except for the short-acting regular insulin, which is clear.
- Never reuse disposable syringes and needles.

When to Consult Your Doctor

- **If after receiving an injection, the PWA has swollen lips or a sensation that his throat is closing, or is experiencing difficulty breathing, CALL AN AMBULANCE.**
- To learn injection techniques, including site selection and rotation (learning and practice sessions with nurses or diabetic educators are also possible).
- Anytime you believe the insulin dose needs to be adjusted on the basis of how the PWA feels or blood sugar readings in the high or low range.
- **If you notice a localized area of redness at the injection site, a total body rash, or hives.** (Rarely, people on insulin derived from the pancreas of an animal develop an allergy or a resistance to the insulin.)
- If you notice that it is taking greater and greater amounts of insulin to achieve good blood glucose control. This may signal that the body is developing a resistance to the insulin and some changes may need to be made.

Injection Site Selection and Rotation

Where to Inject Insulin should be injected under the skin in the layer between fat and muscle tissue to ensure that the insulin will be absorbed in an even and steady manner.

Figure 17.2 indicates the optimal sites. They include the upper, outer arms; the front and side areas of the thighs; the buttocks; and the abdomen. When

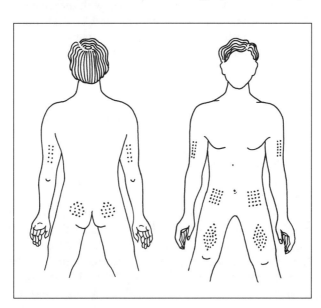

FIGURE 17.2
Injection Site Selection and Rotation (From "Educating the Diabetic Patient" by Charles Kilo. Pfizer Pharmaceuticals, 1982. Reproduced with permission.)

injecting the abdomen, avoid the area around the navel because many blood vessels are located there. In addition, stay away from the waistline; it is a site of many nerve endings, and injections here tend to be more painful.

How to Rotate Sites

Each week, choose a different area of the body to focus on. You can photocopy Figure 17.2 to mark off specific sites within that area injected on particular days. Separate injections by 1 to 1½ inches and don't inject the same site for at least one month.

How to Identify Problems

Occasionally, muscle tissue will become more or less dense than normal from the effects of insulin. Check the injected areas frequently by pressing and running your fingers over the skin. Note any lumps, knots, pits, dimpling, pain, or color change and tell your doctor. Likewise, do not inject these areas until you have consulted her or until the condition resolves.

Nutrition for Diabetics

Nutrition for diabetics is a complex undertaking that frequently requires the services of a registered dietitian to design and teach a special diet tailored to the PWA's likes and dislikes. No one is going to follow a diet if he doesn't like the foods listed—even if it is crucial to his health. Yet, in just about every case of diabetes, *diet is the key*. In time, some people on insulin or oral medications may be able to regulate their disease with diet alone.

For PWAs, diabetes is complicated by their digestive problems. The following discussion provides a broad overview of *diabetic exchange diets*, but it is vital to consult the doctor and nutritionist for specifics on nutrition for diabetics.

Diabetic Exchange Diets

With a few exceptions, a diabetic exchange diet is based on all the ordinary foods a person eats each day. The difference is in the proportions and portion sizes drawn from the basic food groups, the way in which the foods are prepared, and the timing of meals.

The total number of calories suggested for a diabetic PWA depends on the age, sex, and activity level of the individual. It also depends on whether the person needs to lose or gain weight.

You will note that much of what is said next directly contradicts what we discussed in Chapter 15 about nutrition for PWAs. This is because Chapter 15 did not consider the special case of diabetes. People who have both AIDS and diabetes need to balance the two conditions to maintain their weight while stabilizing their blood sugar. You will need expert advice to do this, so see your doctor and registered dietitian.

Managing a Diabetic Diet

What to Do

- Try to serve meals at regular intervals, with snacks spaced in between breakfast, lunch, dinner, and bedtime to keep blood sugar levels relatively stable.
- Have the PWA eat approximately the same amount of food each day, although he should increase his intake slightly on days that he is more active.
- Emphasize more carbohydrates (starches, not sugars) and fiber, with less protein and fat, because it is now believed that complex carbohydrates (bread, cereals, spaghetti dishes) maintain more normal glucose levels in the body in conjunction with fiber. This slows digestion and allows the glucose to enter the bloodstream more gradually.
- Use diabetic exchange lists provided by the doctor, nurse, or registered dietitian. These lists show you how to exchange foods the PWA dislikes for foods he likes and still get the proper proportions of calories and nutrients. It also helps to add variety to the diet by showing which foods are interchangeable with each other.
- Measure portion sizes. Use standard measuring cups and spoons and a kitchen scale. The guidelines and exchange lists set forth by the American Diabetic Association require portions to be
  — level, not rounded or heaping.
  — measured after cooking.
  — measured without fat, skin or bones.
- Prepare foods simply, without sauces, creams, or gravies unless, as is often the case, the PWA needs to gain weight. In that case, the dietitian must tell you how to account for this in your meal plan.
- Bake, broil, boil, roast, or grill foods. It's okay to fry, too, if you use a special vegetable oil spray or take into account the fat you have used to fry the food.
- Avoid foods high in salt, fat, and cholesterol because of their higher risk of cardiovascular disease. However, for PWAs who need to gain weight or who have a poor appetite, you need to balance the relative risks and benefits involved in trying to manage both diabetes and AIDS. Talk to the doctor and/or dietitian about what's best.
- Read food labels carefully and avoid anything that contains corn sweeteners, corn syrup, sugar, honey, fructose, or dextrose as a main ingredient.
- **Be wary of using "dietetic" foods—they are not necessarily also "diabetic" foods.**
- Be careful of artificial sweeteners. Stick to Equal or Sweet 'N Low, in moderation. The chemicals in these are aspartame and saccharin, respectively. Avoid other sweeteners, including fructose, sorbitol, and mannitol, which in large amounts may cause cramping and diarrhea and thus pose special problems for PWAs who may already have these symptoms.
- Encourage the PWA to eat out in restaurants and to eat prepared foods if he likes—he simply must be aware of the contents of what he is eating.
- Ensure that PWAs who are vegetarians get sufficient protein (they can still follow a diabetic diet).

What Not to Do

- Do not skip meals, especially if the PWA is on insulin. When a meal is delayed, give the PWA fruit, some juice, or some graham crackers when you ordinarily would have fed the meal, to prevent blood sugar from dipping.
- Do not serve foods composed mainly of simple sugars, such as candy, jelly, jams, marmalade, molasses, honey, syrups, cake, pie, cookies, sweetened chewing gum, sweetened sodas, condensed milk, or sherbet.
- Do not allow the PWA to drink alcoholic beverages or take over-the-counter cough and cold medicines that contain sugar and alcohol.
- Do not try fad diets or so-called "special diets" for people with AIDS. Discuss them first with the dietitian and doctor.
- Do not serve in between meals, except for allowed snacks.

To the PWA: Diabetic diets are sometimes difficult to understand and follow at first—even for people who don't also have AIDS. See your doctor or nurse and registered dietitian as often as is necessary until you thoroughly understand how to eat. Ask for written materials to supplement your discussions. Make sure the meal plan you receive is one you can comply with. Follow up with your health professionals frequently to let them know how you're doing: if you are tolerating the recommended foods and if your blood sugar is within acceptable limits.

Managing on Days When the Diabetic PWA Feels Ill

People who are HIV positive or who have AIDS are of course more vulnerable to illness, infection, and emotional stressors. All of these, as well as drug interactions, chemotherapy, radiation therapy, accidents, surgery, and pregnancy (which is not recommended for either PWAs or diabetics whose diabetes is not well controlled) can put the diabetic PWA at risk by disrupting the blood glucose/insulin balance.

What to Look For

- Cough, cold, or flu symptoms
- Nausea and/or vomiting
- Diarrhea
- Fever
- Vaginal itching or discharge
- Painful urination, discomfort over the lower abdomen, the urge to urinate more frequently with or without increased urine output
- An infected wound (such as a cut or a bedsore)
- Bleeding gums

What to Do

- Check the PWA's blood sugar at least every four hours.
- Note the body temperature and blood glucose level, and check urine for ketones.
- Check for signs of infection or illness, decreased appetite, vomiting, and diarrhea.
- Stick to the meal plan as much as possible, substituting smaller, more frequent meals for larger meals if necessary.
- Try the "staged" diet described in the box below, advancing to a more complex menu as the PWA begins to feel better.

What Not to Do

- Do not stop insulin, even if the PWA is unable to eat. Instead, ask the doctor if he wants you to switch temporarily to a shorter-acting formulation or a lower dose.
- Do not force the PWA to eat solids if he cannot tolerate them.

A "Staged" Diet for a Diabetic PWA Who Is Ill

If at any time the person's condition deteriorates and he is unable to eat foods from the stage to which you had advanced, drop back one stage until he again feels better.
Note: Some of the foods included in this "sick-day diet" are deliberately high in sugar and should not be eaten under normal circumstances.

Stage 1: Severe nausea, vomiting, diarrhea and fever.
Every 10 to 15 minutes, have the PWA sip a teaspoon of either orange juice, grapefruit juice, tomato juice, soup, broth, tea, coffee, or nondiet cola.

Stage 2: Poor appetite with occasional diarrhea, fever, and fatigue.
Have the PWA eat 1/2 to 1 cup from the following list every one to two hours: bananas, mashed potatoes, creamed soups, hot cereal, plain yogurt, ice cream, jello, broth, juice, nondiet soda. Make sure he also sips nonsweetened fluids every 10 to 15 minutes to replace fluids lost through diarrhea and/or sweating off a high fever.

Stage 3: Slightly improved appetite to the point where small meals are tolerable and the PWA can sit up or walk, although he is still feeling weak and mildly feverish.
Wean the PWA back to the regular diabetic exchange diet, omitting proteins and fats. At this juncture, it might be beneficial to ask the doctor or dietitian for more specific foods to eat and avoid from the various exchange lists.

Stage 4: The person begins to feel better.
Slowly reintroduce proteins, beginning with scrambled eggs, cottage cheese, and broiled fish or chicken. Don't serve heavy or spicy dishes until the PWA is symptom-free for at least two days.

When to Consult Your Doctor

- To report
  - fever
  - infection
  - vomiting
  - diarrhea
  - unstable blood sugar readings
  - high blood sugar readings
  - ketones in the urine
- If the PWA is not better in a few days or if you are having difficulty managing his diabetes under these circumstances. Sometimes temporary hospitalization is the best way to monitor and control the situation.

Routine Health Care for Diabetics

Diabetes can damage blood vessels and nerves in certain target organs of the body, such as the eyes, limbs, and kidneys. Diabetes also decreases the body's ability to fight off infection, a double hazard to an already immunocompromised person. For these reasons, as well as to prevent the long-term complications of diabetes, such as stroke and heart attack, it is important to safeguard the PWA's overall health.

What to Do

- Refer to Chapter 10 regarding how to take care of the person's skin to prevent and care for infections and wounds, to Chapter 13 for information about proper dental care, and to Chapter 19 concerning vaginitis.
- Inspect the PWA's hands and feet daily (see box, page 159) to make sure that any minor problem is taken care of right away. (People with diabetes may have decreased sensation in their extremities, which may cause them to miss injuries and infections.) In addition, be sure not to use very hot water or heating pads due to the danger of causing inadvertent burns.
- Ward off bladder and vaginal infections by encouraging the diabetic PWA to drink six to eight 8-ounce glasses of fluids per day and to empty the bladder every two to four hours. In addition, the PWA should wear loose-fitting cotton clothing (including underwear). If a woman, she should wipe from front to back after going to the bathroom to avoid sweeping bacteria from the rectum into the urethra.
- Apply sunscreen. Even sunburn can elevate blood sugar levels.
- Have blood pressure checked frequently.

Ten Tips for Healthy Feet for PWAs

1. Always wear shoes or slippers.
2. Make sure shoes and socks fit well and are comfortable. Socks should be of a soft cotton or wool material and shoes made of leather or canvas, if possible. Try not to wear either boots or sandals for long periods.
3. Do not wear knee-high stockings or tight garters. Pantyhose is a better choice, although in the summer they trap heat and moisture, predisposing the wearer to vaginal yeast infections.
4. Do not wear socks with holes, patches, or repairs or shoes made of plastic or that cause blisters.
5. Do not wear shoes without socks.
6. Wash your feet with soap and warm (never hot) water. Then pat dry and apply powder to keep them dry. If the skin is cracked or dry, use a lotion, but don't put any between the toes.
7. Cut toenails straight across with clippers or nail scissors, or manicure with an emery board or nail file.
8. Inspect the feet daily for any signs of infection, cuts, blisters, toenail problems, or other abnormalities. Don't forget to check the bottoms of feet. See the doctor right away if you identify a problem.
9. See the podiatrist for treatment of ingrown toenails, calluses, and warts.
10. Avoid being outside for long periods in very cold weather, and apply sunscreen to your feet during the summer.

When to Consult Your Doctor

- For any pain, blood in the urine, sensation that the person has to go to the bathroom but is unable to, abdominal or back pain, vaginal discharge, pelvic pain, unusual vaginal bleeding, or vaginal itching.
- For any decrease in vision, blurred or double vision, pain, or pressure sensation in the eyes.
- For routine health maintenance (this also includes appointments with your internist or endocrinologist, podiatrist, registered dietitian, dentist, and eye doctor).
- For travel advice regarding how the diabetic PWA should eat; how to manage long-distance trips in cars, buses, trains, planes, and boats; insulin storage; special equipment to take with you; and so forth.

CHAPTER **18**

Sexuality and Safe Sex

As we discussed in Chapter 1, HIV is transmitted through the exchange of blood and/or body fluids. Practicing safe sex is one way to prevent transmission and is recommended even if both you and your partner are HIV positive or both of you have AIDS, because **it is possible that one of you may have a stronger strain of the virus that is capable of triggering the other's immunodeficiency**. Safe sex also means not infecting each other with other sexually transmitted diseases that could damage your immunity.

Always keep in mind that HIV is found in the blood (including menstrual blood), vaginal secretions, urine, breast milk, saliva, and semen of infected people and can enter the human body through the mouth (via open cuts or sores), vagina, rectum, or any breach in the skin or mucous membranes (such as a cut or scrape).

Expressing Sexuality

Sexuality is a part of daily life for everyone—male and female, heterosexual, homosexual, and bisexual. Although some medical professionals would advise total abstinence as a way to ensure that transmission does not occur, the decision is yours to make. If you choose to abstain from intercourse, other means of expressing your sexuality are open to you.

You must differentiate between high-risk and low-risk sexual activities. The higher-risk sexual activities include anything that risks the exchange of infected body fluids or blood in any form. They also include engaging in sexual activity while you or the other person are under the influence of mind-altering drugs or alcohol, because these substances can impair your ability to judge which sexual activities are safe and which are not.

What Is Safe?

Here is the lowdown on some specific sexual practices, including some of the more esoteric and exotic practices you may be wondering about. (For more information, contact agencies such as the Gay Men's Health Crisis [GMHC], Planned Parenthood, and other resources to obtain pamphlets, books, and videos and to ask questions regarding safe sex and support groups.)

Okay to Do, but Proceed with Caution

- Bathing or showering together as long as neither partner is incontinent
- Mutual masturbation. No glove is needed if performing masturbation on yourself. Try not to ejaculate onto your partner.
- Rough sex play (spanking, bondage, etc.) as long as the skin isn't broken and no blood is spilled
- "Water sports" (urinating on or using enemas and douches with your partner); they are not the lowest-risk activities but can be engaged in as long as equipment is not shared and waste products do not enter any openings of the body or breaks in the skin. Bathe afterward and do not put soiled fingers in your mouth.
- Body shaving as long as razors are not shared and care is taken not to cause bleeding

What Is Not Recommended

- Piercing or tattooing of the ears, nipples, foreskin, or scrotum. If done, never share needles and always be sure to sterilize them before and after use.
- Nibbling, biting, and deep kissing. If done, engage in with extreme caution so as not to break the skin; do not engage in when there are cuts or open sores in the mouth.
- Pregnancy. When you have AIDS, pregnancy is a very high risk situation for both the mother and the unborn child.

What *Not* to Do

- Never have sex with animals, as animal viruses and bacteria can easily be transmitted. This includes the practice of permitting pet cats or dogs to lick your genitals.
- Never have intercourse under the influence of drugs or alcohol. PWAs should not be drinking or using illicit drugs under *any* circumstances because they may weaken the immune system, somehow function as a cofactor to potentiate the effects of HIV, and/or interfere with the effects of medication being taken.
- Never engage in unprotected sexual activity with anyone—especially intravenous drug users, former users, prostitutes, and individuals who have AIDS or are HIV positive—even if you are already infected. You may contract other sexually transmitted diseases.
- **Never assume that monogamy protects you**. Practice safe sex anyway. You only know that *you* are monogamous. Too many have found out the hard way that their partners were not!
- Never assume that withdrawal before ejaculation is safe. There is enough pre-ejaculatory fluid present on the penis to cause pregnancy and/or infection with HIV.

- Never use douching as a means of protection. In fact, it may push the semen-containing virus and sperm further up into your body.
- Never assume that birth control devices other than condoms will also protect you from HIV. Diaphragms, IUDs, contraceptive foams, films, suppositories, and sponges **do not protect you from infection**—only from pregnancy. Use them for that purpose *in addition to a condom*.
- Never use plastic bags or other makeshift items in place of condoms or dental dams, latex gloves, or finger cots. They have not been demonstrated to protect against the virus.

Practicing Safe Sex

What to Do

Instead of Having Penile/Vaginal or Penile/Anal Intercourse

- Consider engaging in these practices:
  — hugging
  — closed mouth kissing
  — cuddling
  — phone sex
  — talking dirty
  — massage
  — fantasies
  — hand holding
  — role play
  — exhibitionism
  — simulating intercourse without the insertion of body parts or sexual toys
  — use of visual aids such as: sexually oriented magazines, books, and videos
- Talk about sex, instead. The biggest sexual organ is the brain. Discuss your likes and dislikes and experiment with different brands of condoms, different positions, etc. Just be smart and use that brain to be careful not to engage in risky behaviors or overdo things if you are tired, ill, or weak.

If You Engage in Intercourse

Remember that all sex acts are safe as long as both partners agree and are up to the exertion physically, blood isn't drawn, and the following precautions are taken:

- Always use a new latex condom with a water-based lubricant (such as K-Y, ForPlay, H-R, or Surgilube lubricating jellies) **for each act of intercourse**. Condoms treated with nonoxynol-9 *spermicide* are especially recommended, as this spermicide may kill HIV. (There are conflicting reports from studies on this issue.)

    Only latex condoms—not lambskin or natural membrane types— will protect you from HIV. Purchase these at drugstores and supermarkets. Most packages of condoms have expiration dates on them. If there is no date on the package, the rule of thumb is that a condom is good for approximately two years if kept in a dry, cool place and if the package is unbroken. Protect condoms from sunlight and fluorescent light.

- Apply the condom properly and carefully (see box, page 165). You may also want to consider using one condom on top of another to decrease the chance of infection in case one breaks.
- Do not apply baby oil, cooking oils, massage oils, Vaseline petroleum jelly, and fatty or oil-based foods to a condom or to your partner's skin. These fatty foods include peanut butter, whipped cream, chocolate, and liqueurs. Use nonfat or non-oil-based items instead, as they won't damage latex rubber. These foods include honey, jelly, syrups (except chocolate syrup), and confectioner's sugar.
- Use a new latex condom to cover dildos, vibrators, and other sex toys. Wash these items after use with a solution of 1 part bleach to 9 parts water (see Chapter 3 for instructions on using bleach solution).
- Use a new latex condom when performing oral/penile sex. Never allow *ejaculate* to enter your mouth or your partner's.
- Wear latex gloves if you plan to arouse your partner to orgasm using your hand. Licking, sucking, or touching the genitals is safe as long as there is no ejaculate or pre-ejaculatory material present.
- Avoid direct mouth-to-anus contact, not only because of the danger of HIV transmission but because the anus is a portal of entry for hepatitis and parasites as well. This can be accomplished by using a dental dam. *Dental dams* are 6-inch-square pieces of latex that are recommended for use as a barrier during mouth-to-anus contact and for mouth-to-vaginal contact. If a dental dam is not available, an unlubricated condom can be sliced open and spread over the anus or vagina. Both must be held in place by your fingers or a special harness sold in erotica shops. Sometimes using a water-based lubricant over the area increases pleasure. Dental dams and nonlubricated condoms are treated with talc, which can be rinsed off before applying. They are sold in pharmacies and surgical supply outlets. Do not reuse them.
- Don latex gloves or *finger cots* (rubber coverings for a single finger) before inserting fingers or hands into the rectum or vagina. Fingernails should be kept trimmed. This decreases the likelihood of accidentally tearing the glove, scratching your partner, or traumatizing the mucous membranes (sensitive tissue that lines body openings)—all of which provide an entry for HIV.

When to Consult Your Doctor

- If you suspect that you have been exposed to or are experiencing the symptoms of a sexually transmitted disease.

How to Use a Condom in Five Easy Steps

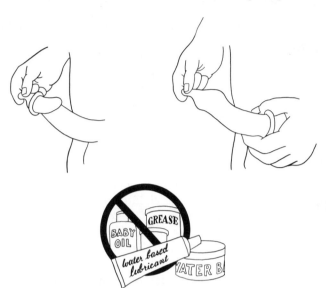

1. Apply the rolled-up condom to the penis when it is erect, leaving space at the tip to act as a reservoir for semen to be collected. If the penis has a foreskin (is not circumcised), pull back the foreskin before putting on the condom.
2. Unroll the condom completely to the base of the penis. (If you decide to lubricate the condom, remember to do so only with water-based lubricants.)

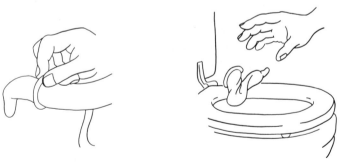

3. Immediately after ejaculation, hold the condom at the base of the penis to secure it in place as you carefully withdraw the penis. Take care not to spill any of the semen inside your partner's body.
4. Dispose of the used condom in the manner in which you dispose of all contaminated waste (see Chapter 3).
5. Wash your penis with soap and water.

Pregnancy and Birth Control

The Transmission of HIV from Mother to Baby

The way in which HIV is passed from mother to baby is uncertain, but it appears that the virus can be acquired in the uterus, from infected maternal blood during delivery, or after delivery. HIV has been found in amniotic fluid, in the blood that travels across the placenta and through the umbilical cord, in vaginal secretions, and in breast milk. It has been isolated from aborted fetuses as well as from children delivered by cesarean section. Thus, we know that babies may be infected while the mother is still pregnant and that there is no advantage to delivering them nonvaginally.

The Implications of Pregnancy for a Person with AIDS

If you are a woman infected with HIV or ill with AIDS, your risk of passing this disease on to a child conceived since you contracted the virus is anywhere from 30 percent to 60 percent. Consider how you feel physically and emotionally right now and decide if you want to take the chance that your baby will have to cope with these same problems.

Children born infected with AIDS must battle the same opportunistic infections and cancers as adult AIDS sufferers. In addition, they don't gain weight or develop normally. Many have brain damage, as well as enlarged livers and spleens. If they live, these children will probably have to face chronic pain and repeated hospitalizations, and they may be ostracized by their teachers, other parents, and their peers.

Furthermore, otherwise well HIV positive women can develop active disease when they become pregnant. Those women who already have AIDS are likely to become sicker during pregnancy because being pregnant adds stress to the body and weakens the immune system.

For all of the preceding reasons, **it is strongly urged that you use a reliable method of birth control to avoid becoming pregnant.** Be sure to discuss your options with your partner so you know who will be responsible for the method you choose and who will pay the costs.

Using Birth Control

What to Do

Use only the methods that have been proven to have lowest failure rate. These are vasectomy, tubal ligation (tied tubes), birth control pills, or a diaphragm with spermicidal jelly used properly.

What Not to Do

- Never rely on methods that have high failure rates. These include the rhythm method and coitus interruptus (withdrawal). It is a good idea, though, to have your partner withdraw just before ejaculating as an additional safeguard (besides condoms) against virus transmission.

- Do *not* consider condoms alone reliable protection against pregnancy. Always use a second method.
- Do not use a diaphragm or vaginal contraceptive sponge during your menstrual period or when you have vaginitis. These devices along with blood (which is a good nutrient source for viruses and bacteria) can provide breeding grounds for opportunistic infections.

When to Consult Your Doctor

- To discuss the various birth control methods. Make your preferences known. Ask for reading materials on your chosen method and others.

Remember, not everyone can use every method. For example, it is recommended that a diaphragm not be used during menstruation. IUDs cannot be inserted when a PWA is taking an anticoagulant. Likewise, these blood thinners pose risks for surgery—vasectomy or tied tubes. Birth control pills may conflict with other medicines that the PWA must take. Therefore, the choice of a contraceptive for PWAs is a highly individualized matter to be decided in consultation with your physician.

Prepare a list of questions to ask and make sure that you fully understand the answers. Some key things you might want to know include:

— How does this method work?
— How effective is it?
— Will it interfere with my medications?
— Will it worsen my disease or put me at risk for other complications?
— What problems and benefits does it possess?

At the same time, ask yourself:

— Will I use this method properly and consistently?
— Will my partner be supportive of this method?
— Will this method interfere with my sense of pleasure and enjoyment?

Make sure you receive a thorough exam and complete instructions on the proper use of the method before you leave the doctor's office.

- If your period is two weeks late or as soon as you suspect that you may be pregnant. (Don't panic. The physical and emotional stressors of AIDS in and of itself may delay your menses—you may not be pregnant.)

If you do become pregnant, either deliberately or accidentally, determine as early on in the pregnancy as possible whether you wish to continue or wish to abort the pregnancy. Delaying a decision may mean a greater chance of abortion-related discomfort and complications. If you decide to continue the pregnancy, start good prenatal care *early*.

Talk to your doctor about what AIDS during pregnancy might mean to you and to the baby. Learn how to take care of yourself to ensure as good an outcome as possible.

Decreased Sexual Desire and Impotence

Remember that for all people with chronic pain or illnesses—male or female—it's perfectly normal for the preoccupations of their day-to-day existence to interfere with such "luxuries" as sexual desire. And while we have by necessity devoted a great deal of attention to safe sex, it is by no means unusual for PWAs to lose their desire and stop having sexual relations. They may be turned off to the idea because of the mode of transmission of the disease or because they are too ill or weak to participate in sex.

What Is Impotence?

Impotence is a catchall phrase often used to describe a man's inability to achieve an erection, to maintain an erection once it is achieved, or to ejaculate after an erection is achieved. In actuality, these problems are different and should not collectively be called impotence. True impotence refers only to a frequent inability to achieve and maintain an erection that is sufficient to permit you to engage in sexual intercourse.

Causes and Psychological Impact of Impotence

Most normal men will occasionally experience the inability to obtain or maintain an erection. This may be due to stress, depression, fatigue, too much alcohol, being distracted, or any number of other temporary causes. PWAs may develop impotence as a result of medications they must take and/or from AIDS-related diabetes, disorders of the nervous system, or emotional factors. Despite the fact that this occasional problem is temporary, many men conclude that they would almost rather die than lose their ability to have intercourse. (It is not unheard of for some men to feel suicidal over the notion of not being able to perform sexually.) It's natural to be distressed and embarrassed—even to overreact—but remember, this is a normal and temporary phenomenon. One unsuccessful attempt at erection can start a vicious cycle of anxiety and depression leading to further difficulties with erections. *Don't let this happen to you!* Don't think that you will suffer from this problem indefinitely. A wide range of treatment options are available to correct the situation.

Diagnosing Impotence

A true diagnosis of impotence is not made until there is a failure to obtain and maintain an erection in at least one out of every four attempts at intercourse. It is usually a gradual, but universal problem. In other words, over time, the PWA will become unable to get an erection regardless of whether he is masturbating or who his partner is. In addition, the erections that naturally occur during sleep and early in the morning, which indicate normal physiological functioning, will disappear. See the box on page 169 for a simple test to determine whether you are having these erections.

Even true impotence may be reversible, depending on its underlying cause. In the meantime, if desire is there, many pleasurable alternatives may be engaged in until the ability to gain an erection returns (see page 163).

Test for Nocturnal Erections

Normally during the sleep cycle, a man will experience one or several erections. To determine whether you are having these erections, glue the ends of a strip of postage stamps together to form a ring. Place this ring around the shaft of the penis (it should fit snugly) before going to sleep. If the ring of stamps is still unbroken in the morning, it is unlikely that you have had an erection.

What to Do

- Try not to feel too embarrassed, ashamed, or unmanly to discuss this problem honestly with your partner. It's very important for the two of you to get it out in the open. Both of you should try to be sympathetic and understanding without sounding condescending or parental.
- Look for possible causes, such as: new stress, new medications, fatigue, worsening illness, alcohol consumption.
- Work on reducing stress, fatigue, alcohol intake, and any other factors you can have influence over.
- Practice other acts of love, sexuality, and sensuality in place of intercourse. You and your partner can satisfy each other in many ways. Do so! You'll both feel better. Don't avoid the sexual side of you because you fear what might or might not happen. Maintain closeness rather than pulling away from each other. Try to understand, not blame or somehow feel responsible and guilty
- Seek out psychotherapy to help overcome emotional causes, to get help for stress and depression, and to help cope with the impotence problem itself. Psychotherapy, meditation, hypnosis, biofeedback, acupuncture, and other treatments have all helped some people (see Appendix C).
- Seek out correct information from reliable sources (e.g., health professionals and organizations). Don't rely on old wives' tales or locker-room stories.
- Confide in only those people you feel you wish to confide in.

What *Not* to Do

- Do not stop taking medications you suspect to be causing impotence. Talk to your doctor first.
- Do not feel pressured to ask or follow advice from friends, coworkers, or magazine articles.
- Do not drink alcohol or use marijuana or other recreational drugs. They have all been implicated in impotence. Alcohol, in particular, can increase your desire but decrease your performance.
- Do not be afraid to bring up this problem when talking to your doctor. Doctors are people, too, and they may be reluctant or forgetful when it comes to raising issues of sexuality.

When to Consult Your Doctor

- If an erection problem occurs more than once. Tell your doctor in some detail exactly what has been occurring. For example, explain whether you have been able to achieve an erection, maintain an erection, and/or ejaculate. Explain whether you are totally lacking in desire or whether it's a case of the mind is willing but the flesh is weak. Are you incapable even when masturbating? Does your performance vary from partner to partner? Are there circumstances that permit you to attain and sustain an erection and those that do not (e.g., stress, depression, alcohol, or drug use)?

What to Expect at the Doctor's Office

After doing a physical exam and possibly some blood and urine tests, the doctor may refer you (and your partner) to a therapist. Sometimes referrals to other specialists are necessary to correct the problem. These may include a urologist, endocrinologist, neurologist, a psychiatrist, or a surgeon (for a penile implant or to correct an anatomical problem).

CHAPTER 19

The Genitourinary System

Menstruation

Every month, a woman releases an egg from her ovary in a process called *ovulation*. If a sperm unites with the egg, that woman becomes pregnant. In preparation for this event, each month there is also a release of hormones that causes a buildup of blood and nutrients within the walls of the uterus to support the fetus. If fertilization does not occur, the hormone levels drop and the lining is shed through the vagina. This normal monthly blood flow is called *menstruation*.

The average cycle of monthly ovulation and buildup and shedding of the uterine lining lasts approximately 28 days. However, this varies greatly from woman to woman. It might be perfectly normal for one woman to experience menstruation every 20 days and another to get her menstrual period every 40 days.

For all women, puberty marks the onset of their periods and menopause the end. Women don't menstruate when they're pregnant. However, menstruation can also stop during times of physical or mental illness. In fact, any significant disruption in a woman's routine or lifestyle can affect her cycle.

Women with AIDS may or may not continue to menstruate depending on how the physical and emotional stressors of the disease have affected their hormonal balance. Very weak, malnourished, and debilitated PWAs most likely will not menstruate. If they do, the possible symptoms are generally the same as for healthy women: lower abdominal cramping, bloating, water retention, acne, cravings for sweet and salty foods, headache, breast tenderness, and/or moodiness. A PWA who is taking an anticoagulant (blood-thinning medication) may bleed a little more than what is usual for her, and the blood may seem thinner with no clots.

What to Do

- Follow instructions given to you by your physician concerning the use of vitamins, acetaminophen, aspirin, ibuprofen, and diuretics ("water pills") for relief of cramps and water retention.
- Tampons should be used only during waking hours and flushed in the toilet for disposal. Change the tampon every two to four hours (or more often, if you need to). Use **only** slender, regular, or small tampons.

- Sanitary napkins should be changed as frequently as is necessary for your flow. To dispose of napkins fold them or roll them and wrap them in paper (newspaper is fine). Place them in a sealed plastic bag and throw this package away with your regular trash. (Check with your local department of sanitation concerning disposal of these and other contaminated wastes, because procedures differ from location to location.)
- Eat sweets or salty snacks if you crave them—it can't hurt!
- Be especially careful if you have intercourse during your period to practice safe sex with latex barriers, because bleeding increases the likelihood of transmission. Consider doubling up condoms. Avoid oral/vaginal contact even with a barrier like a dental dam.
- Keep track of your menses on a calendar so you can inform your doctor of any missed cycles or change in the frequency, flow, or length of your periods.

To the Caregiver

- **Always wear gloves when changing a sanitary napkin for a PWA.**
- Use adult diapers for incapacitated PWAs at this time of the month.

What *Not* to Do

- Never stop taking medication prescribed by your doctor even if you think it is affecting your menstruation. Call and report this suspicion to your doctor.
- Never use "super," "super plus," or other larger-sized tampons. They are too absorbent and don't allow enough air to circulate. The closed, warm, moist environment they provide promotes toxic shock syndrome in an already immunocompromised person.
- Never use a diaphragm or contraceptive sponge during your period. It has to remain in the vagina for at least six hours to be effective and, in combination with the blood that is present at this time, can promote infection.
- Do not douche. Douching is not recommended for any woman. It is simply not necessary and may even promote vaginal infections and irritations by disturbing the normal vaginal balance. If you feel you must douche, douche once (not repeatedly) using plain water or a water and baking soda douche. Be careful of causing an excessively dry condition in the vagina. Furthermore, disinfect your douching equipment carefully and never share it with others. Never reuse disposable douche bottles.

When to Consult Your Doctor

- If there is a change in your flow, the timing of your cycle, or a cessation of your menses.

Vaginitis

Many things can cause *vaginitis,* an inflammation of the vaginal tissue marked by swelling, redness, itching, discharge, and/or a burning discomfort. It may be a result of infections (e.g., gonorrhea, yeast) or irritations (e.g., from foreign objects being inserted into the vagina or frequent douching). Women with AIDS are particularly vulnerable to vaginal infections due to the upset of the normal balance from frequent and/or recent antibiotic use and an altered immune system. A PWA also may be prone to vaginitis if she has recently used new soaps, new spermicides, perfumed bubble baths, or laundry detergents that might cause an allergic reaction within the vagina or had unprotected intercourse.

What to Look For

- Vaginal discharge of any color, consistency, or amount
- Foul-smelling vaginal odor
- Vaginal itching
- Pain with urination or intercourse
- Redness, ulcers, and/or blisters in and around the vagina

What to Do

- Use medications prescribed by your doctor for the vaginitis as directed.
- Clean yourself carefully and gently from front to back with unscented, white toilet tissue or a cotton ball moistened with warm water after using the toilet. Otherwise, you can easily sweep bacteria from the rectum into the vagina or urethra, causing an infection.
- Wear only cotton underwear. Stay away from nylon underwear, pantyhose, or tight pants. These trap moisture and permit the cultivation of bacteria and fungi.
- Stop the use of all sexual toys. Clean them thoroughly with a solution of 1 part bleach to 9 parts water. (See the box on page 46 for instructions on the use of chlorine bleach solution.)
- Stop sexual activity temporarily. You may be uncomfortable while your vagina is inflamed, or you may be at risk of transmitting the infection to your partner. Ask you doctor when you can resume sexual relations.
- Drink at least eight glasses of fluid a day if you can.

What *Not* to Do

- Do not douche unless a doctor advises it.
- Do not self-medicate with over-the-counter products or home remedies unless your doctor says to do so.

- Do not stop taking prescribed vaginal medications before you have completed the full course of therapy. Vaginitis is sometimes difficult to cure and can recur.
- Do not use tampons when you have vaginitis.

When to Consult Your Doctor

- At the first sign of vaginitis. Inform your doctor of the color, consistency, and amount of the discharge along with symptoms such as itching, odor, bleeding, pelvic pain, burning upon urination, vaginal redness, blisters, or ulcerations.

What to Discuss with the Doctor

- Information about any recent sexual activity.
- Whether you've been douching. **Don't douche for at least 24 to 48 hours prior to the exam** (preferably, not at all). Douching is generally not recommended, and in this instance will most certainly wash out any discharge that would be key in diagnosing the problem.

What to Expect at the Doctor's Office

Be prepared for a pelvic exam during which the doctor will use cotton swabs to obtain samples of the discharge. She will send some to the lab to be cultured for common sexually transmitted diseases, such as gonorrhea, chlamydia, or herpes. She may also look at a specimen under the microscope right in the office to check for the presence of yeast, bacteria, or small parasites called *trichomonas*. You may also need blood tests (e.g., to determine if you have been exposed to syphilis).

You will probably be given oral and/or vaginal medications. The vaginal medications may be in the form of creams, ointments, or suppositories—all of which tend to leak and may stain underclothes, so wear a pantyliner.

Painful Urination

A PWA who has painful urination will have to provide a specimen of the urine to test for the presence of bacteria. Cultures may also be taken for venereal diseases. Generally, urinary tract and venereal diseases are treatable with antibiotics. It is also helpful to increase fluid intake to flush out the kidneys. In the case of kidney stones, pain medications will be prescribed. X rays may be taken, and you may be asked to strain the PWA's urine in case a stone is passed so that it can be analyzed at a laboratory.

In Women

Women are particularly vulnerable to urinary tract infections because of their anatomy. The urethra is very close to the vagina and rectum; therefore, bacteria can easily be swept from one of these openings into the bladder (through the urethra), as during sex or when wiping after a bowel movement.

Vaginitis, trauma, and kidney stones may also cause painful urination. Other symptoms that may accompany pain include bleeding, urinating more frequently, or feeling the urge to urinate but not actually being able to. There may be vaginal discharge, pelvic pain, abnormal menses, back or flank pain, fever, nausea, and/or vomiting.

When urinary tract infections are suspected, a specimen of urine will be examined for the presence of bacteria. Antibiotic drugs will usually alleviate the symptoms of bacterial infection within 24 to 48 hours. With this as with any antibiotic regimen, however, it's important to take the medicine as prescribed UNTIL YOU FINISH ALL THE PILLS to prevent complications.

In Men

Pain with urination is a common occurrence with urinary tract infections, sexually transmitted diseases, prostate infections, and kidney stones. There may also be other associated symptoms, such as obvious blood mixed with the urine, the urge to urinate more frequently, difficulties with starting or stopping the urinary stream, incontinence, penile discharge, rectal pain or discharge, back or flank pain, fever, nausea, and/or vomiting. All of these should be brought to the attention of the doctor.

Swelling of the Penis or Scrotum

Scrotal and/or penile swelling, discomfort, and even pain occur now and then in PWAs. The condition may be temporary or permanent, depending on the underlying cause.

Causes of Penile or Scrotal Swelling

For men with AIDS, the underlying causes vary. Cancers (such as Kaposi's sarcoma or lymphoma), infections, injury, and protein imbalances are a few possible causes. Whatever the cause, it is important to identify and treat the problem swiftly because this swelling (also called *edema* or elephantitis) can impair urination, erection, and sexual desire.

Treatment of Penile or Scrotal Swelling

What to Look For

- Enlargement of the scrotum and/or penis that is different from an erection. The penis will seem distorted, especially if uncircumcised. It may appear doughy, pillowlike, or like "an overblown balloon." The skin may appear red and shiny.

- Problems urinating, including difficulty starting the stream, dribbling, or incontinence
- Inability to obtain or maintain an erection
- Pain or discomfort in the genital area, especially when wearing underwear and clothing

What to Do

- Take any medications ordered by your physician as directed.
- Wear only unrestrictive clothing, such as boxer shorts and baggy pants—*not* bikini underwear, spandex tights, or biker's shorts.
- Elevate the scrotum on a folded towel or small cushion for comfort, when sitting or lying down.
- Take a warm bath several times a day. Sit in the tub carefully, and rest the scrotum on a towel.
- Use cool or warm towels over the scrotum and penis to lessen discomfort. Alternate having them on for five minutes, then off for five minutes.
- Keep track of how often you urinate. If instructed to by your doctor, measure urinary output. (Urinals and bedpans often have markings for this purpose.) Note the color of your urine and whether there is an odor, blood, or sediment present.
- Check the penis and scrotum in the morning and evening for the presence of discharge, ulcers, sores, blisters, or discolorations.
- Change positions carefully, but often. Remember that bedsores can form quickly. This is especially true of swollen areas. Use a pillow to separate your legs when lying on your side.
- If your sexual desire or performance has been affected, discuss your feelings with your partner. Think about other ways to attain pleasure. Consider seeing a therapist.

What Not to Do

- Do not drink for at least three hours before going to sleep if you are having urinary problems such as dribbling or incontinence. If you are thirsty, sip a small amount of water.

When to Consult Your Doctor

- **If you do not urinate for more than eight hours, or if your lower abdomen is swollen at the level of your pubic bone, call your doctor immediately.** You may be retaining urine and could need to be catheterized (a thin tube is inserted through the urethra to empty the bladder).

CHAPTER **20**

The Extremities

Swelling

Swelling (edema) is an important symptom in PWAs who have malnutrition, circulatory problems, infections, lymph problems, chemical imbalances, or who are having an allergic reaction to a food or a medication. It can also result from an injury. As you can see, the spectrum of conditions that swelling can represent is broad.

Characteristics of Swelling

Swelling usually occurs in the hands, arms, feet, or legs, but it can appear in any area of the body. When an area becomes swollen, the skin generally changes its appearance in other ways as well. There may be redness, black-and-blue marks, or purplish discolorations. The area also may seem shiny compared with the surrounding skin.

One of the ways swelling or edema is measured is by the presence and extent of pitting. The greater the pitting, the more severe the swelling. It's important for caregivers who are reporting information to the doctor to know how to check for *pitting edema*. To check for pitting, press your finger firmly into the swollen skin. If your finger leaves an indentation, then pitting edema is said to be present.

What to Look For

- Unexplained generalized weight gain. (With a female PWA, note where she is in her menstrual cycles, as bloating and water retention may occur as a result of hormonal influences.)
- A larger appearance to the legs, arms, or other parts of the body; smoothing out of normal creases in the skin
- Recent tightness of shoes and socks beyond what is normal swelling—even under extreme circumstances, such as standing on one's feet on a very hot day
- Tightness of rings, bracelets, wristwatches that leaves temporary imprint on the skin
- Facial puffiness, especially around the eyes or nose
- Shiny, tight, or discolored look to the skin
- Inability to tightly close one's fist, if the hand is swollen
- Pain or itching in the affected area

- An indentation remains in the skin for a few minutes after the swollen area is pressed with one's fingers (pitting)

Treatment of Swelling

What to Do

- Remove all jewelry from affected hands, wrists, and ankles as soon as possible. If this is delayed, swelling may become so severe and the circulation so impaired that jewelry may need to be cut off.
- Remove shoes and socks.
- Elevate the affected limb on a pillow or pillows in a position of comfort **above the level of the heart** for 24 to 36 hours ideally. This can be done with the PWA resting in bed or sitting in a chair.
- Have the PWA rest the swollen area as much as possible.
- Apply an ice pack or plastic bag filled with ice wrapped in a towel **for the first 24 hours.** Leave the ice in place for 15 to 20 minutes, then remove for 5 minutes and repeat.
- Apply moderate heat to the region using a heating pad; warm, moist towels; or warm baths after 24 hours. Be careful not to burn the person, especially if he is diabetic and is therefore less able to detect extremes of temperature. Remember: 15 to 20 minutes on, then 5 minutes off, and repeat.
- *Note:* After the first 24 hours has passed, you can alternate cold and hot applications if the person finds this more effective and comfortable. Always use cold initially (the first day) to keep swelling to a minimum.
- Use anti-inflammatory medications as advised by the doctor.
- Take special care not to injure (or reinjure) the swollen area.
- Help the PWA to walk or have him use a cane or walker if necessary. Take no chance with falls if the PWA is unsteady on his feet or if his legs or ankles are weak.
- Note any additional symptoms, such as discolorations of the skin or shortness of breath. In the latter case, fluid overload in the heart may cause a backup in the body, which may then result not only in swollen ankles, but in shortness of breath from fluid accumulation in the lungs.
- Give diuretics (water pills) only if prescribed by the doctor.

What *Not* to Do

- Never tie or tape hot or cold packs to limbs. Rest them gently on the swollen area and remove them every 15 to 20 minutes. Check the area after each removal.
- Do not apply splints, Ace bandages, slings, or other immobilizing devices to swollen areas without consulting your physician. These can decrease blood circulation and worsen medical problems.
- Do not allow the person to exercise a swollen limb without permission from the doctor. This includes day-to-day activities.

- Do not treat the PWA yourself longer than 24 hours without seeking medical advice.

When to Consult Your Doctor

- If any area of swelling shows no improvement after 24 hours. Swelling can indicate serious medical problems that can be reversed if caught early. Call sooner if the swelling seems to be getting worse or is spreading. Let your doctor know about any pain, known injury, if pitting is present, and/or if there are any other associated symptoms (such as skin discoloration).

What to Expect at the Doctor's Office

The PWA may need to be seen in the office for an examination of the swollen area. Blood or urine samples may be taken to check for the underlying cause of the swelling, such as heart or kidney failure. X rays may be necessary if an injury is involved.

Note: Although most problems with swelling can be taken care of at home with rest, medications, and patience, occasionally hospitalization is required to remove fluid or to administer intravenous antibiotics or other treatments.

Numbness and Tingling Sensations

Numbness and tingling of the legs and feet (beginning usually on the soles) and of the hands (sometimes progressing up the arms) is often described by PWAs as the feeling of "pins and needles" one may experience when a limb "falls asleep." The sensation varies in intensity from merely unpleasant to extremely painful. The effects can last just a short time or be permanent.

Numbness and tingling can make walking painful. The touch of a blanket on the toes can be unbearable. Intricate needlepoint or other close work may become impossible due to an inability to hold a needle. Temperature perception is off. This makes even stepping into a bathtub a dangerous proposition for fear of burns.

Causes of Numbness and Tingling

Causes include the toxic effects of chemotherapeutic drugs like vincristine or vinblastine; medications like AZT (Retrovir); or medical problems such as kidney failure, diabetes, arthritis, and chemical imbalances of calcium or potassium in the bloodstream.

What to Look For

- A sensation of pins and needles in any portion of the extremities: toes, fingers, feet, hands, legs, or arms

- Burning in the extremities that may persist or come and go within a period of 24 hours
- Inability to find a comfortable position for the affected limb
- A change in the way the PWA walks. She may be dragging one foot or stumbling more often.
- Foot drop, e.g., when the ankle extends downward and the entire foot actually appears to have dropped
- A change in the PWA's dexterity; dropping of items from the hands even when the PWA appears to have them firmly in her grasp and the items are not heavy or cumbersome.
- Inability to tell hot from warm or warm from cool. For example, a hot cup of coffee may only feel warm. Or, an ice cube held in the hand may not feel cold—it may feel like it is burning.
- Inability to accurately perceive pain. The PWA may be astonished to see her hand or foot bleeding, because she did not feel the pain of the injury.

Treatment of Numbness and Tingling

What to Do

- Note when the problem started, what part of the body is affected, how it feels, how long the sensation lasts, and what if anything makes it better or worse.
- Be careful of frostbite. The PWA should dress warmly in cold weather (gloves, a hat, and heavy socks) even if she does not feel the cold.
- Take precautions against burns. The PWA should have another person test the water temperature or use a thermometer to check the water temperature for her bath or shower. When she washes dishes she should also use household weight utility gloves to protect her hands from the heat of the running water.
- Turn the hot water heater down in the house so that it is no higher than 120°F.
- Install a bed or foot cradle to keep sheets or blankets from resting on the person's feet and causing discomfort. (See Chapter 2 for information on cradles.)
- Discourage the PWA from impeding her circulation by sitting with her legs crossed or resting with her arms under her body or under a pillow.
- Inspect the PWA's hands and feet at least every morning and evening—more often if you are able. Look for discolorations, sores, cuts, blisters, growths, or ingrown nails that she may not feel due to a diminished ability to perceive pain.

What *Not* to Do

- Do not allow the PWA to place herself in situations where extremes of temperature may be a risk, such as hot tubs, jacuzzis, steam rooms, and saunas.

- Do not allow the PWA to wear tight clothing or jewelry that can impair circulation (e.g., belts, ties, girdles, garters, knee highs, rings, gloves, shoes, bracelets, ankle bracelets).
- Do not allow the PWA to go barefoot.

When to Consult Your Doctor

- If the PWA develops problems with numbness and tingling sensations. She may require nerve conduction studies, an MRI to check for a pinched nerve, or blood tests to check for diabetes or chemical imbalances. She may also need medication or a change in a current drug therapy. (Changes in medication regimens are usually tried before diagnostic testing.)

Difficulty Moving

Many PWAs describe difficulty in moving as one of the most frustrating aspects of their illness. Where previously the PWA was independent, able to get around and do things for himself, now he may be experiencing weakness, fatigue, decreased muscle strength, spastic movements, and unstable joints, making him feel unsure of himself. To make matters worse, the PWA begins (rightly so) to fear becoming dependent on someone else for help with even the simple tasks of everyday existence.

The next section on exercise provides information about passive and active range-of-motion exercises, muscle strengthening, and preventing joint and muscle stiffness (*contractures*) to help the PWA stay active as much as possible for as long as possible. This section describes how you can detect the onset of difficulty moving, and how to manage it.

What to Look For

- An instability at joints, such as a weak ankle or wrist
- A sensation of heaviness in arms or legs that makes lifting them a chore
- Shuffling walk
- Dropping items that are not particularly heavy or bulky
- Inability of the PWA to perform precision work that he could do previously, such as painting or needlepoint
- Difficulty in changing positions, that is, rising from a sitting or lying position
- Aches, pains, or muscle spasms upon initiating movements
- Tremors or jerking motions in lieu of smooth movements
- Slowed reflexes

What to Do

Encourage the PWA to

- Remain as independent as possible without risking injury to himself or others.
- Keep a positive attitude about what he *can* do rather than bemoaning what he can't do.
- Ask for help when needed or when he is unsure if he can safely complete a task alone.
- Walk carefully, lifting the feet, not shuffling. Take extra care with stairs, curbs, hills, and whenever he is on uneven ground. He should look where he is going.
- Use devices to help him maintain his independence, such as a cane, walker, wheelchair, handrails, and specialized utensil handles.
- Make the home safe, by removing potential hazards, such as throw rugs, and by installing safety devices in the bathroom and kitchen. For detailed information on household safety, see Chapter 2.
- Inform friends, family, and volunteers of his limitations, to tell them what they can do to help him.
- Seek referrals to outside agencies that can provide helpful devices, volunteers, and information (see Appendix G).
- Utilize resources in the community. For example, use grocery stores and pharmacies in your area that deliver.
- Take advantage of meal services and take-out food instead of cooking.
- Take rest periods when needed.
- Use public transportation to get around or ask someone else to drive.
- Consider physical, occupational, and/or recreational therapy. These treatment modes are extraordinarily helpful in pain management as well as in training the PWA to adapt to his limitations. Physical and occupational therapy will help him to minimize his discomfort while maximizing his independence. Work with a recreational therapist to seek new hobbies or find ways of adapting old ones.

What *Not* to Do

- Do not let people, however well-intentioned they are, do things for the PWA that he can do for himself. He should be the one in control of asking for help if and when he needs it.
- Do not allow the PWA to lift heavy objects or those that are bulky and cumbersome.
- Do not permit the person to operate a motor vehicle.

When to Consult Your Doctor

- **If the PWA experiences any sudden and complete inability to move a part of the body, CALL AN AMBULANCE.**

- To discuss problems or changes in movement abilities.
- To ask for a referral to physical and/or occupational therapy.
- To inquire about the use of special ambulatory aids, such as canes, walkers, and wheelchairs.
- To ask for a referral to a support group or to psychotherapy if the PWA is having difficulties coping with his limitations.

Exercise

To the PWA: If you have been participating in an organized sports activity or have been working out at your local gym or health spa, it's perfectly all right to continue to do so as long as you have your doctor's consent. Exercise is encouraged. Just know your limitations and don't overdo it. In other words, stop when you are tired or if you begin to feel ill or experience pain of any type.

If you have been part of a group activity such as softball or volleyball and you are concerned about having to attend each game or having to stop halfway through a game, consider switching your activity to a solo sport.

Why Exercise Is Important

Everyone needs a certain amount of daily movement for muscles and joints to remain flexible, strong, and healthy. If a PWA is permitted to remain immobilized, muscles and joints become weak, stiff, shortened, and wasted away. The PWA may develop contractures; that is, muscle fibers become shortened and resist stretching. Eventually, movements become limited and painful. *Ankylosis* is the fixation of a joint into one position. This can also be painful and restrict motion. An immobile joint can show changes in as little as four days! Once these problems occur, they are to some degree permanent. Therefore, prevention of muscle immobility and weakening is the key—through active and passive range-of-motion (ROM) exercises and frequent position changes for those who are restricted to a chair or bed.

Range-of-Motion Exercises

Active and passive range-of-motion exercises are for PWAs who can no longer participate in regular exercise regimens (sports, workouts, etc.). Active range of motion (AROM) entails putting joints and muscles through a range of movements that will help to maintain muscle tone and to prevent joint immobility and stiffness. If the PWA is confined to bed most of the time, AROM prevents some of the common problems associated with immobility, including foot and wrist drop and abnormal hip positions.

Passive range of motion (PROM) performs the same function, but it is carried out for the PWA by the caregiver. The caregiver takes over range-of-motion exercises for a PWA who is very weak, partially or completely paralyzed, or comatose. The caregiver supports the weight of the PWA's limbs and helps him to move his joints.

Candidates for ROM Exercises

- A PWA not participating in organized sports, working out in a gym, or exercising on his own (walking briskly, bicycle riding, swimming, etc.)
- A PWA who is paralyzed or partially paralyzed
- A PWA confined to the bed or chair, especially one who relies on caregivers to transfer him from bed to chair or turn him from side to side
- A PWA who uses a wheelchair, cane, or walker
- A PWA who has a weak grip
- A PWA who has joint stiffness, decreased muscle tone, and lessened strength and/or endurance
- A PWA with any suggestion of a foot drop, wrist drop, or abnormal hip rotation
- A PWA who is comatose

What to Do

- Get permission from the doctor before beginning any exercise program including AROM or PROM. Have a nurse or physical therapist instruct you first in the proper method of performing ROM exercises and demonstrate them to you before attempting on your own.
- Start ROM exercises as soon as possible, especially if the PWA is confined to a chair or bed. The key is to start *before* contractures, ankylosis, stiffness, and foot drop or wrist drop have developed.
- Maintain a dialogue with the PWA when performing ROM as to what is to be done. If the PWA is comatose, the caregiver should still state out loud beforehand what she is going to do.
- Determine the joints to be exercised first and the positions to be used.
- Provide for the comfort and safety of both the PWA and the caregiver. Wear loose clothing and select a place that has ample room to perform the exercise. Maintain a comfortable room temperature.
- Keep fluids on hand so that dehydration doesn't occur.
- Maintain proper posture and body alignment for the PWA and good body mechanics for the caregiver.
- Watch for fatigue, pain, spasm. Stop the exercises if any of these develop.
- Support the PWA's limbs while putting them through movements during PROM exercises. Each joint should be moved carefully, in a way that is comfortable for the caregiver. Movements should be slow, rhythmical, and repetitive. Flex and extend each joint completely in each direction as it would normally move.
- Put each joint through the complete range of motion cycle six times in both AROM and PROM. Repeat the exercise cycle two to three times a day if possible.
- Have the PWA wear shoes as much as possible (even in bed) and install a footboard on the bed to prevent foot drop. When seated, the PWA should place his feet flat on the floor now and then.

What Not to Do

- Never exercise or do ROM on any area with a torn ligament, fracture, joint dislocation, swelling, or suspected injury.
- Never initiate or continue ROM when there is pain, fatigue, or muscle tremors or spasms (sudden involuntary quivering or contractions of the muscle) in an area to be exercised.
- Never force an alert PWA to participate in AROM or PROM exercises. Discuss the pros and cons, but permit him to make the decision. (For example, ROM exercises might result in exhaustion, injury, pain, or muscle spasms.)
- Never ignore safety. For example, be sure not to engage in exercises too close to the edge of the bed.
- Do not become discouraged early on if the PWA tires easily. Strength, tolerance, and endurance will build.
- Do not rush the ROM exercises. Avoid jerky, fast movements.

Falls

To help decrease the likelihood of a fall, it is important to identify risk factors. Anyone who is weak, fatigued, or confused or has poor vision or mobility problems is at risk for falling. Sedation from medications, diarrhea, a cluttered environment, and/or a PWA's desire to act independently in all things even if physically or mentally unable can also contribute to the probability of falling.

To minimize falls, floors should be uncluttered, rooms and hallways well lit, and all high-risk areas identified and made safe (see Chapter 2). All PWAs should be encouraged to call for assistance when necessary. Confused, agitated, or sedated PWAs should never be left alone.

Even if all precautions are taken, falls can still occur. Some falls are witnessed but cannot be stopped in time. In other cases, a PWA may be found on the floor after having fallen.

What to Do

- Try to assist a PWA who is falling if you are present. Lower him to the ground slowly by sliding him down the length of your own body while protecting his head at all times. If you cannot reach the PWA in time, try to move obstacles out of the way so he does not hit them as he falls.
- Try to observe carefully if you are present but are too far away to help the PWA to the ground or to remove dangerous obstacles. Note if the PWA hits any areas of his body, especially his head.
- Allow the person who has fallen to remain on the ground in the position he assumes, whether you witnessed the accident or merely found him on the floor.

- **Make sure he is breathing and has a pulse. If not, begin CPR if you have been trained to do so. Check the person for injury and bleeding _without_ moving him.**
  - Put on gloves if the PWA is bleeding, and assess whether the wound is major or minor. Keep him lying on the floor during this evaluation. Minor facial cuts can bleed profusely even when they are not deep. Major lacerations require an emergency room trip for suturing, a tetanus shot, and X rays.
  - Apply direct pressure to a minor bleeding wound with gauze pads, a clean towel, paper towels, or a sanitary napkin. Bleeding should stop shortly. Bandage the area with sterile gauze and paper tape or an adhesive bandage. Apply ice to minimize swelling. If the wound begins to bleed again, it may be an indication that sutures are needed. Apply pressure again and if ineffective, go to the emergency room.

  Note: If the PWA has been taking a medication such as coumadin or heparin, which thins the blood, remember that bleeding will be more prolonged and profuse. In addition, more black-and-blue areas will occur. Professional assistance may be needed under these circumstances to stop bleeding.

- Determine if the PWA can speak if he is conscious and whether he has had a change in his mental status (e.g., confusion in a previously lucid person).
- Watch minor injuries, such as bumps, bruises, or scrapes, over the course of several days to make sure that they are healing.
- Apply ice for minor swelling during the first 24 hours and heat after that. Always elevate the affected part of the body.
- Wash minor scrapes with soap and water and apply a bandage, if necessary. Wear gloves.
- Help the PWA to a sitting position if he tells you that he's not hurt and you see no outward signs of injury. Insist that he remain there resting for several minutes before attempting to move. Then help him to his feet and then directly into a bed or chair, whichever is closest. This may require that you pull a chair over to where he has fallen.
- Call for assistance if the PWA cannot help himself up or help you to help him. While waiting for help make him comfortable on the floor with pillows and blankets.
- Determine the reason for the fall and correct the problem, if possible.
- Reassure the PWA and try to minimize his embarrassment over falling.
- Assess the PWA every 20 to 30 minutes for six to eight hours after the fall, especially if he struck his head (see box, page 187). Check for changes in vision, mental status, bruising, and swelling.

What Not to Do

- **Do not immediately move a PWA who has fallen,** even if you saw the accident and he says he is not hurt. **Moving a person improperly can cause permanent paralysis.**

Head Injury Warning Signs

In the case of falls resulting in head injury, follow the doctor's instructions regarding observation and care. In addition, here are some general guidelines to follow:

- Observe for disorientation, lethargy, and mood or personality change.
- Ask the PWA if he is experiencing blurry vision, double vision, headache, nausea, dizziness, and numbness or weakness in the extremities.
- Watch for unequal pupil size; loss of consciousness; seizures; forceful vomiting; leakage of clear or blood-tinged fluid from the ears, nose, or mouth; slowing of the pulse; fever higher than 101°F; difficulty walking or talking.
- Briefly awaken the person every three to four hours to make sure he is easily aroused and not confused. Do this for at least 24 hours—longer if any doubt exists.

Note: Sometimes a head injury will not become apparent for several hours— in rare instances, even several days—after a fall, so be alert to any unusual symptoms or behaviors during this period.

- Do not hurt yourself trying to help someone else. If, when it is proper to do so, you cannot move the person who has fallen, call for assistance.

Emergencies

- **CALL AN AMBULANCE**
  - —In the case of major trauma, like a protruding bone.
  - —If the person is unconscious, even if only briefly. Any loss of consciousness is serious and requires immediate medical assistance.
  - —If you are unsure as to how serious an injury is, or if you suspect a concussion or other major problem.
- **GO TO THE EMERGENCY ROOM**
  - —If the person has a major laceration.
  - —If the person is confused and the confusion is a new symptom.

When to Consult Your Doctor

- To report all falls, those with and without injury. The doctor may determine that X rays are needed to rule out more serious internal injuries.
- To report any changes in vision, mental status, bruising, or swelling.

CHAPTER <u>**21**</u>

The Brain

Headaches

Contrary to what some people believe, a headache is not an illness or a disease. It is a symptom. As for other people who suffer from headaches, for PWAs, the pain can be a sign of any one of many problems, some minor and some very serious. Headaches can be classified into three broad categories, muscle contraction or tension headaches; vascular or *migraine* headaches; and organic or pathological headaches. The location, duration, severity, and accompanying signs and symptoms, as well as the nature of the pain and what relieves or worsens it all vary according to headache type.

Tension Headaches

Tension headaches comprise the majority of ordinary, everyday headache pain. They stem from spasm of the muscles that surround the skull and thus often feel like a band tightening around the scalp or a pressurelike sensation across the forehead, at the temples, on the top of the head, or in the back of the head. This type of headache is particularly prevalent in PWAs (and caregivers) because of the emotional trauma (anxiety and depression) associated with AIDS. Most tension headaches will fade with rest and over-the-counter pain medication, such as Tylenol (acetaminophen). They generally do not have any other associated symptoms. If other symptoms are present (e.g., fever or vision changes) or if the pain is unresponsive to pain medicine, there may be another cause for the headache and it should be investigated further. Tension headaches will occasionally be very severe, very prolonged, and accompanied by nausea or even neck pain, so don't become alarmed, but be sure to notify the doctor.

Migraine Headaches

Migraines are a very specific throbbing type of headache (usually on one side of the head) whose cause is still a mystery. It is believed that biochemical influences may negatively affect the blood vessels in the head, causing them to become inflamed and to contract and expand abnormally. Aside from the characteristic severe, throbbing pain, migraines may cause visual disturbances before the pain begins. These range from temporary blind spots in the field of vision to flashes of color to the appearance of strange, wiggly lines. There may also be sensitivity to light, nausea, and vomiting. In fact, the migraine is a syndrome (a set of symptoms that occur together), not merely a headache. For

PWAs, the problem (already a treatment challenge) is compounded by the fact that the symptoms may mimic those for the organic lesions (i.e., brain tumors, brain infections [encephalitis]) that also cause headaches in PWAs. If the PWA has been given medication to treat his migraines and gets no relief, or if atypical symptoms (symptoms not normal for the individual PWA when he gets a migraine) appear, it is vital to let the doctor know.

Organic Headaches

The type of headache that it is most important to diagnose in a PWA is an organic or pathological headache—that is, one caused by a brain lesion—either from an opportunistic infection or a cancer. The symptoms may be very vague in the beginning, much like those of a tension headache. But if the pain is persistent, localized to one spot, and seems to build in frequency and intensity over time, don't ignore it.

Organic headaches are caused by an underlying structural dysfunction. In PWAs, these headaches can also be from something as commonplace as sinusitis or as rare as cryptococcal meningitis or a brain lymphoma. A sinus headache is usually across the forehead and face (over the cheekbones) and is accompanied by nasal congestion and greenish discharge; the headache often worsens as the day goes on or if the person bends forward. There may be other symptoms of an upper respiratory infection, such as a fever, earache, or sore throat. Sinus infections are more serious in PWAs than in otherwise healthy persons, because PWAs don't have the capacity to fight off the infection.

A pathological headache may also be marked by fever, stiff neck, sore throat (with meningitis), nausea, vomiting (especially projectile), visual changes, dizziness, and confusion. It may be described as the "worst headache ever." **These headaches require immediate attention.**

Finally, PWAs may have headaches from a variety of causes requiring one to be a detective at times. For example, the PWA who suddenly develops headaches upon admission to the hospital may be getting them because of the steam heat or because he is not receiving his usual six cups of coffee a day. Or, a PWA may develop medical-induced headaches from a spinal tap (see Appendix A) or after receiving *intrathecal* chemotherapy (see Chapter 22).

What to Look For

- Pain of any type located anywhere in the head
- Head pain that seems particularly severe, comes on suddenly, or lasts an unusually long time
- Worsening of the head pain with stress, with certain activities, when taking certain medications, and so forth
- Accompanying symptoms: nausea, vomiting, dizziness, loss of consciousness, confusion, stiff neck, fever, sore throat, vision changes, and development of weakness or numbness in an extremity

What to Do

- Carefully evaluate the PWA for signs and symptoms as discussed, and get to an emergency room if the symptoms call for that.
- Administer medication if the PWA has had it prescribed for headaches such as these in the past and the situation has been discussed with the doctor.
- Monitor the PWA over a minimum period of 24 hours for any worsening or improvement in the headache (with rest, medication, and/or distraction, as from an activity).
- Allow the PWA to rest in a quiet, darkened, comfortable environment until the pain has passed.
- Consider some of the alternative therapies described in Appendix C (e.g., biofeedback and relaxation exercises) to help allay the pain.

What *Not* to Do

- Do not over- or underestimate the meaning of a headache. Seek medical attention for **any** of the headache danger signs (see box below).
- Do not administer medication for any headache except what is clearly a tension headache without first consulting the doctor. You may mask vital symptoms such as fever or worsening pain, making it possible for a diagnosis to be missed or delayed.

When to Consult Your Doctor

- If any of the signs of a serious headache are noted (see box below), **GO TO AN EMERGENCY ROOM.**
- To discuss a particular drug that you suspect is causing headaches as a side effect.

Headache Danger Signs

GO TO THE EMERGENCY ROOM FOR:

- Sudden, excruciating pain that is like nothing ever experienced before. This may be a sign of a *subarachnoid hemorrhage.*
- Any headache associated with neurological symptoms, such as: weakness, numbness, confusion, excessive sleepiness, dizziness, seizures, or visual impairment.
- Head pain accompanied by any other symptoms, particularly fever, shortness of breath, or symptoms affecting the ears, nose, or throat. This may mean anything from meningitis to heart failure.
- Any headache associated with or arising from a head injury, such as can occur if the PWA has a fall.

- To discuss any severe or prolonged headache as well as one with the accompanying symptoms mentioned. The PWA may need to see a neurologist and/or undergo *CAT* or *MRI scanning* (see Appendix A).
- To get authorization to administer medications for the pain.
- To schedule at least yearly visits to the ophthalmologist for eye exams, as vision problems can also lead to headaches.
- To ask about counseling for headaches that are of a psychological nature.

Seizures

A seizure (also known as a fit or convulsion) sometimes accompanies the brain infections or tumors that occur in AIDS. During a seizure, the body's muscles undergo involuntary contractions that appear as *spasms* or contortions of the face, torso, arms, and/or legs.

AIDS patients may experience various types of seizures, ranging from a barely noticeable twitch of the face, fluttering of the eyelids, and momentary lapse in attention span (known as a *petit mal* attack) to a full-blown *grand mal,* or *tonic clonic,* seizure.

Grand Mal Seizures

These seizures involve the entire body, with movements of the arms and legs, shaking of the body, loss of consciousness and possibly biting of the tongue, abnormal breathing, and/or loss of control of the bladder and bowels. After a grand mal seizure has passed, (usually two to five minutes, although the event may seem longer to an observer), the PWA may sleep or appear disoriented for a period. He may not be able to speak properly for several moments to hours after an attack. This ability will return, however.

Partial or Focal Seizures

Rarely, a PWA whose brain dysfunction is localized to one specific site may experience *focal,* or *partial,* seizures. In this case, the PWA may have only localized twitching or numbness of one muscle, or he may exhibit bizarre behavior, such as lip smacking, hallucinations, or staggering. He will be unresponsive to you, although he appears conscious, and may move around purposefully, uttering unintelligible sounds.

Any infection or cancer that infiltrates the brain of a PWA may set off a seizure, as can a very high fever (in an adult, body temperatures exceeding 104°F) or a severe drop in blood sugar. This last case may occur in PWAs who take insulin for AIDS-related diabetes (see Chapter 17). It is important to note that **seizures in PWAs are not epilepsy**, which is a completely different disease entity.

Various anticonvulsant medications, such as Dilantin (phenytoin sodium), Tegretol (carbamazepine), and phenobarbital, are the mainstay of prevention and treatment.

What to Look For

- A sudden loss of consciousness with a rolling of the eyes back into the head
- "Crying out" as air is pushed out of the lungs past the vocal cords
- Stiffness followed by involuntary twitching or shaking that may start on one side of the head or body and then progress to the entire body
- Repetitive flexing and extending of the neck, arms, and legs
- Irregular breathing with a bluish tinge to the skin from a decrease in oxygen
- Saliva accumulation in the mouth ("foaming of the mouth")
- Blood in the mouth from tongue biting
- Vomiting
- Loss of bladder and/or bowel control
- Excessive sleepiness and/or disorientation following the convulsive event

What to Do

During the Seizure

- Help the PWA into a lying position if he is standing or sitting.
- Place a pillow, a sweater, or something else soft that is available (without having to leave the PWA to obtain it), under his head.
- Remove eyeglasses and loosen tight clothing.
- Move away sharp objects and furniture so that the convulsing PWA will not injure himself by striking against it.
- Monitor the PWA's breathing and pulse, if able.
- Hold the PWA's head to the side if he has blood or saliva in his mouth or if he is vomiting, to prevent him from accidentally inhaling this fluid into the lungs. This is important to prevent complications such as pneumonia. It may be difficult to keep a seizing person's head turned. The best method is to place the palm of your hand firmly against his forehead. You may have to exert moderate pressure. If you think that he may injure his neck under the force of your resistance, occasionally release your hand and let his head turn, and then resume applying pressure.
- Observe the events carefully so that you will be able to provide information to the doctor. The PWA will not remember anything about the attack.

After the Seizure

- Turn the PWA onto his side to allow drainage of fluids from his mouth.
- Stay with the person until he is fully awake, alert, and oriented.

What Not to Do

- Never attempt to force something into the PWA's mouth. Very rapidly after the onset of a convulsion, the jaw clamps tightly shut and rarely will you have time to prevent him from biting his tongue (which rarely happens in any case). Furthermore, you may be injured yourself in the attempt. It is a myth that he will "swallow his tongue"—this is physiologically impossible.

- Do not panic! A seizure is a frightening thing to watch, but it is generally not a medical emergency in a person with a known history of seizures.
- Do not attempt to restrain the PWA. You cannot stop a seizure.
- Do not offer the PWA anything to eat or drink after a seizure until you are certain that he is awake and not in danger of having another seizure. Otherwise he could choke and aspirate (inhale) the liquids, foods, or vomit into the lungs—a condition that could cause a serious pneumonia to develop.
- Do not try to clean up a person too soon after he has had a seizure, and don't try to wake him up afterward if he is sleepy. He may need to recover for several minutes or for several hours. The time frame is very variable. Use the time following the seizure to make sure he is breathing, to note that his skin color returns, and to call for help.

When to Consult Your Doctor

- If the person is not breathing or is injured, or if you cannot detect a pulse, **CALL AN AMBULANCE**.
- If this is the PWA's first seizure or if he has prolonged (longer than five minutes) or multiple attacks, **CALL AN AMBULANCE**. Long seizures or seizures that follow one after the other can cause brain damage.
- After any type of seizure. The doctor will need to know what happened in detail and what you suspect may have brought on the episode. He may need to adjust the PWA's medication, obtain tests, or hospitalize him.

Dizziness and Fainting

Dizziness can describe several distinct entities. Often, a PWA will say she is dizzy when in fact she is light-headed or feeling faint. This is not the same as true dizziness, which is an actual spinning sensation. When the PWA feels as if she herself is spinning, she is said to be dizzy, which is in contrast to a sensation that the room is spinning around her. The latter condition is often called *vertigo*. Light-headedness, dizziness, and vertigo can have similar or very different causes.

Causes and Characteristics of Vertigo, Dizziness, and Light-Headedness

Vertigo signals a disturbance in a person's equilibrium apparatus, which is located in the inner ears, eyes, and brain. With vertigo, the PWA may also have ringing in the ears, decreased hearing, nausea, and vomiting. Medications (particularly narcotics) and alcohol can cause vertigo, as can encephalitis (an infection of the brain caused by opportunistic infections) and brain cancers.

Like vertigo, light-headedness and dizziness may also stem from narcotics. In addition, two drugs frequently used to treat AIDS, ganciclovir and pentamidine, can cause a dramatic drop in blood pressure, inducing light-headedness and dizziness. Furthermore, pentamidine is also noted to affect a PWA's blood sugar, causing both hyper- and hypoglycemia, depending on the individual (see Chapter 17). Both of these blood sugar conditions can cause dizziness.

Starvation (PWAs sometimes don't eat because of severe nausea, vomiting, and diarrhea), dehydration (from the same causes), and changes in position (spending a long time lying in bed and then suddenly attempting to sit or stand) can all cause light-headedness and dizziness.

Loss of Consciousness

On occasion, these symptoms can progress to loss of consciousness (also called *syncope,* or a fainting spell). Usually, the PWA and caregiver will be warned by other accompanying symptoms, such as blurred or double vision, pallor, sweating, nausea, palpitations, chest pain, shortness of breath, feeling flushed, and feeling weak in the knees. The PWA may not be able to walk straight, or she may seem confused and disoriented.

A more serious type of loss of consciousness occurs with no warning signs at all. Some have described the sensation as standing up and being engaged in an activity one minute and waking up on the floor or in a hospital bed the next.

Syncope occurs when the blood supply to the brain is temporarily decreased. Although it doesn't have to be, it *can* be as a result of a serious neurological or cardiac condition and requires immediate medical attention.

What to Do

For Dizziness

- Get the PWA to a safe place. Lie her down, if possible, and open a window to let in some fresh air.
- If infusing (see Chapter 22 for information on infusion) ganciclovir, pentamidine, or other medications known to cause dizziness or sudden drops in blood pressure, slow the drip rate and give her fluids. **Do not give anything by mouth to a PWA who seems confused or about to lose consciousness, since choking is a serious threat.**
- Administer dizziness medication if prescribed.
- Stay with the person and monitor her pulse, respiration, and blood pressure.

For Fainting Spells

- Carefully monitor the events before, during, and after. For example, the doctor may want to know what brought on the spell or if there was any seizure activity.
- Lay the unconscious person on her back. **Check for pulse and breathing (see page 59). If none are present, begin CPR if you have been trained to do so. CALL AN AMBULANCE.** If pulse and respiration are stable, ele-

vate the PWA's legs so that they are higher than the level of her head. This will usually arouse her.

- Ascertain, once the person is conscious, if there were or are any other symptoms accompanying the fainting spell, such as chest pain, palpitations, headache, loss of sensation on one side of the body, difficulty breathing or speaking.

What Not to Do

- Never leave a dizzy or light-headed person alone. She might fall and injure herself.
- Do not give alcohol to someone who has just regained consciousness. Alcohol is a depressant drug that would be dangerous to administer without knowing the underlying cause of the fainting spell and might even induce another loss of consciousness.

When to Consult Your Doctor

- **If the PWA has a syncopal episode, complains of chest pain or shortness of breath, or has a severe headache with fever and other neurological symptoms, CALL AN AMBULANCE.**

Memory Lapses, Delirium, and Dementia

It is part of the tragedy of AIDS that vital, intelligent people often fall prey to a sudden or gradual deterioration in mental functioning. To add to the insult, PWAs are often very much aware (in the beginning) that they are confused and feel frustrated and helpless to control it. Often, a reason (sometimes reversible) can be pinpointed and treated; other times the exact cause is never discovered.

Note: PWAs who are not technically delirious or demented also may have very limited attention spans. This may be due to a preoccuption with their illness, transient confusion, too much sensory stimuli in the environment, medication side effects, or an overwhelming experience, such as a dramatic shift from being in the home to being in the intensive care unit. Some of the following information will apply equally to them. The main thing to keep in mind is to maintain orientation (i.e., remind the PWA of who he is, where he is and what the time and date are), to engage the PWA in simple tasks and short activities, and to limit visitors.

Characteristics of Delirium and Dementia

In both delirium and *dementia,* there is confused behavior. The crucial difference is that **delirium is completely reversible.** Delirium appears suddenly (often having its acute onset at night) and disappears just as suddenly (usually within a month). **Dementia is a chronic, gradually worsening condition.**

Both are marked by memory impairment (especially in short-term memory). The confused person may remember clearly things that occurred 20 years ago but may not be able to tell you what he ate for breakfast. See Table 21.1 for a comparison of delirium and dementia. Other symptoms of dementia and delirium include intellectual decline leading to an inability to understand concepts, disorientation, and poor judgment that often puts his safety in jeopardy. For instance, the confused PWA may not understand when to turn off the stove or whether it is safe to cross the street. He may have disruptions in his sleep cycle.

As part of this condition, the PWA suffering from an organic problem in his brain leading to either dementia or delirium may also display dramatic mood swings—from inappropriately happy to melancholy. His thoughts and actions may run the gamut from extreme lethargy to not being able to keep still; he may be fearful, apathetic, or full of rage.

It is crucial to keep in mind that PWAs with these conditions have no control over their behaviors (which may be bizarre—occasionally even violent). It is also important to realize that dementia and delirium are not exclusive of each other. If a person with dementia suddenly becomes dramatically worse, he may be delirious as well, from an acute, usually reversible cause.

Causes of Delirium and Dementia

The possible causes of delirium in PWAs include illicit and prescription drug use, alcohol intoxication or withdrawal, cardiovascular disorders, metabolic disorders (very high fevers, dehydration, malnutrition, liver or kidney failure, diabetes, thyroid disease, and anemia), head injury from falls, and, of course, cancerous brain tumors and infections (toxoplasmosis of the brain, neurosyphilis, tuberculosis, meningitis, and encephalitis from various causes).

Delirium, but not dementia, may be caused by a psychiatric illness, although severe depression and schizophrenia can mimic some of the symptoms of dementia—particularly disorientation, mood swings, and a decline in attentiveness to one's appearance and personal hygiene.

The causes of HIV-associated dementia are less clear. Whatever the underlying problem (research indicates that a "slow virus" may be implicated), the PWA has a chronic, gradual, but global and irreversible decline in intelli-

---

TABLE 21.1   *How to Distinguish Delirium from Dementia*

	Delirium	**Dementia**
Onset	Abrupt	Gradual
Duration	Short-lived	Irreversible
Course	Fluctuates over 24 hours	Relatively stable
Awareness of Surroundings	Impaired	Normal
Thinking	Dreamlike	Poor abstraction
Prognosis	Good	Poor

gence and his ability to function in daily life, including the loss of mathematical aptitude, vocabulary, abstract and analytical thinking, and coordination.

What to Look For

- Worsening forgetfulness—especially forgetting simple tasks or events that are usually familiar to the PWA, sometimes putting his safety in jeopardy
- Disorientation (not being able to tell you who he is, where he is, or what day time of day it is)
- Sudden and dramatic onset of confusion—this is usually from an acute and reversible cause
- Decline in personal hygiene and appearance
- Restlessness and agitation
- Aggressive or violent behaviors
- Decline in mental abilities: inability to exercise judgment, to reason, to think abstractly, to comprehend simple concepts or instructions
- Severe depression
- Shallow emotions with mood swings, from very happy to sad
- Disruption in normal sleep patterns
- Loss of bladder and bowel control

What to Do

- Gently and repeatedly remind the PWA of who and where he is and what time of day it is.
- Use concrete reminders to trigger a weak memory. For example, for a PWA who insists that you have not given him his medication, design a chart on which you can demonstrate by pointing to check marks that he has indeed received his medicines.
- Be patient and understanding.
- Repeat instructions multiple times, in simple language.
- Always approach a confused or agitated PWA from the front.
- Speak slowly and calmly.
- Keep the atmosphere quiet, with few sensory stimuli. Limit loud music. The less going on in the place where the person is, the better.
- Try to reassure a confused person who is hallucinating and neither argue with nor feed into the imaginary imagery. For example, if the person thinks that he is in a jungle with giant spiders hanging from the ceiling, you might say something like, "I'm sure that you see spiders on the ceiling right now, but I don't see them."
- Find the cause of the PWA's agitation. Is he frightened or in pain?
- Keep the home environment safe by providing good lighting, childproof locks on cabinets, covering exposed outlets, installing special devices for bathroom fixtures, and so forth (see Chapter 2). Keep medications, poisons, and matches out of reach.

- Keep the daily routine of a confused PWA simple and consistent. He will feel more secure if he knows what to expect in terms of meals, naps, bedtime, and activities. If there has to be a deviation from the routine (e.g., a doctor's visit), explain what's going to happen.
- Make sure the PWA has a Medic Alert tag on at all times.
- Be present at mealtimes to assist the confused PWA. If necessary, cut up his food for him to prevent injury and/or choking.
- Keep bathroom activities as private as possible, but never leave the PWA alone when he is in the bathtub. Bathing may be a frightening experience to a confused individual. You should never force the person to bathe, but encourage it by diminishing the sources of the fear. For example, prefill the tub with a few inches of warm water and never drain it while he is present. Try not to get soap or water in his eyes. Sponge bathing may be necessary.
- Keep the telephone number for the poison control center on hand. A confused person might inadvertently overdose on a medication or ingest a poison.
- Minimize embarrassment to the person. Especially early on, the PWA may be aware that he is confused. He may say something like, "I'm a bit muddled today, aren't I?" Acknowledge the feeling, if it's true, and then get on with things. Don't deny or dwell on the fact.
- Limit the number of visitors who may call on the PWA at the same time to prevent sensory overload.

What *Not* to Do

- **Never put your own safety in jeopardy if a confused PWA does something dangerous or becomes violent.** Get help—by summoning the police if necessary.
- **Never leave a confused person alone—either at home or in a car.**
- Never let a confused person be in charge of his medications, meals, bathing, or other critical or potentially dangerous activities.
- Do not talk about a confused person to others in his presence.
- Do not allow a confused person to indulge in any alcohol or caffeine.
- Do not argue with a confused PWA. If he is engaged in inappropriate or unsafe behaviors, divert his attention by giving him a simple task to do or distract him by putting on the television or some soothing music.

When to Consult Your Doctor

- If there was an event that precipitated the confusion, such as a blow to the head from a fall or a seizure, **GO TO THE EMERGENCY ROOM.**
- For any acute onset of confusion or for any dramatic worsening of the condition in an already confused PWA.

What to Discuss with the Doctor

- Any noticeable decline in mental abilities or any change in personality or behavior.
- A change in any medications you suspect to be causing disorientation or dulling of mental powers.
- If you feel that you need additional help managing the care of a confused PWA.

Insomnia

Insomnia is the most common sleep disorder suffered by the ill, the hospitalized, and those in pain—that is, PWAs. Insomnia can encompass difficulties falling asleep, as well as difficulties sleeping through the night and the perception of not having slept deeply and restfully.

Causes of Insomnia

There are many causes of insomnia in PWAs, of course, aside from pain and physical symptoms (e.g., needing to get up several times a night to urinate or defecate). Other causes include anxiety, depression, worries about financial or other practical matters, medications, caffeine, alcohol, or a disruption in one's normal routine, as during hospitalization.

Not getting a good night's sleep can affect one's outlook and ability to cope with the stressors of daily life. People who suffer from insomnia are sleepy during the day, feel clumsy, and cannot concentrate well.

What to Do

- Have a consistent schedule for going to bed and waking up each day.
- Make sure the bedroom is quiet and that the bed and room temperature are comfortable.
- "Wind down" at the end of the day. Engage in a quiet activity, such as reading, doing a handicraft, watching television (something relaxing), or listening to soothing music.
- Have a light snack rather than a heavy meal just before turning in.
- Drink a glass of warm milk before going to bed.
- If you cannot fall asleep after a half hour, get out of bed (if able) and read or do another quiet, relaxing activity. Return to bed when you feel tired and ready to try again.
- Try to get exercise during the day, if you are able. This tires you and releases tensions, facilitating sleep.
- Use your bed only for sleeping (if you are physically up to it)—not for working, for watching television, or for other waking activities.

- Try using the relaxation techniques described in Appendix C if worry is at the core of sleep problems, and/or consider seeing a therapist for help.

What *Not* to Do

- Do not use caffeine, tobacco, or alcohol.
- Do not turn on the light or look to see what time it is if you awaken during the night. This may stimulate you and prevent you from drifting back to sleep.
- Do not use sleeping pills unless prescribed by your physician. Even then, limit their use lest your body becomes too accustomed to them and you cannot sleep without them. After repeated use, sleeping pills disrupt the deepest form of sleeping called "REM" or "rapid eye movement" sleep and thus don't allow refreshing sleep.
- Do not drink a lot of fluids before going to bed, as you will undoubtedly have to get up during the night to urinate.
- Do not take naps during the day.
- Do not engage in strenuous exercise in the hours before bedtime.
- Do not make insomnia a vicious cycle by worrying about falling asleep. This fuels anxiety and makes it even harder to relax and sleep.

When to Consult Your Doctor

- If a specific medication you are taking disrupts sleep—either because of its side effects or because you must wake up in the middle of the night to take it.
- To ask about the occasional use of a sleeping pill to relax you and reestablish your sleep routine.
- To request an increase in pain medication if pain is keeping you awake.
- To ask about a referral to a therapist or biofeedback specialist and about other nonpharmacological measures to restore sleep.

CHAPTER **22**

Chemotherapy and Radiation

Chemotherapy

The term chemotherapy is familiar to most people within the context of cancer treatment. More broadly defined, chemotherapy can mean any kind of treatment with drugs. For PWAs, chemotherapy is used to manage primary Kaposi's sarcoma and lymphomas (see Chapter 1 for explanations of these illnesses).

In general, chemotherapy of varying types is used to prevent the multiplication of rapidly growing cells. Chemotherapy can be prescribed prior to surgery to help shrink tumors (making them easier to remove), or postoperatively to ensure that any remaining malignant cells (not excised surgically) are destroyed. Chemotherapy is also used in nonsurgical cases—alone, or in conjunction with radiation therapy (see page 205)—as a means of killing off malignant cells.

Chemotherapy is sometimes used as a *palliative* measure; that is, not to cure or treat, but to alleviate pain. It accomplishes this by shrinking the tumor and therefore increasing the person's comfort.

Delivery Methods

Chemotherapy can be delivered to the bloodstream in many ways. Some chemotherapeutic agents are taken in pill form; others are given as an intravenous (IV) *infusion* into a peripheral IV (e.g., the needle is inserted into an arm) or a central venous access device (see Chapter 23). Infusions can last as little as 5 or 10 minutes or can run continuously over a 24-hour period, depending upon the specific type of medication being administered. Chemotherapy can also be given by "IV push." This means that a doctor introduces the medication via a syringe into an intravenous line slowly over a few minutes.

In cases of brain or spinal cancer, chemotherapy can also be delivered intrathecally—that is, into the tissues surrounding the spine. This procedure is performed by a physician and is similar to a spinal tap. Chemotherapy can also be delivered into a reservoir previously implanted surgically into the PWA's skull.

Chemotherapy can be given via a single drug regimen, or in combination, using two or more drugs that may be administered in several different ways. Sometimes a "rescue" drug called leukovorin is given to help rescue normal, healthy cells from the damaging effects of the chemotherapy. **It is very important that this medication be taken at the specified times and in the specific dose ordered for the PWA.**

Delivery Settings

Chemotherapy can be administered in many settings. Initially, most PWAs will be hospitalized for evaluation, administration of the regimen, and close monitoring. After the first course of the drug(s), some PWAs will be able to receive their chemotherapy at home if a venous access device is in place. In these cases, an IV- and chemotherapy-certified registered nurse will visit the home and administer the medication. In other cases, chemotherapy can be administered in a doctor's office, an outpatient clinic, a day infusion center, or, as stated, in the hospital.

Side Effects of Chemotherapy

Regardless of the medication used or how it is delivered, healthy cells will, to some degree, be attacked along with the cancer cells because the chemotherapeutic drug cannot distinguish between them. It is for this reason that side effects occur.

The most common side effects from chemotherapy include: hair loss, mouth ulcers, lowered blood cell counts, nausea, vomiting, diarrhea, fatigue, loss of appetite, fever, numbness and tingling in the fingers, and, sometimes, impotence. These side effects are difficult to adjust to but are usually not permanent. Side effects resolve in varying amounts of time, depending on the specific drug used and how often it is given.

You may have heard that receiving chemotherapy can compromise the immune system. This is especially true for PWAs, who are already immunosuppressed to varying degrees. Therefore, the use of chemotherapeutic agents must be weighed against the possible harmful effects. In most cases, the potential benefits outweigh the risks and chemotherapy is tried. Once chemotherapy has been initiated, the PWA's condition is carefully monitored by means of daily blood tests, physical exams, and reports from the PWA as to how he feels.

Aside from the possibility of side effects, other potential dangers occur during infusion. *Extravasation,* which is the leakage of the chemotherapeutic agents from the vein into the surrounding tissue, can occur if the chemotherapy is not properly and carefully administered by a qualified medical professional. Great care must be taken to ensure that the IV site is properly established in a vein and is open before any medication is given. If leakage occurs, there can be tissue irritation from the drug being infused. This irritation can be minor, causing some discomfort, or it can be more serious, leading to inflammation, ulcers, and necrosis (tissue death). The latter requires surgery, including cleaning out of the dead and damaged tissue and other debris (e.g., pus, bacteria) and even a skin graft in some cases. This occurs rarely, but it is always a potential danger.

What to Do

- Read all you can about chemotherapy and its side effects.
- Consider attending support groups for those undergoing chemotherapy.

- Be sure the registered nurse used for home infusion of chemotherapy is from a reputable agency and is certified in both chemotherapy (*oncology*) and intravenous therapy.
- Arrange in advance for transportation to and from the doctor's office, hospital, or clinic for outpatient administration. Be sure someone always accompanies the PWA.

When to Consult Your Doctor

- If the PWA is sent home on chemotherapy. Discuss any side effects or problems the PWA is having. For example, report to the doctor or nurse any difficulties with IVs or central access devices. Let her know immediately of any redness, swelling, or pain at the IV site after chemotherapy is given.
- If the PWA is unable to eat due to side effects, or if you feel he is losing weight, discuss this with the doctor, nurse, or dietitian.
- To inquire about referrals to support groups, individual counseling, and cancer organizations.

What to Discuss with Your Doctor

- Possible side effects of the agents used. Request that they be planned for; for example, if it is known that nausea is a common side effect of the treatment, then request that antinausea medications be ordered in case they are needed.
- The possibility of placing a venous access device to prevent the need for peripheral IVs and blood drawing.

What to Expect at the Doctor's Office

When the PWA first begins chemotherapy, he should be prepared for a hospital stay. He may actually need to be hospitalized for several courses, depending on his body's reaction to the drug(s). While there he may have blood drawn daily as well as X rays and other diagnostic tests. Anticipate that changes and adjustments may be needed in the therapeutic regimen.

Radiation Therapy

Radiation therapy, using either cobalt or electron beams, is used to treat tumors by either shrinking or eliminating them. Sometimes, radiation is intended to control disease; other times it is used as a palliative measure to give relief of pain and other symptoms. Radiation is often used prior to surgery to reduce tumor size and make it easier to remove. It is also used after surgery to kill off any remaining cancer cells. Chemotherapy and radiation therapy are sometimes used together for this purpose. Sometimes radiation to shrink a tumor is done for cosmetic effect, such as when a tumor is on the face. Often, it is done to shrink painful lesions pressing on other areas, especially if the tumor is interfering with the function of a vital organ.

Delivery Settings

Radiation treatments are administered by the department of nuclear medicine in a hospital or in another radiation facility. They can be done on an inpatient or outpatient basis. Treatments are usually performed five times a week, but this does vary case by case. The amount of radiation used is prescribed by a *radiologist,* and the radiation beam is directed only at the malignancy. Marks are usually made on the PWA's skin to indicate where the beam is to be aimed. **These markers are *not* to be washed off.**

Often, the amount of radiation used depends on the tolerance of the organs that surround the malignancy. Radiation in improper doses can damage other organs, such as the heart, liver, intestines, bone marrow, kidneys, and lungs. Lead aprons are usually used to cover parts of the body not to be *irradiated.*

Side Effects of Radiation

As is the case with chemotherapy, radiation treatments are not specific to cancer cells. Therefore, healthy cells are also attacked. Side effects of radiation are similar to those of chemotherapy: hair loss, mouth sores, lowered blood cell counts, nausea, vomiting, diarrhea, fatigue, loss of appetite, and fever. In addition, in contrast to chemotherapy, radiation can cause skin changes. These are most often described as red, dry, orange-peel looking areas at the irradiated site.

What to Do

- Have someone accompany the PWA and assist him with his transportation if he is to receive radiation therapy as an outpatient.
- Practice meticulous skin care. Carefully wash the area to be irradiated (inside the marks) with mild soap and water. Apply a moisturizer. Use products that contain no perfumes or alcohol.
- To protect radiation markers from accidentally being wiped off, either by washing or by clothing, avoid tub baths if the radiation marks are on the extremities or torso. Cover them with plastic wrap when showering, or sponge bathe. Wear loose clothing instead of girdles, tight belts, and so on.
- Remind the PWA to ask to be protected with lead aprons and blankets during treatments so that only the cancerous area is irradiated.

When to Consult Your Doctor

- To report any side effects, skin changes, or accidentally removed radiation marks.
- To ask for referrals and information about support groups and cancer organizations that may be helpful to you.

What to Expect at the Doctor's Office

All or some of the radiation treatments will be done while the PWA is hospitalized. During this time, there may be changes in the amount or number of treatments. This may depend on blood test results, X rays, and scans, which will probably be performed to track the PWA's progress.

CHAPTER 23

Home Administration of Nutritional and Medical Therapies

Gavage (Tube Feedings)

Gavage, also known as tube feedings or *enteral* nutrition, is the administration of nutritionally balanced liquid food via a tube that has been surgically placed into the stomach or small intestine. It can also refer to the use of a *nasogastric* tube that is inserted by a doctor or nurse into the nostril, down the throat and esophagus until it reaches the stomach. A nasogastric tube is placed by a doctor or nurse at the hospital bedside. It is a temporary measure, used primarily while in the hospital, because nasogastric tubes are smaller and therefore can clog and become dislodged more easily than the larger tubes placed by a surgeon for use on a more long-term basis. A PWA can be sent home with a larger gavage tube in place in the abdomen or intestine.

Gavage is used when a person cannot eat enough to sustain life. In cases of PWAs in a coma or who have swallowing problems, the use of tube feedings is common. These larger tubes can also be used to administer medications—either liquids or pills that have been crushed, mixed with water, and injected with a syringe. Problems with gavage feedings include stomach cramps, bloating, gas, diarrhea and/or constipation, nausea, and vomiting.

Methods of Tube Feeding

There are three methods of administering tube feedings at home. Either the physician will order a particular method according to the tolerance of a PWA for his feedings or the nurse and/or caregiver will choose a delivery method which best fits into the PWA's lifestyle.

Bolus

In the *bolus* method, a syringe (minus the needle) is filled with the liquid food as prescribed by the doctor or dietitian and is injected slowly into the tube on a specific, predetermined schedule. This is often done four times a day, to simulate breakfast, lunch, dinner, and a bedtime snack. Problems with accidental injection of air into the tube are common. This can result in bloating and passage of gas rectally or orally.

Gravity Infusion

Here, a disposable bag, which must be changed daily and washed between uses, is filled with the liquid food as prescribed. The bag comes with tubing that connects to the gavage tube. It is hung on an IV pole and the drip rate is regulated by hand, or by a clamp or dial. Feeding is done several times a day in small amounts, or only once a day in a larger amount. Though this method is relatively simple, regulating the flow is usually an imprecise science at best and, if the flow slows too much, it is possible for the gavage tube to become clogged.

Pump Infusion

In this case, a small pump is used to infuse the feeding at a prescribed rate for a specific amount of time. Many types of pumps are available, and there is usually a disposable bag and tubing that fits the particular pump being used. It is connected to the gavage tube. This method allows for exact measurement of feedings, and the pump has an alarm that signals when the bag is empty or there is a blockage in the system. Feedings can be given over 24 hours or cycled for a prescribed amount of time.

Liquid Nutritional Supplements

The particular liquid food substance used for tube feedings and/or as an oral supplement is prescribed on an individual basis by a doctor, usually in conjunction with a dietitian. These liquids are nutritionally complete and must meet the PWA's needs for calories, nutrients, vitamins, and minerals. Taken into consideration are: fluid loss (from vomiting and diarrhea), the need for electrolytes and protein (to aid in tissue growth and repair), individual tolerance, and other medical problems (such as allergies or diabetes).

Liquid food substances can be purchased commercially in a ready-to-feed preparation (such as Ensure or Sustacal), or they may be mixed at home using a blender and by following a recipe provided by a dietitian. There are many different types: milk-based, low residue (bulk), high nitrogen, and semi-synthetic.

Administering Food and Drugs via Gavage

What to Do

- Store liquid food mixtures properly.
- Follow directions regarding *aspiration* of stomach contents to check placement and infusion of feedings. This will be taught to you by a hospital or home care nurse before the PWA leaves the hospital.
- Monitoring tolerance to feeding. Assess the PWA for bloating, belching, or passage of gas via the rectum, which indicates a buildup of air in the stomach.
- Flush the tube with water as taught. This includes flushing it after medications are instilled to ensure that the medicine is in and the tube is not clogged.
- Make sure that air is not also injected when injecting medications into the tube with a syringe, as this can result in bloating, cramps, and gas.

- Keep track of the amount of food introduced and the amount of urine produced. Roughly half of the amount of the feeding should be excreted as urine.
- Assess the PWA for signs and symptoms of dehydration (see Chapter 16); you may need to give water as well as supplements.
- Monitor the site of the gavage tube insertion for signs of poor healing or infection: redness, swelling, pain, or foul drainage.
- Be sure visits from home care nurses are arranged and all the necessary equipment is available before taking a PWA home from the hospital with a gavage tube in place.
- Always have the PWA in a sitting position for at least 30 minutes during the infusion and for 30 minutes after the infusion is completed. If the PWA is comatose, prop him up in bed (to at least a 30° to 45° angle) using pillows or foam wedges, or, if he is in a hospital bed, use the bed controls to put him in a sitting position.
- Administer liquid foods at room temperature.
- Start feedings slowly and in small amounts to offset diarrhea; increase the rate as tolerance builds.
- Increase the amount as ordered by the doctor or dietitian.
- Avoid infusion of air into the stomach, as this will cause bloating, cramps, and gas, as would occur when bottle feeding a baby.

When to Consult Your Doctor

- To report any signs of poor healing or infection, such as redness, swelling, pain, or foul drainage.
- To report diarrhea, constipation, nausea, vomiting, or dehydration.
- To talk about gavage tubes and the various methods and types of feeding products available.
- To inquire about home care nurses to assist with the initial transition from hospital to home.
- To report the PWA's tolerance of the feedings as well as problems. If nausea or diarrhea are a problem, ask about medicines to manage these symptoms.

Total Parenteral Nutrition (TPN)

Parenteral nutrition, also called *hyperalimentation,* is used when food and fluids cannot be absorbed, tolerated, or consumed in amounts adequate to maintain weight and sustain life for a lengthy period of time. The individual may be in a coma or may be suffering from malnutrition (as many PWAs do, because of their various intestinal problems).

TPN Prescriptions

Total parenteral nutrition (TPN)—when given with *lipids* (fats)—provides the total daily nutritional requirements for a PWA and allows him to maintain his weight. It provides the fluid, electrolytes, calories, protein, vitamins, and minerals that are needed daily. Lipids can be added in separately to add calories and essential fatty acids.

TPN must be ordered by a doctor, aided in some cases by a registered dietitian. Each mixture is tailored to the person who will be receiving it. The prescription is changed as the individual's needs change. For example, if the PWA has high blood sugar, insulin may be added until his blood sugar levels return to normal.

TPN is mixed under sterile conditions in a pharmacy by a specially trained pharmacist. Improperly mixed TPN can cause illness. Because of the chemical properties of the solution, TPN is given only via a central *venous access device.* TPN can be given at home when a person has a central venous access device *implanted.* The infusion is regulated by a pump that is programmed to deliver a specific amount of TPN over a specified time period. TPN can be given as a 24-hour infusion or cycled for 8, 10, or 12 hours to be given while the person is asleep.

Complications of TPN and Venous Access Devices

There are several potentially serious complications that can arise during home infusion of TPN. It is therefore extremely important that PWAs receiving TPN infusions comply with blood testing to monitor for infections, glucose and electrolyte levels, and so on. Early detection of a problem usually leads to early and easy solutions.

Infection

Infection can occur because the device provides a direct route for bacteria and fungi to enter the bloodstream; in addition, the TPN itself, with its high sugar content, is a good medium for bacterial growth. Infection most frequently results from improper care of the device—if, for example, the person caring for the device has poor handwashing techniques, does not don **sterile** (not just clean) gloves when changing the dressing, does not carefully assess the insertion site, ignores the signs of infection, or gives contaminated fluid. In some cases, intraveous antibiotics are given to kill the germs causing the infection; more often the device must be removed as well.

Occlusion

Occlusion of the device means that the venous access device has become clogged and no fluid can be infused, nor can any blood be removed. This can happen if the device is not properly flushed with normal saline and heparin as ordered by the doctor and when not in use. The device can also become clogged if the flow rate of the fluid is very slow, usually below 30 cc per hour. This can often be reversed by adding *urokinase* or *streptokinase* (enzymes used therapeutically to dissolve blood clots) into the device to eat away the clotted material and once again open up the catheter. This is done by doctor's order only.

Air Embolus

An air *embolus*, that is, an air bubble, can enter the bloodstream via the device and travel to vital organs, where it can cause new medical problems. To avoid this, the catheter must be properly clamped when not in use. Air emboli can also form if IV tubing is not properly primed, that is, if fluid has not been run through the tubing before connecting it to the access device. This can be prevented (although it is not a common occurrence) through careful learning of catheter care.

Blood Sugar Imbalance

Hypoglycemia or hyperglycemia (see Chapter 17) can occur if the rate of glucose (sugar) infusion does not match the rate of insulin production. Sometimes it is necessary to add insulin to the TPN, administer insulin injections, and/or perform home glucose monitoring to make sure a proper blood sugar is maintained.

Triglyceride, Electrolyte, and Calcium Imbalances

Recipients of TPN may also suffer from an elevated triglyceride level, which indicates lipids need to be stopped at least temporarily. Electrolyte imbalances can occur, requiring a change in TPN formulation as well. Excess calcium within the body can cause inflammation of the pancreas, which puts a halt to TPN infusions for a period of time.

Types of Venous Access Devices

The types of venous access devices discussed here are those intended for long-term use. They allow for safe administration of TPN, chemotherapy, medications, blood, and blood products. They can also be used by trained medical personnel to draw blood specimens instead of using a peripheral vein.

These devices are usually surgically implanted under local anesthesia while the PWA is in the hospital. The PWA then goes home with this venous access device in place. The PWA, the caregiver, and most often a home care registered nurse together care for the device, use it to infuse what is prescribed, and assess it for signs of infection, which are then immediately reported to the doctor.

There are three types of venous acess devices currently available: *nontunneled; tunneled;* and *implanted ports* (see Figure 23.1).

Nontunneled Catheters

These devices come in single, double, or triple *lumen* types and are usually made of silicone or polyurethane. Venous access devices may be inserted centrally into a neck vein or into an arm. They often can be inserted into the PWAs arm in a clinic, a physician's office, or even a PWA's home. This is because they are threaded into the arm in a manner similar to the insertion of an ordinary intravenous line. Central sites require surgical insertion under local anesthesia.

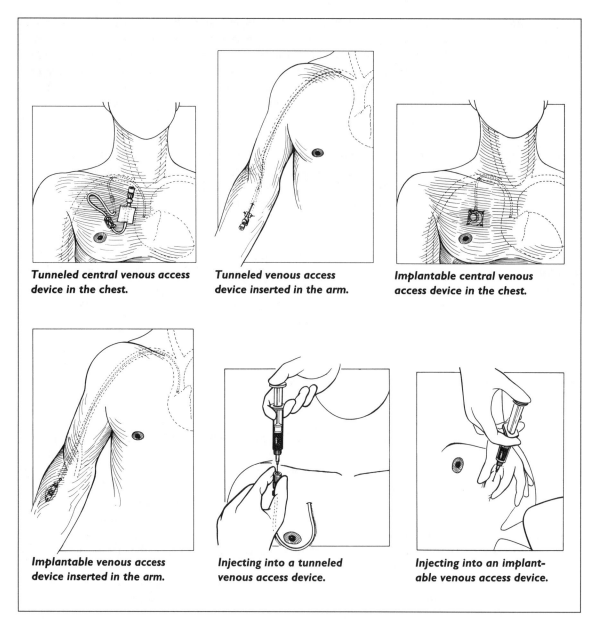

Tunneled central venous access device in the chest.

Tunneled venous access device inserted in the arm.

Implantable central venous access device in the chest.

Implantable venous access device inserted in the arm.

Injecting into a tunneled venous access device.

Injecting into an implantable venous access device.

FIGURE 23.1   ***Venous Access Devices*** (Illustrations © 1990 by Pharmacia Deltec Inc., St. Paul, Minnesota. Reprinted with permission.)

When this device is inserted into an arm, a common problem is positioning, meaning that if the PWA bends his elbow, the vein bends, too, causing the IV flow to slow down and the alarm on the pump to sound off. This can be remedied by unbending the arm and keeping it out straight until the infusion is finished.

In most cases, these devices can be hidden under a shirt. They have "tails" (also known as a catheter, a pigtail, a lumen, or a port) hanging externally from the body. **The device must always be covered with a sterile dressing over the insertion site.** Unused lumens must be flushed to prevent them from becoming clogged.

Tunneled Catheters

These are available in single, double, or triple lumen types. They are made of silicone and are always surgically implanted under local anesthesia. Two surgical sites are created. The first is a small (approximately 1 to 1½ inch) incision at the collarbone. The second is an exit site for the actual catheter. It is lower down, either at the level of the nipple or in the abdominal region. Again, as with nontunneled devices, a dressing must remain in place at all times over the insertion site; a catheter will always exit the body, and unused lumens must be flushed to keep them open. As with the nontunneled venous access devices, a shirt will usually cover the device. Tunneled catheters are often favored because they are usually not influenced by the PWA's position.

Both tunneled and nontunneled devices have the advantage that the skin never needs to be pierced for blood drawing, injections, administration of medications, and so on once they are in place. When hooking the device to an infusion, only the external catheter is pierced with the needle. This is a big plus for those who fear needles, or don't feel they can pierce their own skin. On the negative side, a sterile dressing must always be present over the insertion site. Dressing changes must be performed as ordered, even when the device is not in use.

Implanted Ports

These devices are available in a single or double lumen and are made of either silicone or polyurethane. They are always implanted surgically, usually under local anesthesia. With these devices, two surgical sites are used—one small area (1 to 1½ inch) at the collarbone and another where the actual port is implanted, also about an inch long. The port, about the size of the face of a wristwatch, is implanted under the skin. Double lumen ports look like two watch faces side by side. (Unused ports must be kept open by flushing them.)

After implantation, the port can't be used for approximately ten days while the surgical site heals. By contrast, tunneled and nontunneled devices can be used immediately after surgery because no piercing of the skin is needed. When the surgeon says it's okay to use the port, it is accessed with a special needle—usually a huber needle, which is a curved needle with tubing attached. This needle and tubing can then be hooked to the IV tubing for infusion. When ports are accessed with a needle, a sterile dressing must be applied and changed as ordered. When the port is not in use, however, no dressing is necessary. Port devices are easily hidden under a shirt and are less noticeable if there is no clothing covering them than are the tunneled and nontunneled devices.

When in constant use, the huber needle must be changed as frequently as your doctor advises. This can vary from daily to every seven days. A larger-sized needle is used for blood administration than for other intravenous infusions. Often, blood administration takes longer than other infusions, too.

If the needle has been inserted too deeply, it may touch the stainless steel or titanium bottom of the port. In this case, the needle must be gently lifted so that it no longer is in contact with the base of the port. If the needle isn't in far enough to pierce the port diaphragm (as can happen with overweight people), fluid may be infusing under the skin instead of into the port. This can be avoided by using good technique and obtaining a blood return upon accessing the device. This should be taught to you by your home care nurse.

When using a multilumen device, a PWA can receive several fluids (e.g., blood and medications) simultaneously. Remember to flush each lumen separately after use.

What to Do

Before Getting a Venous Access Device

- Obtain information about all the venous access devices available to you and discuss with your doctor the type of device that she recommends.
- PWA and caregiver should discuss the pros and cons of each device.
- Consult with nurses, too, as they most often care for these devices.
- Discuss the subject with others who already have venous access devices.
- Prior to surgery, the PWA should read and sign both the surgical and anesthesia informed-consent forms and be sure they are witnessed. He should not do so until he is comfortable with his decision and has had all of his questions answered to his satisfaction.
- Ask about the postoperative period: what pain medication will be ordered; how soon can your device be used; who will perform the initial dressing changes, and when will they need to be done?

   Note: Most PWAs have only minor discomfort after placement of a device. Most often they are eating, out of bed, and back to normal only hours after placement.

When a Venous Access Device Is in Place

- Enlist the aid of a home care nurse after the PWA has the central venous access device placed, to teach you to infuse the TPN, use the pump, and care for the venous access device.
- Be sure all the necessary equipment is in the home prior to discharge from the hospital.
- Be prepared to follow up on TPN formula or equipment deliveries to your home and on the scheduling of home care nursing visits.
- Provide the PWA with any foods he normally would eat, when he is able—in any amount he can tolerate.
- Monitor the PWA's weight as ordered or at least twice a week.

- Monitor the PWA's blood sugar if you have been so advised. (Follow the instructions of your doctor, nurse, or diabetic educator, or see Chapter 17 for assistance.)
- Learn the signs and symptoms of hyper- and hypoglycemia (see Chapter 17) and infection (see Chapter 10). Learn what to do if these problems develop.

Care and Use of a Venous Access Device

- Be prepared to learn how to use the device, change dressings, hang IV fluid, and use an IV pump. Take notes, ask questions, and practice—both before and after the PWA leaves the hospital.
- A home care nurse will usually be arranged for by the social worker or by the physician. He will often do things slightly differently than the hospital staff does. Be prepared for this and be adaptable. The only thing that matters is that there be good sterile technique. These nurses usually bring supplies with them, or the supplies are delivered to your home separately. Be aware of the need to be available to receive these visits/deliveries.
- Carefully assess the insertion site for signs of problems and notify the doctor as soon as possible.
- Maintain good hygiene and skin care to avoid infection (see Chapter 10).
- Flush the device as ordered to ensure that unused lumens or ports do not become blocked.

When to Consult Your Doctor

- If you suspect that there is an infection, an occlusion, or other problems with your catheter or infusion. The PWA may need hospitalization, medications, blood tests, X rays, and even catheter removal.

Sterile Dressing Changes for Venous Access Devices

All of the venous access devices require sterile dressings when in use, and only the port type can remain uncovered when no needle is present.

In general, sterile dressing kits include the following items:

- Sterile gloves. **These must be used without exception.** Note that these differ from the clean gloves used for blood and body fluid precautions.
- Alcohol wipes, swabs, or sticks
- Povidone iodine (often called Betadine) swabs, wipes, or sticks
- Povidone iodine ointment. This comes in a tube. (Not included in some kits.)
- Tincture of benzoin wipes, swabs, or sticks. These are to coat the skin around the insertion site to help the outer dressing to adhere. (Not included in some kits.)
- Occlusive outer dressing. This can be clear or opaque.
- Tape. This is used to seal the outer edges of the outer dressing.

To Change a Sterile Dressing for a Venous Access Device

Note: Determine if you need to change the needles or catheter caps (usually according to a schedule provided by the doctor). If these must be changed, the infusion must be stopped and then restarted once the changes are complete. Otherwise, the infusion can continue during the dressing change.

1. Wash your hands thoroughly and dry them.
2. Remove the old dressing if one is in place by touching only the outer layer, if possible, to avoid infection. If the old dressing is expected to be bloody, wear clean gloves for your own protection.
3. Carefully inspect the catheter site for redness, swelling, odor, drainage, soreness to the touch, and general skin condition. Remember that recently inserted devices may cause the insertion site to appear pink or puffy.
4. Put on sterile gloves as taught to you previously by your nurse. (You can also refer to Chapter 10.)
5. Open the kit as you were taught, to avoid contaminating the sterile items inside.
6. If you were taught to use an adhesive remover, do so now to clean the skin of old tape, tincture of benzoin, and bacteria.
7. Use alcohol swabs, wipes, or sticks in the amount taught (usually three) to clean the area. Always begin on top of the insertion site, wiping in a circular motion and widening the circle until you are approximately 1 inch away from the insertion site. Make wider and wider circles, being careful not to go over a circle already made. Repeat the process in the same way as many times as you were taught, always beginning at the insertion site and ending approximately 1 inch from it.
8. Follow the same procedure as above, now using the povidone iodine swabs, wipes, or sticks.
9. If povidone iodine ointment is included in your regimen, this step is next. Never

(continued)

- Gauze. This is used to cover the insertion site and/or to fold and place under the huber needle in port-type devices as a support.
- Adhesive remover. This facilitates removal of previous dressing remnants and helps clean the skin. (Not included in some kits.)
- Catheter cap. This covers the needle insertion site on the catheter when not in use and needs to be changed when the dressing is changed.

The contents of sterile dressing kits vary from company to company. Some items may be part of a particular kit, but the hospital or home care agency policy may be to exclude their use. Often what is the hospital policy is not the home care agency's policy. Neither is right or wrong. Policies differ based on a facility's experience, interpretation of research, and fiscal needs.

While in the hospital you will be taught according to hospital policy, including the use of their equipment (such as IV pumps). Upon returning home,

(continued)

touch the tube or package to the skin. Squeeze out a ribbon of ointment and allow it to drop onto the insertion site.

10. Next, cover the site with gauze and/or place a folded gauze pad under the huber needle (in a port) to lend it support, according to the method you were taught.

11. Use tincture of benzoin to coat the skin area approximately an inch away from the insertion site. Paint a square box around the area. This will protect the skin and increase adherence of the dressing. (In some cases, this step is omitted. As always, follow the directions given by your doctor or nurse.)

12. Cover the entire area with the occlusive dressing from the kit. This takes practice to avoid wrinkling or improper placement.

13. Secure the outer edges with tape.

Additional Notes

- If you have external lumens, change the catheter caps: Shut off the infusion, clamp the catheter, remove the needle (and discard it properly), twist off the old cap, twist on a new cap, and insert a new sterile needle into the cap. Then open the clamp and set the infusion rate.

- If you have an unused lumen or port, remember that you must flush it with the prescribed amount of normal saline and heparin to keep it open.

- If you have an implanted port, remember to change the huber needle as ordered, usually daily to every seven days. Replace the old needle with the proper needle size.

- Always change IV tubing as ordered and on schedule.

- Avoid comparing notes with other PWAs who have venous access devices. Different devices call for different dressings on varying schedules. Use the preceding information as a general guide, but always follow the instructions and advice of the nurse or doctor. They know what's best in your case.

the visiting nurse will teach you her way of doing things and how to use her equipment. Often, the home care nurse will visit you while you are still in the hospital to begin the teaching process. It is vital that you be sure to understand what is taught and to ask questions and practice. If the method taught by the home nurse is different from the one used in the hospital, adapt to the new method, but don't be afraid to ask why there is a difference.

The box on pages 218–219 details the basic procedure for changing a sterile venous access device dressing. The procedure is not difficult or complicated, but it often seems that way in the beginning. Good manual dexterity comes with practice. Most PWAs and their caregivers find that putting on sterile gloves properly without contaminating them is the most difficult part of the task to master. Practice is the only solution to that problem.

Remember: It is very difficult to learn by simply reading instructions. A demonstration by a registered nurse is a much better way to learn. This section is designed as more of a refresher for you to use as a reference when you are finally on your own.

PART IV

Psychological Issues

CHAPTER 24

The Emotional Toll on the PWA

Anxiety

Think of the times that you have experienced anxiety—that feeling of worry, upset, and uncertainty that stems from a perceived threat or danger that is *usually* more imaginary than real. Perhaps it was the night before an exam you were sure you hadn't studied hard enough for or the time you had the lead in the school play. Maybe you were anxious when you went for your road test or you flew in an airplane for the first time. You might have suffered from anxiety when you asked the person you love to marry you or when you presented yourself to your doctor to receive the results of your HIV test.

People who are HIV positive and those who have AIDS often live in a nearly constant state of anxiety, especially early on in their disease. This is of course due to conflicts that PWAs have about their abilities to maintain certain values and achieve certain goals in life. It occurs because they perceive that being infected with this disease will cause a change (for the worse) in their health, income, friendships, sexuality, home life, and work role. And while anxiety usually stems more from imagined fears than from reality, being HIV positive is a very legitimate reason for being anxious.

In addition, the people who develop AIDS are in many ways the least prepared for the shock of a serious and sometimes terminal illness. Most often they are the young and previously healthy members of society, many of whom were meticulous about their bodies. People in their twenties, thirties, and forties don't normally contemplate death or try to come to grips with their mortality. They are not reflecting back on their lives and what they have accomplished but are looking ahead to what they hope to achieve.

The frequently targeted homosexual and intravenous drug–using populations are already often abandoned by society as being somehow unworthy of help and caring. Now, they may face even more ostracism and discrimination—even if they are only HIV positive and have no symptoms to indicate a progression of their disease. In some ways, being HIV positive and well is worse than being ill, because you never know when you wake up in the morning if this will be the day you are going to get "it"—a cancer; an opportunistic infection. Finally, the very treatments used to try to control AIDS can contribute to discomfort and anxiety.

Caregivers, too, experience extreme anxiety. You yourself may be HIV positive and a look at your friend or lover may be a frightening look into what your own future may hold. Even if you are not HIV positive, you will no doubt be faced with the day-to-day anxieties of taking care of someone who is profoundly ill or dying. How will you pay the bills? What should you say to avoid upsetting the individual? Will you have the strength to withhold life support if that is the person's wish? Will you have the will to go on after she is gone?

Differences in Coping with Anxiety

Although nearly everyone has experienced anxiety, not everyone deals with it in exactly the same way. For the insecure and isolated person, feelings of anxiety may be much more pronounced, and much more support may be needed to assist that person in coping with her anxiety. On the contrary, those who have always handled change and stress well and who have good communication skills—those who can clearly identify their needs—are usually able to keep anxiety to a tolerable level. In fact, anxiety has been known to spur people into taking positive action and gaining a sense of purpose and direction in their lives. Along those lines, the discovery of HIV infection can actually be transformed into a constructive experience for some people. It may be an opportunity to become closer to friends and family by coming to terms with their alternative lifestyle choices and healing old wounds. Because of the realization that the life we cling to is so tenuous, it may be a time of discovering and developing strengths we never had to call upon before in ourselves and others.

What to Look For

- Nervous, restless, jittery behavior
- Insomnia
- Change in appetite
- Episodes (sometimes called "anxiety attacks") during which the person is short of breath, sweating, dizzy; feels faint; or has the sensation that her heart is pounding or skipping beats. The person may tremble or complain of tightness in her chest or a sense that her throat is closing. She may have trouble catching her breath and seem to gasp for air. Her pulse and breathing may be rapid when measured. She may experience diarrhea or have the need to urinate frequently.
- Ambivalence; inability to make decisions
- Becoming easily angered and short-tempered
- Complaint of feeling out of control
- Sense of dread or of impending doom

What to Do

- Remain with anyone suspected of having an episode of acute anxiety.
- Offer reassurance calmly and confidently.

- Encourage her to discuss her thoughts and feelings. Try to communicate your thoughts and feelings even if the PWA seems confused and irrational or is not able to listen or concentrate.
- Remember that anxiety is a universal feeling, but not everyone expresses it in exactly the same way or handles it in exactly the same way.
- Encourage the anxious person, when calm, to keep a journal—to write out her thoughts and feelings in an effort to pinpoint the exact cause of the anxiety and perhaps to develop some solutions and coping mechanisms.
- Administer antianxiety medications if prescribed by the doctor and log their effectiveness.
- Encourage the PWA to learn and practice relaxation techniques, such as meditation, biofeedback, self-hypnosis, or listening to tapes (see Appendix C).
- Urge the PWA to seek therapy with a trained professional—a psychiatrist, psychologist, social worker, or nurse therapist.
- Explore various support groups for PWAs or caregivers.
- Try distractions. Being preoccupied with hobbies, watching television, or reading often aid in relaxation and getting through anxious moments.

What *Not* to Do

- Do not panic in the presence of someone having an anxious episode. It will only worsen the situation. Anxiety attacks are usually short-lived, and the sufferer is usually not in any danger.
- Do not medicate the PWA without consulting a doctor first.
- Do not provide the PWA with recreational drugs or alcohol to calm or soothe her. They will only worsen the anxiety. These substances also pose special risks to PWAs due to the effects they may have on the immune system and their potential interactions with prescribed medications.

When to Consult Your Doctor

- **If someone with a history of cardiac or respiratory illness is experiencing anxiety attack symptoms, these symptoms may be of a physical, not a psychological, nature. In this situation, take no chances. CALL AN AMBULANCE.**
- To inform the doctor of any anxiety the PWA may be experiencing; or discuss this issue with her at your next office visit. You will need to describe the nature of the anxiety attacks in as much detail as possible, including how often they occur, how long they last, what provokes them, and so on.

What to Expect at the Doctor's Office

The PWA may need a physical exam including blood work to rule out any physical cause for the symptoms.

Medications may be prescribed to help decrease and deter the anxiety or to aid with sleeping difficulties. Be careful to give them as directed and to follow the precautions given to you by the doctor, nurse, or pharmacist. Many have potentially dangerous sedating qualities or must be taken with care when mixed with certain other drugs or substances.

Depression

Depression is common among those who are ill, especially among those who are terminally ill. It is equally common in those who care for others and see the changes in their health, hope, and quality of life.

Confucius said of depression, "We should feel sorrow, but not sink under its oppression; the heart of a wise man should resemble a mirror, which reflects every object without being sullied by any." This, of course, is wise advice, but difficult to follow. Despite that, try to keep it as a creed. Be sad. That's only natural under the circumstances. But try to get beyond the sadness so that whatever remains of the quality and quantity of your life is not tarnished by the stain of depression. Many people affected by chronic or terminal illness have demonstrated that if depression is allowed to cloak your every waking moment, your life is guaranteed to be miserable and may even be cut shorter by your negative outlook.

Characteristics of Depression

Depression is manifested by physical as well as emotional and behavioral changes. Often noted are feelings of low self-esteem, irritability, social withdrawal, helplessness, hopelessness, decreased energy level, decreased sexual desire, inability to concentrate, feelings of fatigue, changes in sleep habits, changes in appetite, feelings of dejection and worthlessness, decreased motivation, and slowed speech and movement. Many of the symptoms of depression are difficult to distinguish from the vague symptoms of early AIDS or AIDS-related dementia.

Some have summed up depression as a feeling of emptiness, as life oozing out of their bodies. Associated with depression are anxiety, guilt, and fear. A depressed person may be unable to experience pleasure. She may engage in self-pity to the ultimate level of contemplating or attempting suicide.

For some, depression can be a short-term problem. It may pass, given time; a compassionate, empathetic ear to listen; accurate and current information about the problem troubling the PWA; and an opportunity to work through her thoughts and feelings. Others grapple with severe, lifelong depression, which may even have a biochemical component to it; that is, the feelings are in part due to chemical imbalances within the brain. Finally, some medications used to treat certain AIDS-related conditions may precipitate depression. These include steroid drugs; some high blood pressure and heart medicines; tranquilizers; and alcohol.

Risk Factors for Depression

- Recent upsetting news or changes in levels of health, social status, or relationships
- Use of medications known to cause depression

- Depression, suicide attempts, or psychiatric illness in the PWA's own past or among close family members

What to Look For

- Changes in sleep patterns—either insomnia or increased sleeping hours
- Changes in appetite—lacking the desire to eat or the other extreme of compulsive overeating or binging
- Overindulgence in alcohol or recreational drugs as a means of escape or as a daily routine
- Self-demeaning comments or behaviors
- Social withdrawal—even from those closest to the person
- Laziness or decreased energy level and interest in those around the PWA
- Absence of laughter and smiles in a previously happy person

What to Do

- Remain with the depressed person even if she doesn't interact with you. Don't allow the person to be alone, even if she would prefer it. Observe her for any physical, behavioral, or emotional changes that you should bring to the attention of her physician or therapist.
- Encourage the depressed PWA to verbalize her thoughts and feelings to someone she trusts and feels comfortable talking to. If you are the recipient of these thoughts and feelings, try to listen with an open mind. Remain nonjudgmental. Offer support, understanding, and hope.
- Allow the PWA to cry if she wants to. It often makes one feel better.
- Administer any medications as previously prescribed for depression and note their effectiveness.
- Consider therapy or a support group.
- **Take seriously all mention of suicide or attempts at committing suicide.** Ask the depressed person for details of any plan she may have, however impossible it may seem. **Remain at all times with the person who expresses thoughts of suicide.**

It is important to differentiate the rash, suicidal thoughts or actions of a depressed person from the calm, well-planned suicide of a terminally ill person who wishes to put an end to her misery (see box, page 228, and Chapter 26). Although some might condone suicide under certain circumstances, certainly a person should be restrained from self-destructive behaviors when she is not thinking clearly. Two such instances may be when the person first hears the news that she has AIDS (she may be far from terminal at this stage), or perhaps when she is taking medications that may cause depression.

Treat suicide attempts or talk of committing suicide as an emergency. Notify the doctor immediately. **Remember that sometimes a person is most at risk of committing suicide after a paralyzing depression lifts.** For example, a person may be so immobilized by her depression that she is incapable

---

How to Recognize High-Risk People and Suicidal Behaviors

Consider that a person may be contemplating suicide if she

seems profoundly depressed.

has experienced a loss of self-esteem.

is restless, agitated, and anxious.

expresses feelings of guilt and hopelessness.

is demonstrating self-denigrating or self-destructive behaviors.

tells you that she feels isolated, unloved, and incapable of loving others.

seems to have lost touch with reality and the ability to put things into perspective.

becomes sloppy about her appearance, her job, or other obligations.

talks openly about "doing away with herself" or begins to give away cherished possessions to others.

These individuals are known to be at greater suicide risk:

Anyone with a history of prior attempts

Individuals who have family members who have attempted or committed suicide

Depressed people—including those not clinically diagnosed by a therapist as being depressed

Abusers of alcohol and/or drugs

People who live alone

People who have never been married are at highest risk, followed by those widowed, separated, divorced, married without children, and married with children.

Unemployed individuals

Ill individuals—especially those experiencing chronic pain, chronic disease, recent surgery, or those who are terminally ill

Women make more suicide attempts, but men are more successful.

Remember: Always ask if a suspected suicidal person has a plan for committing suicide. **Even if the plan seems far-fetched, or no plan exists, take the person seriously.** She is crying out for help.

---

of acting. Once she is helped a little bit by medication or therapy, she may actually be able to muster the energy to harm herself. So be on guard! This is a very high-risk time.

What Not to Do

- **Never ignore suicidal thoughts or actions.** Don't assume an attempt won't be made. Remain with the person at risk and protect her from harm. Notify the doctor as soon as possible.
- Never tease a depressed person in an effort to "snap them out of it."

When to Consult Your doctor

- If the depressed person verbalizes suicidal ideas or makes a suicide attempt (however half-hearted or inept), this is a psychiatric emergency. **GO TO THE EMERGENCY ROOM.**
- To inform the physician of any changes in physical or emotional state. Discuss the possibility of depression.

What to Expect at the Doctor's Office

A thorough physical exam and blood work may be necessary to determine any underlying physical cause. Antidepressant medications, psychotherapy, support groups, and/or hospitalization may be necessary to deal with the problem.

Fear

In the award-winning Broadway play *Conversations with My Father,* a character comments on FDR's famous quote: "We have nothing to fear but fear itself," saying, "Isn't that enough?" Fear can be a formidable enemy. It can immobilize one. Often, life cannot go on until fear is conquered.

Characteristics of Fear

Fear is closely tied to anxiety in that many of the physical symptoms are the same. Palpitations, rapid heartbeat, sweating, and dry mouth are common. In contrast to anxiety, however, fear is less vague—more centered. It constitutes an emotional reaction (a dread) to a real or imagined threat. When we are anxious, we often feel agitated and afraid, but the specific cause cannot be pinpointed. Fear has an object, be it a medical procedure, a change in lifestyle—even the unknown.

Fear occurs when one feels she cannot control a given situation or her own reaction to that situation. Often, on some level, people are aware that their fears are unfounded and exaggerated, yet this has little influence on their ability to manage the fear. It is very much like this when one is afraid of the dark. You know there's nothing out there. You can process this on an intellectual level. Yet, you remain afraid.

Confronting Medically Related Fears

In the throes of fear, one's ability to hear and process information is disturbed, causing one to hear only what one chooses to—usually what is most threatening or upsetting rather than what would help one to understand and cope. This is vital for caregivers to comprehend and keep in mind when dealing with PWAs. Chronically, seriously ill people may frequently be confronted with frightening news, events, and situations. They may be unable at the time of the news to completely process and follow instructions or information.

It may be very helpful under these circumstances for caregivers to be present at doctor's appointments, for medical tests, and during hospital rounds when at all possible—both to offer support and to be the listener and advocate for a PWA disabled by her fears.

Encourage the PWA to discuss all of her questions and fears with her health care team. Doctors must be encouraged to fully explain anything that is unclear, confusing, or potentially frightening. Fear of the unknown or un-realistic fears associated with illness and medical procedures may easily be put to rest just by knowing what to expect and by being armed with information. Likewise, if you as the caregiver are attempting to accomplish a task that the PWA fears, remember that you must devote time and patience to the task and must expect that you may have to repeat and reinforce your instructions several times.

What to Look For

- Rapid heartbeat and palpitations
- Clinging behavior
- Crying
- Diarrhea
- Rapid speech, stuttering; repeating oneself
- Shortness of breath; hyperventilation
- Feeling of tightness in the throat or chest
- Inability to remain alone
- Dry mouth
- Dilated pupils, darting eyes (lack of eye contact)
- Inability to sit still; rocking back and forth

What to Do

- Remain with the fearful PWA until she is calm and in control.
- Encourage the fearful PWA to verbalize her thoughts and feelings in as much detail as possible.
- Assist the fearful PWA to see reality and to fully hear and process factual information. Repeat what you are saying if necessary.
- Seek out information to clarify a situation that may be causing fear because there are unknowns. Deliver information slowly and repeat it as often as necessary until the PWA seems to be retaining it. Avoid overwhelming her with a truckload of information that she can't hear or process.
- Allow the PWA to cry if it helps.
- Allow the PWA to be in control as much as possible. Encourage her to make her own decisions. This helps to allay fears.
- Remain supportive, thoughtful, empathetic, and hopeful. She has to believe that her feelings are legitimate and that they can be expressed in a non-judgmental atmosphere.

- Draw upon the assistance of therapists, support groups, relaxation techniques, and antianxiety medications to help the PWA come to terms with and cope with her fears.

What *Not* to Do

- Never administer medications not prescribed for the PWA for this specific problem.
- Do not make light of fears even if they seem irrational or childish to you.
- Do not treat a fearful PWA like a child. Encourage her to be in control and make her own decisions as much as possible.
- Do not feed into a fearful PWA's fantasies or unrealistic views. Be honest, realistic, and factual.
- Do not try to calm the PWA with alcohol, over-the-counter medications, or illicit substances.

Anger

Anger is one of the most powerful of all emotions. Like love, it can spur one into action. It can cause one to fight back against all odds, rather than meekly surrendering and waiting for impending doom. Often anger is a reaction to feeling vulnerable or powerless. For many people, anger is a way to sidestep anxiety, to stop their feelings of impotence. In other words, anger is a means of feeling powerful even if you are powerless in a situation. It may be a part of the grieving process or a reaction to the loss of rights or opinions.

Expressing Anger

For most people, anger is difficult to express in a calm, controlled manner. Often, there is the expression of hostility and rage. Unrestrained anger can lead to physical violence and injury to oneself and/or others.

It is vital for caregivers to understand and remember that anger is frequently misdirected at those closest to us when there is no one else to be angry at or when we are angry at the fates or our higher power for "making" us ill or for making us feel helpless and hopeless. Anger is taken out on those with whom we feel safest or those we feel will still love us and accept us unconditionally—even if we treat them badly.

What to Look For

- Clenched teeth and tight jaw
- Hostile facial expression and stance
- Clenched fists
- Raised voice
- Verbalization of displeasure—often in a hostile manner

- Verbal abuse (cursing and swearing)
- Physical violence
- Inappropriate actions, such as noncompliance with or sabotage of one's medical treatments
- Thwarting authority
- Bitter communications with loved ones—even severing communications or relationships with friends, lovers, and family, temporarily
- Turning on caregivers—laying blame for problems and circumstances on them even when completely unrelated
- Sarcasm
- Criticism of others, especially health care professionals

What to Do

- Try to put yourself in the PWA's place. Be understanding, empathetic, gentle, and patient.
- Encourage the angry PWA to verbalize, even yell and scream if she feels it is necessary, unless she is out of control and seems violent.
- Discuss her thoughts and feelings seriously, placing an emphasis on reality and how the angry person may regain control of herself. Help her to put things into perspective.
- Encourage the PWA to carefully think through any decision to end medical therapy when that is the object of her rage. Encourage compliance while allowing the PWA to question her treatment and to express her displeasure and frustration. Suggest she discuss with her doctor the addition of new modes of treatment.
- Ask family, friends, and lovers to try and maintain contact with the PWA despite her angry mood. Help each other to deal with the anger.
- Seek professional help in dealing with hostility and share that information with other involved persons if necessary.
- Encourage the angry PWA to join a support group to seek psychotherapy.
- Treat the PWA who is angry as an adult, not as a child. This includes holding her responsible and accountable for her words and actions.
- Accept apologies gracefully and encourage the discussion of hurt feelings and important issues.

What *Not* to Do

- Never pressure an angry and confused person into making poorly thought out and quick decisions.
- Never abandon an angry PWA or retaliate for an angry outburst. Don't give her the "cold shoulder" or the silent treatment. Try to discuss the problem honestly and completely after things have calmed down.
- Never assist the angry PWA to be noncompliant or to sabotage her own treatment. Discuss changes in treatment when she is calm and rational. Let the doctor know what she would like to do.

- Never help or encourage a PWA to displace her anger onto others, including health professionals.
- **Never remain in a physically dangerous situation or allow yourself to be physically abused.**
- Do not inflame a volatile situation by feeding into it, that is, fighting back, calling names, saying the PWA is ungrateful, or threatening to leave. Matters will only worsen.
- Do not medicate the angry person to sedate her unless you have been directed to do so by a doctor.
- Do not physically restrain an angry PWA, as it can injure her.
- Do not trivialize the anger or the situation that prompted the anger. Take it seriously and encourage discussion.
- Do not make decisions for the angry person as if she were an unruly child.
- Do not make it difficult or uncomfortable for the PWA to change her mind or to apologize.
- Do not automatically assume that just because the anger is quick or extreme the issue causing the anger is not justified.

When to Consult Your Doctor

- To discuss the PWA's doctor-directed anger; encourage the PWA to do the same. Remind the PWA to try to remain as calm as possible and to try to listen to the doctor's responses. The PWA should feel free to question the doctor. Expect precise answers in most cases, but also be prepared for the doctor to say she doesn't know the answer when this is the honest truth. The PWA has to be prepared when the doctor has no precise answer or solution to offer.
- To ask for healthy ways to express anger and to deal with it, such as: exercise, therapy, or keeping a journal in which one records thoughts and feelings, including anger. And, again, don't forget about support groups, therapy, and relaxation techniques.

Guilt

Guilt is everywhere for PWAs and their caregivers. It seems at times to be inescapable. The PWA has guilt over causing those who care about her to watch her become ill and even die. There is guilt over how she contracted AIDS, guilt over unkept promises, guilt over bad behavior—guilt caused by selfishness or martyrdom. Caregivers feel guilty over anticipatory grief. Parents experience guilt out of a sense that they did a bad job rearing their children. Others are guilty about not being able to visit the PWA in the hospital. The list goes on and on.

Characteristics of Guilt

Guilt is a global feeling of self-blame generated by the acceptance of personal responsibility for supposed wrongdoing. Often a person feeling guilty judges herself by unrealistic criteria—criteria she would never apply to others in a like situation. And if self-blame isn't bad enough, guilt is often caused by accusations made against one by others whether they are accurate or not. We are all, at one time or another, quickly willing to take blame, find fault or accept culpability, but we are very slow to forgive—ourselves or others.

Guilt can eat away at a person, bite after bite, until there is nothing left but an empty shell where once a person lived. This is the true danger of guilt. It is easily avoided via the simple apology, discussing the situation honestly, and exploring each other's thoughts and feelings. Bringing what makes us feel guilty into the light is like exposing a vampire or a demon to that light. Once out in the open—in the light of day, so to speak—the guilt doesn't survive for long.

An excellent therapist we know once said that there are two categories of guilt: "real guilt" and "false guilt." Real guilt is guilt that a moral person feels when she has said or done something truly immoral, damaging, or denigrating to another individual. For example, it is appropriate to feel guilty after committing a crime or deliberately hurting someone else.

False guilt is simply everything else. You feel guilty about not settling things with your mother before she passed away. You feel guilty because you were in St. Louis on business when your lover received the news that she is HIV positive. You are not responsible, nor have you done anything wrong. Yet, somehow you feel guilty.

Real guilt must be faced, acknowledged, and somehow made right—by apologizing to the wronged individual, for example. False guilt must be eliminated, simply by exposing it for the impostor that it is, and then *letting it go.*

What to Look For

- Avoidance of the subject, person, or place involved
- Inability to look others in the eye
- Tearful behavior
- Occasional angry outbursts, especially if the subject of the guilt arises. It is easier to express anger than to admit guilt, therefore guilt is often transformed into anger.
- Verbal admission of guilt
- Verbalizing blame or being blamed
- Pervasive sense of being wrong
- Suicide-related comments or incidents
- Unrealistic expectations for yourself and/or others
- Insomnia
- Changes in appetite
- Nail biting
- Diarrhea
- Trembling

What to Do

- Encourage the PWA to discuss the situation and her feelings and thoughts honestly, openly, and as calmly and completely as she can with those involved. Likewise, encourage others to express and explore their thoughts.
- Try to be nonjudgmental. Give your opinion only if it is asked for.
- Provide reassurance, apologize when called for (even if you're shy or embarrassed), and accept the apologies of others where appropriate. Then let the incidents in question fade into oblivion.
- Avoid placing blame on anyone (including yourself).
- Seek out support groups and therapy, or call upon your religious beliefs to assist in eliminating guilt-ridden feelings and behaviors.
- Observe the guilt-ridden person for suicidal thoughts, comments, or attempts. Always inquire as to whether a person expressing thoughts of suicide has an actual plan. Ascertain details of the plan and report them to the doctor.

What *Not* to Do

- Never tell someone that her view is wrong or worthless. Each person is allowed her opinion, just as she is allowed to disagree with yours.
- Do not lie or exaggerate.
- Do not indulge in the "should haves" and "shouldn't haves" or the "what if's."
- Do not judge yourself or others by unrealistic criteria.
- Do not be unforgiving, condescending, or self-righteous. Put the past behind you and go on—life and the energy to live it are a precious commodity.

When to Consult Your Doctor

- As with all emotional turmoil, feelings of guilt should be relayed to the doctor.
- To report the PWA's suicidal thoughts and deeds; **they must be addressed as an emergency.**

Dependency

Being ill is never easy. To some degree, the sick role means changing or surrendering our role in our family, business, or even society. With the increasing severity of illness, our tendency to rely on others increases. We seek their advice, guidance, support, and care. Often, this extends to such a degree that we find ourselves thinking that we require the assistance and support of others for our every need, then asking for and even imploring others for it. Depending on our individual personalities and styles, we either tend to regress and become dependent on our caregiver, or we become demanding and manipulative, resenting the need to be assisted. Ambivalence abounds. We have mixed thoughts and send ambiguous signals: "I want to be cared for, but don't help me."

Repercussions of Dependency

As time passes, many PWAs feel less and less competent to care for themselves or to make decisions. They begin to feel helpless and eventually hopeless. Unfortunately, the caregiver's strong feelings of caring, being needed, and protectiveness often occur when the PWA is least in need of them, when they may not even be in the best interests of the PWA or the caregiver. Eventually, the caregiver can grow tired, annoyed, and resentful—even if she fostered the dependency and once enjoyed it.

A new facet emerges in the sick role when hospitalization occurs. PWAs and significant others may feel the need to tolerate invasions of privacy, decreased self-determination, decreased autonomy, and changes in personal habits and lifestyle within the hospital environment without complaint. In becoming a patient, the PWA may become meek, passive, and dependent. On the other hand, if it has been her lifelong personality, the PWA may become argumentative, controlling, and rarely willing to compromise, thereby becoming labeled as uncooperative and noncompliant.

What to Look For

- Increasing weakness on the part of the PWA, causing decreasing ability to care for herself independently
- Passivity
- Inability to correctly judge what she can and cannot physically accomplish without assistance
- Regressive behavior
- Seeking assistance from others before trying to do for herself
- Ambivalence about needing help

What to Do

- Assess the PWA's ability to perform tasks without assistance realistically.
- Encourage the PWA to ask for help only when she needs it.
- Assist the PWA only when you are asked to do so. You may also offer help if you anticipate a need.
- Reinforce the PWA's strengths. Be supportive. Emphasize what she can, not what she cannot, do.
- Discuss decisions with the PWA and provide information as needed. However, encourage the PWA to make her own decisions.
- Discuss self-deprecating statements with the PWA when they are made. Foster a positive self-image.

- Facilitate adjustments to hospitalizations by asking questions, noting answers, and remembering to compromise. Remember that doctors and nurses are medical professionals, not maids or babysitters.
- Your "tough guy" approach may be surprising to other loved ones. Explain and reinforce to the PWA and to significant others that you are not being uncaring when you encourage the ill person to do for herself.

What *Not* to Do

- Never infantilize the PWA by doing things for her or making decisions for her if she is capable of doing these things for herself.
- Do not label someone as uncooperative or noncompliant. Labels never help anybody. Talk things over openly and honestly.
- Do not assume that being sick makes the PWA in any way incompetent.

When to Consult Your Doctor

- To discuss obtaining a home health aide or other help at home, if needed.
- To discuss questions and answers regarding hospital routines if hospitalization becomes necessary. Also discuss with both your doctor and your caregivers (including hospital staff) ways in which you can retain more control.

CHAPTER **25**

Emotional First Aid for Caregivers

Being a Friend

It has been said that when bad things happen, or a crisis occurs, you can find out who your friends are. Being a friend to someone who is terminally ill is difficult. It is emotionally painful, physically exhausting, and mentally trying. Significant others go through all of the stages discussed in the next chapter on death and dying. They feel helpless, inadequate, and overwhelmingly sad. Some avoid the PWA out of a sense of guilt for some past incident, because of discomfort over knowing that the PWA is terminally ill, or out of fear that they may be next. Some don't know what to say, how to act, or what to do. Often, the PWA will feel abandoned, punished for being sick, and angry at the rejection.

We cannot emphasize strongly enough the importance of maintaining friendships with PWAs. Now more than ever it is important to stay in touch, say what you feel must be said, do the things you always wanted to do, and be open, honest, and *normal*. Yes, normal! Be who you are. Be the way you are. Treat one another as you always have.

One cautionary footnote needs to be added about being honest and saying what you feel you need to say. Closing relationships and setting things right between individuals is vital so that everyone can feel as much at peace with impending death as is humanly possible. It is not necessary, however, to talk of painful things that are in the past and are of little consequence now just to get them off your chest and put them onto the terminal person. She has enough to deal with already.

What to Do

- Be there. Be the friend you always have been—now more than ever.
- Touch your friend. Hug and kiss—no more and no less than usual.
- Respond to the PWA's questions with candor.
- Display your emotions openly and respond to the PWA's emotions honestly. Laugh and cry together.

239

- Go out together in public, but keep in mind the possibility of the PWA's fatigue. There will be limitations. Try not to show your disappointment if evenings are cut short, or plans are canceled altogether.
- Celebrate holidays, birthdays, and anniversaries as usual.
- Offer to help with children or parents—possibly acting as a liaison.
- Give her a massage, read to her, or engage in similar quiet activities on bad days.
- Allow the PWA to ventilate fears, thoughts, and plans. If you are uncomfortable with this, say so. Offer opinions as they are solicited.
- Keep your promises. This means a lot to a PWA.
- Take anger in stride. Often, PWAs displace their anger onto caregivers, friends, and family. Point out calmly that it is not you she is angry at. Be understanding.
- Have a positive, but not false, attitude.
- Take care of yourself. Seek out support groups for caregivers and friends of PWAs. Maintain your own health.
- Be an advocate for your friend and others with this disease. Learn all you can about AIDS.

What Not to Do

- Do not force the PWA to discuss her illness, health, or state of mind. Listen to what she says she wants or needs.
- Do not lie. The PWA won't believe comments like, "You look wonderful," anyway. Be gentle, but honest.
- Do not be afraid to tell the PWA bad news of either a current event or a personal nature (unless she is confused). Present the information in a tactful way.
- Do not force religion on the PWA. If she asks you to pray with her or to arrange for a visit from a clergy member, assist her.
- Do not lecture about eating habits, exercise, and the like. She's doing the best that she can. The PWA needs your support, not your criticism, no matter how well intended it is.
- Do not confuse acceptance of illness or impending death with defeat.

Help for Caregivers

Agreeing to be the caregiver for anyone who is ill is a huge responsibility. More and more often, family members, lovers, spouses, and friends of PWAs are agreeing to undertake this endeavor. Most caregivers are mature, educated, intelligent, and sensitive people with a great desire and capability to help.

Caregivers are often selfless people who need support—in dealing with their emotions, their own health, and their loss of the ability to freely plan their time. Who cares for the caregiver, especially as the PWA becomes more ill and dependent?

Following are some suggestions for helping the caregiver. In addition, consult the resource and referral lists in the back of the book.

What to Look For

- The realization by you, the caregiver, that you need help or time for yourself
- Increasing impatience
- Feeling tired more often, insomnia, or lack of restful sleep
- Inability to take care of personal matters, usually due to a lack of time to yourself
- Feeling neglected by others or as if you are neglecting yourself
- Being past due for doctor or dental visits. Realizing that you haven't felt well lately
- Realizing that you haven't been alone or socialized with anyone but the person you care for
- Inability to keep abreast of business or family matters

What to Do

- Utilize all formal resources, such as hiring a home health aide for one or more days a week, if this is acceptable to the PWA. Honestly discuss why you feel that this is necessary.
- Seek out and participate in support groups for caregivers. Likewise, try to contact another caregiver in your community with whom you can make friends and share feelings. Chances are that person is going through what you are going through.
- Take time out for yourself if the PWA is independent enough. Go shopping, get a manicure or a massage, visit the gym and work out, or have lunch with friends or family.
- See if you can set up a PWA-sitting circle. Obtain phone numbers of the family members and friends of other PWAs who are willing to be substitute caregivers for a few hours a week on a steady or as-needed basis. Use this time to go to the doctor, the dentist, or a movie. Clear this beforehand with the PWA. Share opinions and be willing to compromise.
- Be honest with the PWA. If you feel claustrophobic and need to be alone to clear your head, say so honestly but gently. In most cases, he will understand. He may be tired of your company, too.
- Write a list of chores that must be done and prioritize them if you feel overwhelmed by what has to be done. Be willing to amend the list as needed.
- Remember that one of the goals of caregiving is to maximize autonomy for both you and the PWA.

What *Not* to Do

- **Never ignore your own needs**. They are legitimate, worthwhile, and important, especially to your physical and mental health.
- Do not feel guilty. Your needs are important, too. Take care of yourself physically and emotionally. The better you feel, the better caregiver you will be.
- Do not feel the PWA needs you and only you 24 hours a day. Both of you can benefit from time apart. Substitute caregivers may not do things the way you do, but they can be perfectly competent and caring.
- Do not be afraid to accept the offers of others to help. They may need to do this for themselves.

Managing Day-to-Day Stress

We all know the detrimental effects that stress can have on the body. Stress can induce illness and decrease one's ability to concentrate and to cope. Although stress in small doses may be motivating, large amounts of stress can be immobilizing. The daily stress of living with AIDS affects PWA and caregiver, friends and family—in fact, all concerned. Therefore, learning to manage stress is a crucial part of living with AIDS.

What to Look For

- Physical symptoms such as tension headache; tight neck, shoulders, or back; eyestrain; changes in sleep patterns (most commonly, insomnia); abdominal problems (like diarrhea or cramps); rash; hyperventilation; going to the bathroom often; and trembling hands
- Inability to concentrate; disorganized thinking
- Being easily distracted
- Change in one's desire, willingness, or ability to engage in sexual activity
- Expressions of feeling tense, edgy, short-tempered, or impatient

What to Do

- Try the following stress management techniques. Do them alone or in combination; with a friend or by yourself.
  - **Self-hypnosis.** This can be learned via books, audiocassettes, or videocassettes, through a therapist (see the accompanying box for information on selecting a therapist), and/or by taking classes.
  - **Biofeedback.** Attend a local biofeedback center.
  - **Meditation.** A variety of techniques can be learned from books and video- or audiotapes.

—**Guided Imagery.** Learn this via audio- or videocassettes, in therapy, or within a support group.

—**Deep-Breathing Exercises.** This is also known as diaphragmatic breathing; most doctors are familiar with the techniques. These exercises may also be learned through books and tapes.

—**Progressive Deep Muscle Relaxation.** This is a systematic method of focusing your attention on specific muscle groups, alternately tensing, then relaxing, them to accomplish relaxation. Again, this can be learned through books, tapes, or with the guidance of medical personnel.

—**Autogenic Training.** These exercises are intended to induce a feeling of heaviness and warmth in muscles via mental imagery. This can be learned via audio- or videocassettes or from a therapist.

- Exercise if possible. Go to a gym, jog, swim, ride a bike, hike, or take a long walk. Work off the stress.
- Occupy your mind with other things, such as books, television, plays, movies, board games, or cards.
- Take a warm, relaxing bath.
- Talk things out with friends, family members, or others within a support group or network.
- Write. Keep a journal listing your concerns and what you can do about them. Often this helps to put the source of the stress into perspective.
- Laugh. Old, funny movies, jokes, and tickling all relieve stress.
- Think positively. Focus on the good in your life and on those things which are within your control.
- Get a massage.
- Consider talking to a therapist (see box, pages 244–245), or to a member of the clergy, if you are religious.

What Not to Do

- Never turn to alcohol or drugs for stress relief.
- Do not self-medicate with others' medications or with drugs given to you to treat a prior problem. Ask the doctor.

What to Discuss with Your Doctor

- Stress and your reactions to it. Describe any physical symptoms you may be experiencing and what you have done to help yourself.
- The benefits of antianxiety medicines.

How to Choose a Therapist

Many PWAs, their caregivers, and their loved ones may desire and benefit from some form of counseling or psychotherapy. However, you may be unsure of how to locate a therapist who best suits your needs. Here are some tips to help guide you.

- Check credentials. There are a myriad of titles and levels of training to sift through when trying to find an appropriate match for your particular wants and needs. The following list includes the most commonly used titles and their definitions.
  - **Psychotherapist.** A *psychotherapist* may imply any level of training drawn from a variety of backgrounds. There are no laws governing who may use this title; it is a self-designated label. Therefore, a psychotherapist may be a psychiatric nurse specialist, a social worker, or even someone with a college degree is psychology. Although it's most important that the individual you consult has experience in your problem and that you feel comfortable with her, this is a case of caveat emptor (let the buyer beware). Be sure that your psychotherapist has the proper training and qualifications.
  - **Psychologist.** Anyone using the title *psychologist* must have a doctoral degree (Ph.D.). These individuals undergo approximately five years of postgraduate work and their specialty is "talk therapy." There are two types of psychologists; they have equal levels of training but with a differing focus. A "clinical psychologist" has the title "Psy.D." Her training emphasizes more clinical experience than that of the traditional "Ph.D.," whose training is divided between clinical aspects and academic research.
  - **Psychiatrist.** A *psychiatrist* is a physician who specializes in emotional illness. She has gone through medical school and completed a residency in psychiatry. Unlike other types of therapists, she alone (except for, in some states, psychiatric nurse practitioners) is licensed to prescribe and dispense medications. Therefore, if you require antidepressants, antianxiety medicines, or sleeping aids, a psychiatrist is a good choice.

    Because they are physicians, psychiatrists may be better equipped to understand the physical aspects of a PWA's illness and how AIDS affects the brain (AIDS dementia, for example). Psychiatrists may also be in a better position to manage the interactions of the multitude of medications a PWA takes along with any psychiatric medicines that may be needed.

    Remember that a reputable psychotherapist or psychologist who determines that your problem requires medication will refer you to a psychiatrist with whom she collaborates. You can then continue to see your nonphysician provider for talk therapy and the doctor for medication.
- Check costs. Psychotherapy can be an expensive undertaking that is not always covered by medical insurance. For PWAs who are already extremely burdened by medical costs, it is worth looking into community mental health centers. They usually offer low-cost counseling or have a sliding-fee scale based on your ability to pay.

(continued)

(continued)

- Get referrals from your health care professional, a reliable friend, or a colleague. This is preferable to leafing through the yellow pages. Remember that a therapist may consider that working with you is a conflict of interest if she is also seeing your friend. However, even if this therapist can't take you on as a client, she can refer you to someone else.
- Interview the therapist. Call to make an appointment with one or more therapists that you are considering. Honestly explain that you wish to have a trial session with them to see if they can help you with your problem. In the trial session, go with your gut feeling about this person. Consider the following questions:
  — Do you feel at ease with this person? Although there is always a certain amount of unease during your first interaction with a stranger, a good therapist will recognize this and should be able to put you at ease.
  — Is the therapist talking too much? In the first one or two sessions, you should be doing the bulk of the talking. Early on, it is the role of the therapist to be the interviewer. She should be eliciting information about you and the details of the problem by asking questions. Beware if she is talking more than she is listening.
  — Do you feel as though this person really "hears" you? In other words, does the therapist seem to understand and empathize? You should feel that a strong alliance is possible with this individual—that she will be helpful and trustworthy.
  — Do you perceive that the two of you have the same or similar value systems? This is especially important when choosing a therapist for a situation like AIDS. Many people (even therapists) may have uncomfortable or even discriminatory feelings toward certain groups who contract this disease. Therefore, you must feel that the therapist is not fearful of treating someone with AIDS, or an AIDS caregiver, and that she is not being judgmental, so that you can be totally open and honest.
  — What is the therapist's clinical orientation or vision of psychotherapy? In other words, does the therapist's mode of treatment gel with what your needs are? For example, long-term commitments to psychoanalysis might not be appropriate for a person in a crisis over being terminally ill.
- Consider someone who is gay or has experience working with PWAs if you are homosexual. Asking others in your circle may lead to excellent referrals.
- Once in therapy, evaluate the following:
  — Are you making progress? Remember that change doesn't happen overnight, but you should get a sense that things are moving forward. If they are not, honestly consider whether it's because of you or the therapist. Don't hesitate to bring it up in your sessions—this may certainly change the pace of things.
  — Is the therapist acting appropriately? If you feel that the therapist's behavior is somehow improper, discontinue seeing the therapist. Never feel that you can't make a change in therapists for whatever reason.

CHAPTER 26

Death and Dying

Do not stand by my grave and weep.
I am not there. I do not sleep.
I am a thousand winds that blow.
I am a diamond glint of snow.
I am the sunlight on ripened grain.
I am the gentle autumn rain.
When you awake in the morning hush,
I am the swift, uplifting rush
of quiet birds in circling flight.
I am the soft starshine at night.
Do not stand by my grave and cry.
I am not there . . . I did not die.
—ANONYMOUS

Issues of death and dying are faced by all of us at some time in our lives, but rarely is it as traumatic as when a young person is told he has an incurable illness. In this age of medicine, we associate death with old age. Very few young people die, as they once did of infectious diseases or in childbirth.

Thoughts of Death

Thoughts of death invade the consciousness of the PWA and all of those who are connected to him long before his illness reaches the terminal stages. This period between the knowledge of impending death and actual death is often referred to as the "living–dying phase." This time is overshadowed by fears of leaving one's loved ones, losing one's possessions, not realizing one's dreams or aspirations in life, loneliness, sorrow, loss of self-esteem, loss of self-control, changed body image, pain, suffering, and mental regression. These fears are experienced by the dying person as well as by those persons who are significant in his life.

The Stages of Dying

Elisabeth Kübler-Ross has described various stages passed through by terminally ill people and their loved ones upon recognizing that death is near. They are denial, anger, bargaining, loss and depression, and finally acceptance. These stages don't necessarily occur sequentially, and often stages are skipped altogether. Peoples' responses to knowing that death is imminent are certainly not uniform or predictable. The uniqueness of each PWA, family member, caregiver, lover, and friend provides each with an individual way of working through the dying process. No one way is wrong, right, or the best.

Denial

Denial occurs because reality is seen as threatening. Denial helps us to exclude frightening reality from our awareness. We can selectively shut out bad news, thereby protecting ourselves from anxiety and allowing ourselves to participate in other areas of living. Denial permits a gradual management of a crisis and usually leads to the mobilization of more effective coping mechanisms.

In this stage, a PWA may say, "No, not me!" Doctor shopping is common as the individual seeks out a second, third, even fourth opinion in the hope that the diagnosis can be changed. People who know and care about the person also experience denial in much the same way, by saying things like, "It can't be true"; "He looks so healthy"; or, "He's too young to die." Often, relationships between the dying person and his friends and family members improve during the denial phase as each tries to reassure the other that nothing is wrong.

Anger

Anger occurs when denial is no longer possible. Often this happens when the dying person begins to display signs of illness. An outpouring of envy, resentment, and grief may be directed against caregivers, doctors, nurses, family members—even the person's surroundings. It's important to realize that all grieving has an element of anger to it, and one should not feel guilty about being angry. Yet, significant others try to hold back displays of anger toward the PWA, because no one likes to admit to anger toward a dying person. However, not expressing honest emotions can adversely affect relationships. Some caregivers and loved ones try to disguise their anger, even from themselves. They may repress it to the point of causing physical illness, such as headaches, abdominal pain, or high blood pressure.

Anger mounts for the PWA with the experiences of dehumanizing therapies, repeated hospitalizations, changes in lifestyle, loss of control over bodily functions, and loss of one's independence. Strong sentiments of "Why me?" pervade this period. For caregivers, it is a difficult time, but it is important to remember that angry outbursts are not intended to be personal assaults.

Bargaining

Bargaining starts as anger lessens. It is an attempt to postpone pain or death by offering good behavior in exchange for a return to health. The bargains are usually made with God and are kept secret from others. Even atheists and those who are not religious are known to bargain. The dying and their loved ones realize that there is only a slim chance that bargaining will accomplish something, but it's worth a try. Soon bargaining ends. Typically, it is followed by a period of loss and depression.

Loss and
Depression

During this stage, anger, bargaining, and stoic behavior are replaced by a period of deep depression. The PWA is silent or not very verbal, and often introspective and sad.

This stage is very difficult for others to accept and deal with. It is instinctive for loved ones to try to cheer up the PWA. But all attempts to do so have a hollow ring. These efforts to "put on a happy face" are a means to disguise the anxiety of significant others. In reality, the PWA would be better served if friends and family were to simply sit quietly at his side, hold his hand, and even, if asked, to pray with him. If the PWA chooses to talk, just listen and be there.

Loved ones also experience the loss and depression stage, but in a milder form. They experience it more deeply after the death occurs.

Acceptance

Given enough time, a kind of acceptance of impending death develops. This is a state almost void of feelings. Survival becomes no longer necessary, although hope still exists. There is a sense of closure, especially if the PWA has been able to get his affairs in order. Business such as the drawing up of wills, discussion of funeral arrangements, and closing relationships to the PWA's satisfaction will bring a sense of peace.

Any unfinished business no longer matters. The PWA is physically weak, sleeps a lot, and is only minimally verbal. Often loved ones need more attention and support now than does the dying person. This is not to be mistaken for a happy stage. It is, however, peaceful for the PWA, and this often brings a sense of calm to those around him.

Some individuals never reach this stage of acceptance. They fight to the end—struggling, usually angry. Fighting is often viewed by those who care for them as a good and hopeful sign. However, these PWAs often suddenly give up the fight and they, too, die.

Supporting the PWA during the Dying Process

All significant others in the life of a person dying of AIDS parallel the psychological reactions and resolutions of the dying person in their own time and in their own ways. They may or may not be in synchrony with the PWA.

Often, one loved one will attempt to protect another or even the PWA from the truth. This can be disastrous, leading to mistrust, rejection, anger, and playacting in relationships; honesty becomes lost in the mire. Open relationships should be attempted, giving all of those involved a chance to separate in a meaningful and supportive manner.

At the terminal phase, the dying person usually knows that death is near, even if he was never explicitly told. He often comes to the awareness and then seeks verification from those he trusts. It is important to be gently honest, leaving the door open for hope. This removes the PWA's fear of deceit.

It seems that the more medical advances made, the more we seem to fear and deny the reality and inevitability of death. Doctors are trained to devote their energies, attention, and skills to healing and "saving lives." Many are acutely uncomfortable with helping people through the dying process. Yet, they could contribute so much in permitting death with dignity and without pain. Perhaps it is because doctors may themselves fear death or are unable to cope with confronting a patient whom they have failed—or who they subconsciously may be angry and disappointed with for failing them by not getting well.

Whatever the case, dying in our culture has become impersonal and lonely. When a person is severely ill, he is often treated like a person without a right to an opinion, without a right to make decisions, or even to know the simple truth. Others take over, often protectively and with good intentions. It would take so little to remember that the PWA has feelings, wishes, and opinions and that the dying have a right to be heard.

What to Do

- Live one day at a time.
- Be honest and open regarding issues of death and dying. Try to discuss it freely.
- Talk honestly about the future, what will happen upon the person's death (and afterward, if appropriate).
- Say the things to each other that you rarely say, or haven't said. Equally important, listen—without feeling that you need to discuss or converse.
- Allow for sadness, tears, and hugs—no false brightness. Face reality as it is and enjoy moments of laughter (there will be some) as they come. Nothing is truly inappropriate if it is real.
- Allow yourselves to walk in the other's shoes. Try to understand what the other person is going through, feeling, and thinking. Be supportive of one another. Console one another.
- Encourage the PWA to be as independent as possible both physically and in decision making for as long as he is able. Help him to live, not vegetate, until his final breath.
- Assist the PWA to complete the business of dying, such as drawing up a will, establishing a *health care proxy* (see page 256), discussing funeral arrangements, and making peace with others. Encourage him to let his wishes be clearly known to all significant others.
- Allow the PWA to die his own way—at home, in a hospice, or in a hospital—accepting death or fighting it.

What *Not* to Do

- Never lie. Even the most anxious PWA will figure out the truth eventually. Be gentle, maintain hope, but be honest.

- Do not avoid the PWA. You need one another's support—now more than ever. Do not hesitate to visit—just call first and agree to follow the PWA's lead.
- Do not avoid discussions of death, dying, or plans such as funeral arrangements. Bring up the subject gently and pursue it only if the PWA indicates he wants to talk about it. Follow his lead. Note his wishes and assure him they will be followed.
- Do not dehumanize the dying person or treat a dying person like an object. Remember the person in the body.

What to Discuss with Your Doctor

To the PWA: Discuss face to face with your doctor all aspects of death and dying, including the use of pain and antianxiety medications to ease suffering; the decision to be resuscitated or not; and whether you would like to die at home, in a hospice, or in a hospital.

Hospices

Hospices offer a good compromise for people who do not want to die at home or who cannot, for various reasons. Maybe the caregiver is too elderly to be able to manage the needs of a terminally ill person. Maybe the caregiver has to work and cannot afford skilled nursing care during the hours he will not be available. Maybe it is too frightening or sad for either the PWA or the caregiver to consider allowing the person to die at home.

By contrast, a PWA may not want to live out his last days in the sterile, impersonal environment of a hospital or may fear that his wishes (such as no heroic measures) will not be honored. (Although this is not necessarily the case in a hospital, whether or not the PWA's feelings are founded in reality is not the issue—they must be respected and considered legitimate for him.)

Hospices offer a place where a dying person can stay to receive **care, not cure, and not treatment**. The emphasis is on allowing the person to live out his life in the most pain-free, comfortable, and loving environment possible outside of the home and under the circumstances. The main difficulty with hospice care is that there are not enough beds available. There are also home hospice programs available for PWAs who are expected to live only 3 to 6 months longer and wish to die at home. These programs essentially provide for pain control only.

Check with religious and community organizations as well as your doctor for programs and locations near you, or refer to Appendix G.

Dying at Home

Up until about 50 or 60 years ago, most people in North America died at home. Then, with increasing medical advances, there was a shift to hospitalization to manage the critically ill, and most deaths began to occur there. The dying became surrounded by machines, hospital staff, and other patients. Gone were the days when a person was allowed to die in peace and dignity in his own bed, with those who loved him surrounding and comforting him. Even the most loving and caring of hospital staff cannot replace a person's family, his friends, his own bed, and familiar surroundings.

Today, there is a recognition that a person may desire to reach the end of his life in a familiar and beloved environment. If this is his choice (and his caregivers are willing and able to accommodate him), wouldn't it require less adjustment for him, aid in his acceptance of death, and be more physically comfortable? In modern society, we have the technology and the resources to achieve this. Often the planning is time consuming, and sometimes time runs out before the goal can be reached, but isn't it still worth a try?

Preparation for Dying at Home

Granting the wish of a terminally ill person to die at home is often a frustrating and difficult process. The planning can be tedious: preparing the home with the necessary equipment and help in the form of nurses or nursing attendants; obtaining instructions from doctors and the like. However, the most difficult part of the process for caregivers and loved ones is adjusting to the fact that someone you care about is returning home to die and that you will be there to watch it happen.

In addition, loved ones and others often have concerns about returning to the home after someone has died there. Fears that these feelings are selfish abound, leading to feelings of guilt. Much of this can be worked through prior to the PWA returning home. Talking it out with each other, with doctors, nurses, social workers, therapists, or within the context of a support group is helpful and may be all that is necessary. In most cases, the overwhelming desire to grant the PWA's last wish eases the way, allowing for significant others to adjust their thinking and begin to set plans in motion. Often, this is seen as a last gift to the dying person, a final gesture of love.

What to Do

- Discuss the issues involved in dying at home with the PWA, caregiver, loved ones, medical personnel, and social workers.
- Set plans in motion. Follow up on necessary telephone calls. Be sure all equipment is in the home prior to the PWA's return.
- Make the arrangements needed with the funeral home and your physician before taking the PWA home.

- Be sure to obtain information about whom to contact when the time comes if the PWA has no private doctor—paramedics or a physician.
- Keep the necessary telephone numbers at hand to ease the logistical process after death occurs.
- Call the paramedics after the PWA dies *only* if you are told to do so, as for example if you have no private doctor, no doctor is on call at your clinic, and the police tell you to do so. Be sure that the paramedics know that this death was expected and that the PWA is *not* to be resuscitated.
- Relish every single moment of your time together—don't waste it! Take photos, videos, tape-record conversations if you and the PWA want to and it is appropriate.
- Encourage significant others to call and come visit—to help out. Be one another's support group before, during, and after the PWA's death.
- Make simple but honest explanations to children who are involved. Include them in plans. They know something is going on. Children will be more afraid of the unknown than of the known. Consult professional help (pediatricians, books, child psychologists) to understand what a child's view of death is at different developmental stages so that they can be helped to understand and cope with the loss in age-appropriate ways.
- Take care of yourself as the caregiver at this time. Maintain your own physical and mental health.
- Look to your spiritual beliefs for solace if you are religious.
- Take time out to let the hospital staff know of the PWA's death. They care.

What *Not* to Do

- Never rush in your preparations to allow a PWA to come home to die. Time is of the essence, but this must be done right. Planning is the key to a smooth transition from hospital to home.
- Do not close your mind to the possibility of death at home. It is nothing to be afraid of. Often it benefits not only the dying but also loved ones, who can have a more quiet and personal good-bye.
- Do not assume anything. Double-check arrangements. Get things in writing from the funeral home.
- Do not call 911 (or your local emergency number) if someone is expected to die and dies. This service is for emergencies, and an anticipated death is not an emergency.

When to Consult Your Doctor

- To discuss the possibility of allowing the PWA to die at home. If the doctor agrees, enlist his help in planning. Obtain additional assistance from social workers, clergy, and nurses, including referrals for support groups and places to secure needed equipment and services.

- To inform your doctor of the name of the funeral home.
- To call the doctor when you believe death has occurred.

Steps to Take after the PWA's Death at Home

Laws vary from state to state regarding the required procedure after someone has died at home. In general, if the person has been under the care of a private doctor and was discharged from the hospital knowing death was imminent, this is what should take place:

1. Upon death (see box below), contact the doctor's office or service. If another physician is covering for your physician, he is informed. Emergency personnel (911) should not be contacted in the event of an expected death.
2. Call the funeral home when the actual death has taken place. (A funeral home should have been contacted prior to the PWA's return home and should be aware that the person was expected to die at home. Prior to the PWA's death, leave the private doctor's name with the funeral home and make arrangements regarding the casket, cremation, and so on.) Ensure that the funeral home knows your doctor's name, address, and telephone number or that of the covering doctor. The funeral home will come to the home to obtain the body and take it to the funeral home. They will follow any previously made arrangements. The funeral home will provide a death certificate to the doctor for signing.
3. If there is no private physician (e.g., if the PWA was a clinic patient) things are more complicated. In some cases, a clinic will have a doctor on call 24 hours a day, seven days a week, and this will be the person to be contacted in place of a private doctor. This person would be the one informed of the death and the one to sign the death certificate.

   If this is not the case, often the paramedics must be called to officially pronounce death. This can be done by calling your local police precinct and explaining the situation. The police will dispatch a paramedic unit to your home as soon as possible. Often it takes time because this is not seen as an emergency.
4. In rare instances, when a PWA has not been under a doctor's care for an extended period of time, or if it is thought that he died under suspicious circumstances, the medical examiner is called and the death is investigated

---

How to Know If Death Has Occurred

Death may be assumed to have occurred if all efforts to arouse the person have no effect, if the pupils do not shrink when a flashlight is shined directly in the eyes, and if the person has no detectable pulse and seems not to be breathing. Check for a pulse by placing your fingers on the side of the neck or on the wrist beneath the thumb. Listen and feel for breathing by positioning your ear above the person's mouth and nose; look for the rhythmic rise and fall of the chest wall.

prior to the issuance of a death certificate. An *autopsy* may be performed. (If you have religious or other objections to this, make them known.) After the investigation is concluded, the body is released.

Suicide and Assisted Suicide for the Terminally Ill

We hope that the information provided in this section will not be misconstrued. We neither sanction nor censure these practices. However, we recognize that the issue of suicide and so-called assisted suicide (helping a person to end his life) may arise for the terminally ill PWA and therefore should be addressed. Near the end of life, a PWA may rationally feel that it is preferable to cut short his existence—choose his own time to die—rather than to live on for the sake of living, when the meaning and the quality of his life no longer exist.

We are speaking here only of suicide—not the discontinuation of life support, living wills, or any of the other medical/legal/ethical issues covered later. If suicide (or assisted suicide) is under consideration, it is important to remember certain key issues.

Suicide and attempted suicide are not illegal anywhere in the United States. However, there may be religious or practical consequences that you should take into serious consideration. For example, if you commit suicide, you may not be permitted to receive last rites or be buried in hallowed ground. Your family may undergo tremendous shock and psychic pain because of their views on suicide, and/or they may not be able to collect on your life insurance policy. Your suicide attempt may fail or you may suffer considerably before you succumb to death.

Before committing the act, you should be absolutely certain that you

- are in a lucid, nondepressed state of mind when you make the decision and that you are not under the influence of drugs that may be affecting your judgment or state of mind.
- have exhausted all other options or possibilities.
- have transacted any final business.
- have brought a peaceful closure to your relationships.
- have absolutely and unmistakably no will or desire to continue your life.

Legal Issues Concerning Assisted Suicide

In bold contrast to suicide, helping another person to commit suicide is against the laws of every state and nation of the world except for the Netherlands, where physicians alone have been able to perform euthanasia since the 1970s. This is vitally important to understand, because no matter whether you are a doctor, a nurse, or an ordinary citizen; whether the person was your intimate partner in life for 50 years; and whether he was suffering terribly and would have died anyway within hours, the law is the law.

We quote from *Final Exit*, which is perhaps the best known "how to" book on the process of what its author, Derek Humphry, calls "self-deliverance" and assisted suicide for the dying:

> If you are asked by a loved one to assist in death, consider the following:
>
> 1. In terms of personal philosophy, and your relationship to this person, is it the right thing to do?
> 2. Who else knows, or might get to know, about this, and will they keep it a secret?
> 3. If the law enforcement authorities find out, are you prepared to take the consequences, whatever they may be? (P. 15)

We refer you to the works of Derek Humphry and the Hemlock Society (both listed in the back of this book), and to Appendix G for further information about pain, suicide, and death and dying.

Durable Medical Power of Attorney, Health Care Proxies, and Living Wills

The following information on legal issues is only a general guide. Laws vary from state to state and from country to country. It is hoped that the following information will induce you to think, make decisions, seek out the laws particular to where you live, and be an agent for change if you believe those laws to be inadequate. We encourage you to use the law to your advantage. Protect yourself by knowing your legal rights and fight for them.

A durable medical *power of attorney* or health care proxy gives decision-making rights, usually within the guidelines provided by the PWA, to anyone named by the PWA—partner, spouse, friend, family member, or any other loved one. These documents are signed by the PWA and the person he chooses while he is still alert, oriented, and competent to make decisions. These documents are executed only if the PWA becomes unable to make decisions due to confusion, increasing illness, or coma—or if no living will exists.

The person designated to act on the PWA's behalf must agree to this responsibility and must follow any clearly expressed or written wishes made by the PWA while he was competent. If no wishes were made known, then the significant other named must make decisions and act in the best interests of the ill person.

Durable power of attorney and health care proxy are legal documents that must be signed by witnesses in addition to the PWA and the significant other. In most states they must also be notarized. Generally, this can be done without an attorney, by obtaining blank forms (such as those given as examples in Figure 26.1) and completing them. These forms can usually be obtained at the

POWER OF ATTORNEY FOR HEALTH CARE INSTRUCTIONS

CAUTION:

THE ATTACHED POWER OF ATTORNEY FOR HEALTH CARE IS PROVIDED FOR YOUR CONVENIENCE. IT MAY OR MAY NOT FIT THE REQUIREMENTS OF YOUR PARTICULAR STATE. A GROWING NUMBER OF STATES HAVE SPECIAL FORMS OR SPECIAL PROCEDURES FOR CREATING HEALTH CARE POWERS OF ATTORNEY. IF POSSIBLE, SEEK LEGAL ADVICE BEFORE SIGNING ANY POWER OF ATTORNEY. IF NOT CLEARLY RECOGNIZED BY LAW IN YOUR STATE, THE DOCUMENT MAY STILL PROVIDE THE BEST EVIDENCE OF YOUR WISHES IF YOU SHOULD BECOME UNABLE TO SPEAK FOR YOURSELF.

Section 1—DESIGNATION OF HEALTH CARE AGENT:
Print your full name here as the "principal" or creator of the power of attorney.

Print the full name, address and telephone number of the person (over age 18) you appoint as your health care "attorney-in-fact" or "agent." Appoint *only* a person whom you trust to understand and carry out your values and wishes. Do not name any of your health care providers as your agent, since some states prohibit them acting as your agent.

Section 2—EFFECTIVE DATE AND DURABILITY: The sample document is effective if and when you become unable to make health care decisions. That point in time is determined by your agent and your doctor. You can, if you wish, specify other effective dates or other criteria for incapacity (such as requiring two physicians to evaluate your capacity). You can also specify that the power will end at some later date or event before death. In any case, you have the *right to revoke* the agent's authority at any time by notifying your agent or health care provider orally or in writing. If you revoke, it is best to notify both your agent and physician in writing and to destroy the power of attorney document itself.

Section 3—AGENT'S POWERS: This grant of power is intended to be as broad as possible so that your agent will have authority to make any decision you could make to obtain or terminate any type of health care. Even under this broad grant of authority, your agent still must follow your desires and directions, communicated by you in any manner now or in the future. You can specifically limit or direct your agent's power, if you wish, in Section 4.

POWER OF ATTORNEY FOR HEALTH CARE

1. DESIGNATION OF HEALTH CARE AGENT

I, _____ hereby appoint:
(principal)

_____
(Attorney-in-fact's name)

_____
(Address)

_____

Home: _____ Work: _____

as my attorney-in-fact (or "Agent") to make health and personal care decisions for me as authorized in this document.

2. EFFECTIVE DATE AND DURABILITY

By this document I intend to create a durable power of attorney effective upon, and only during, any period of incapacity in which, in the opinion of my agent and attending physician, I am unable to make or communicate a choice regarding a particular health care decision.

3. AGENT'S POWERS

I grant to my Agent full authority to make decisions for me regarding my health care. In exercising this authority, my Agent shall follow my desires as stated in this document or otherwise known to my Agent. In making any decision, my Agent shall attempt to discuss the proposed decision with me to determine my desires if I am able to communicate in any way. If my Agent cannot determine the choice I would want made, then my Agent shall make a choice for me based upon what my Agent believes to be in my best interests. My Agent's authority to interpret my desires is intended to be as broad as possible, except for any limitations I may state below. Accordingly, unless specifically limited by Section 4, below, my Agent is authorized as follows:

A. To consent, refuse, or withdraw consent to any and all types of medical care, treatment, surgical procedures, diagnostic procedures, medication, and the use of mechanical or other procedures that affect any bodily function, including (but not limited to) artificial respiration, nutritional support and hydration, and cardiopulmonary resuscitation;

B. To have access to medical records and information to the same extent that I am entitled to, including the right to disclose the contents to others;

C. To authorize my admission to or discharge (even against medical advice) from any hospital, nursing home, residential care, assisted living or similar facility or service;

D. To contract on my behalf for any health care related service or facility on my behalf, without my Agent incurring personal financial liability for such contracts;

E. To hire and fire medical, social service, and other support personnel responsible for my care;

F. To authorize, or refuse to authorize, any medication or procedure intended to relieve pain, even though such

(continued)

FIGURE 26.1 **Sample Health Care Power of Attorney** (Copyright 1990 American Bar Association. Reprinted by permission of the American Bar Association and in cooperation with the ABA Commission on Legal Problems of the Elderly.)

use may loead to physical damage, addiction, or hasten the moment of (but not intentionally cause) my death;

G. To make anatomical gifts of part or all of my body for medical purposes, authorize an autopsy, and direct the disposition of my remains, to the extent permitted by law;

H. To take any other action necessary to do what I authorize here, including (but not limited to) granting any waiver or release from liability required by any hospital, physician, or other health care provider; signing any documents related to refusals of treatment or the leaving of a facility against medical advice, and pursing any legal action in my name, and at the expense of my estate to force compliance with my wishes as determined by my Agent, or to seek actual or punitive damages for the failure to comply.

4. STATEMENT OF DESIRES, SPECIAL PROVISIONS, AND LIMITATIONS

A. The powers granted above do not include the following powers or are subject to the following rules or limitations:

_____
_____
_____
_____
_____

B. With respect to any Life-Sustaining Treatment, I direct the following: (INITIAL ONLY ONE OF THE FOLLOWING PARAGRAPHS)

☐ REFERENCE TO LIVING WILL. I specifically direct my Agent to follow any health care declaration or "living will" executed by me.

☐ GRANT OF DISCRETION TO AGENT. I do not want my life to be prolonged nor do I want life-sustaining treatment to be provided or continued if my Agent believes the burdens of the treatment outweigh the expected benefits. I want my Agent to consider the relief of suffering, the expense involved and the quality as well as the possible extension of my life in making decisions concerning life-sustaining treatment.

☐ DIRECTIVE TO WITHHOLD OR WITHDRAW TREATMENT. I do not want my life to be prolonged and I do not want life-sustaining treatment:
a. if I have a condition that is incurable or irreversible and, without the administration of life-sustaining treatment, expected to result in death within a relatively short time; or
b. if I am in a coma or persistent vegetative state which is reasonably concluded to be irreversible.

☐ DIRECTIVE FOR MAXIMUM TREATMENT. I want my life to be prolonged to the greatest extent possible without regard to my condition, the chances I have for recovery, or the cost of the procedures.

☐ DIRECTIVE IN MY OWN WORDS: _____
_____
_____
_____
_____

Section 4—STATEMENT OF DESIRES, SPECIAL PROVISIONS, AND LIMITATIONS:

Paragraph A: Here you may include any limitations you think are appropriate, such as instructions to refuse any specific types of treatment that are against your religious beliefs or unacceptable to you for any other reasons, such as blood transfusions, electro-convulsive therapy, sterilization, abortion, amputation, psychosurgery, admission to a mental institution, etc. State law may not allow your agent to consent to some of these procedures, regardless of your health care power of attorney. Be very careful about stating limitations, because the specific circumstances surrounding a future health care decision are impossible to predict. If you do not want any limitations, simply write in "No limitations."

Paragraph B: Because the subject of "life-sustaining treatment" is particularly important to many people, this paragraph provides a place for you to give general or specific directions on the subject, if you want to do so. The different paragraphs are options—choose only *one*, or write your desires or instructions in your own words (in the last option). If you already have a "Living Will", you can simply refer to it by choosing the first option. Or, the instructions you provide here can do what a Living Will would do.

Paragraph C: Because people differ widely on whether nutrition and hydration is something that ought to be refused or stopped under certain circumstances, it is important to make your wishes clear on this topic. Nutrition and hydration means food and fluids provided by a nasogastric tube or tube into the stomach, intestines, or veins. This paragraph allows you to include or not include these procedures among those that may be withheld or withdrawn under the circumstances described in the preceding paragraph. Either choice still permits non-intrusive efforts such as spoon feeding or moistening of lips and mouth.

(continued)

FIGURE 26.1 **(continued)**

Section 5—SUCCESSORS: If you wish to name alternate agents in case your first agent becomes unavailable, print the appropriate information in this paragraph. You can name as many successors in the order you wish.

Section 6—PROTECTION OF THIRD PARTIES WHO RELY ON MY AGENT: In most states, health care providers cannot be compelled to follow the directions of your agent, although in some states, they may be obligated to transfer your care to another provider who is willing to comply. This paragraph is intended to encourage compliance with the power of attorney by waiving potential civil liability for good faith reliance on the agent's statements and decisions.

Section 7—NOMINATION OF GUARDIAN: The use of a health care power of attorney is intended to *prevent* the need for a court-appointed guardian for health care decision-making. However, if for any reason, court involvement becomes necessary, this paragraph expressly names your Agent to serve as guardian. A court does not have to follow your nomination, but it will normally comply with your wishes unless there is good reason not to.

Section 8—ADMINISTRATIVE PROVISIONS: These items address miscellaneous matters that could affect the implementation of your power of attorney.

SIGNING THE DOCUMENT: Required procedures for signing this kind of document vary from signature only to very detailed witnessing requirements, or, in some cases, simply notarization. The suggested procedure here is intended to meet most of the various state requirements for signing by non-institutionalized persons. The procedure here is likely to be more detailed than is required under your own state's law, but it will help ensure that your Health Care Power is recognized in other states, too. First, sign and date the document in front of *two witnesses.* Your witnesses should know your identity personally and be able to declare that you appear to be of sound mind and under no duress or undue influence. Further, your witnesses should not be:

C. With respect to Nutrition and Hydration provided by means of a nasogastric tube or tube into the stomach, intestines, or veins, I wish to make clear that . . .
(INITIAL ONLY ONE)
☐ I *intend* to include these procedures among the "life-sustaining procedures" that may be withheld or withdrawn under the conditions given above.
☐ I *do not intend* to include these procedures among "life-sustaining procedures" that may be withheld or withdrawn.

5. SUCCESSORS
If any Agent names by me shall die, become legally disabled, resign, refuse to act, be unavailable, or (if any Agent is my spouse) be legally separated or divorced from me, I name the following (each to act alone and successively, in the order named) as successors to my Agent:
A. First Alternate Agent_____
   Address: _____
   Telephone: _____
B. Second Alternate Agent_____
   Address: _____
   Telephone: _____

6. PROTECTION OF THIRD PARTIES WHO RELY ON MY AGENT
No person who relies in good faith upon any representations by my Agent or Successor Agent shall be liable to me, my estate, my heirs or assigns, for recognizing the Agent's authority.

7. NOMINATION OF GUARDIAN
If a guardian of my person should for any reason be appointed, I nominate my Agent (or his or her successor), named above.

8. ADMINISTRATIVE PROVISIONS
A. I revoke any prior power of attorney for health care.
B. This power of attorney is intended to be valid in any jurisdiction in which it is presented.
C. My Agent shall not be entitled to compensation for services performed under this power of attorney, but he or she shall be entitled to reimbursement for all reasonable expenses incurred as a result of carrying out any provision of this power of attorney.
D. The powers delegated under this power of attorney are separable, so that the invalidity of one or more powers shall not affect any others.

BY SIGNING HERE I INDICATE THAT I UNDERSTAND THE CONTENTS OF THIS DOCUMENT AND THE EFFECT OF THIS GRANT OF POWERS TO MY AGENT.
I sign my name to this Health Care Power of Attorney on this _____ day of _____, 19_____.
My current home address is:_____
_____
   Signature:_____
   Name:_____

WITNESS STATEMENT
I declare that the person who signed or acknowledged this document is personally known to me, that he/she signed or acknowledged this durable power of attorney in my presence, and that he/she appears to be of sound mind and under no duress, fraud, or undue influence. I am not the person appointed as agent by this document, nor am I the patient's health

(continued)

FIGURE 26.1   **(continued)**

- Your treating physician, health care provider, or health facility operator, nor an employee of any of these.
- Anyone related to you by blood, marriage, or adoption.
- Anyone entitled to any part of your estate under an existing will or by operation of law. Even a creditor of yours should not be used under these guidelines.

If you are in a nursing home or other institution, be sure to consult state law, because a few states require that an ombudsman or patient advocate be one of your witnesses.

Second, have your signature *notarized*. Some states permit notarization as an alternative to witnessing. Others may simply apply the rules for signing ordinary durable powers of attorney. Ordinary durable powers of attorney are usually notarized. This form includes a relatively typical notary statement, but here again, it is wise to check state law in case a special form of notary acknowledgement is required.

care provider, or an employee of the patient's health care provider. I further declare that I am not related to the principal by blood, marriage, or adoption, and, to the best of my knowledge, I am not a creditor of the principal nor entitled to any part of his/her estate under a will now existing or by operation of law.

Witness #1:
Signature: _____ Date: _____
Print Name: _____ Telephone: _____
Residence Address: _____
_____

Witness #2:
Signature: _____ Date: _____
Print Name: _____ Telephone: _____
Residence Address: _____
_____

NOTARIZATION

STATE OF _____)
) ss.
COUNTY OF _____)

On this _____ day of _____, 19____, the said _____, known to me (or satisfactorily proven) to be the person named in the foregoing instrument, personally appearing before me, a Notary Public, within and for the State and County aforesaid, and acknowledged that he or she freely and voluntarily executed the same for the purposes stated therein.

My Commission Expires: _____
_____   NOTARY PUBLIC

FIGURE 26.1   **(continued)**

hospital when you are admitted, or from social workers, lawyers, and/or AIDS organizations.

Durable power of attorney for health care and the health care proxy are generally regarded as more comprehensive and more flexible than a *living will*. Living wills are usually focused on limiting treatments in the case of terminal illness. In other words, the living will spells out the PWA's wishes as to the type of treatments, lifesaving measures, and so forth, that he wishes to undergo or forgo. It usually doesn't name a person who is responsible for decision making if the PWA is unable to do so. Living wills are also legal documents required to be witnessed and notarized. As of this writing, the living will has been recognized by statute or case law everywhere in the United States except for Massachusetts, Michigan, and New York.

These documents fall under the Patient Self-Determination Act (PSDA) passed into law in 1991 by the federal government. This law in essence says that health care consumers can initiate advanced directives regarding treatments they do and do not want to receive. Under the PSDA, all health care facilities receiving funds under Medicare or Medicaid must comply with state laws regarding the regulation of advanced directives. Each state law is different (see Table 26.1). Some recognize living wills; others, durable medical power of attorney. You must know the law in your state and take advantage of it.

It is unfortunate that the majority of people (PWAs included), do not take advantage of their right to prepare a living will, name a health care proxy, or assign durable medical power of attorney. Use of these tools is the best way to exercise your freedom of choice, maintain your autonomy, and make your decisions known and binding.

TABLE 26.1   *State Statutes Governing Living Wills and Appointment of Health Care Agents (as of June 1993)*

Jurisdictions with legislation that authorizes both living wills and the appointment of a health care agent

Arizona	Louisiana	Oklahoma
Arkansas	Maine	Oregon
California	Maryland	Pennsylvania
Colorado	Minnesota	Rhode Island
Connecticut	Mississippi	South Carolina
Delaware	Missouri	South Dakota
District of Columbia	Montana	Tennessee
Florida	Nebraska	Texas
Georgia	Nevada	Utah
Hawaii	New Hampshire	Vermont
Idaho	New Jersey	Virginia
Illinois	New Mexico	Washington
Indiana	North Carolina	West Virginia
Iowa	North Dakota	Wisconsin
Kansas	Ohio	Wyoming
Kentucky		

States with legislation that authorizes only living wills

Alabama
Alaska

States with legislation that authorizes only the appointment of a health care agent

Massachusetts
Michigan
New York

Note: The specifics of living will and health care agent legislation vary greatly from state to state. In addition, many states also have court-made law that affects resident's rights. For information about specific state laws, contact Choice In Dying (see Appendix A).

Source: Choice In Dying, Inc. (formerly Concern for Dying/Society for the Right to Die)

Reasons to Consider Making a Living Will or Health Care Proxy

- Recent or current hospitalization
- Indications of increasing illness or nearing end-stage disease

---

What to Do

- Carefully and thoroughly seek out your options. Be sure you understand them clearly. Avoid rushing into decisions or bending to others' wishes. Periodically reassess your options. Explore thoughts and feelings, and change things if you desire.
- Discuss your thoughts with loved ones, and seek out theirs. Try to discover who most closely thinks the way you do. Learn their biases. Then choose someone to be your health care proxy or medical power of attorney, and ask if he consents to the responsibility.
- Know the laws of your state. Write out documents according to these laws. Remember to obtain the proper witnesses, notarizations, and so on. Prepare these legal documents by following procedures to the letter.
- Inform your significant others of your decision, as well as of the location of these documents.
- Inform your doctor, and bring copies of these documents with you if you are admitted to the hospital. Be certain that they appear on your medical record. This must be done for each hospitalization. Ask your physician about his feelings concerning compliance with living wills and about working with a health care proxy or a medical power of attorney.

Do Not Resuscitate (DNR) Orders

A *DNR order* is an order written into a patient's medical chart by his doctor that instructs the hospital or nursing home staff not to try to revive a person who has stopped breathing or has no heartbeat. This means that doctors, nurses, nursing attendants, and others will not perform cardiopulmonary *resuscitation* (CPR), mouth-to-mouth resuscitation, electric shock, insertion of tubes to open the airway (*intubation*), injection of medication into the person's heart, or open chest heart massage. In nursing homes, it also means staff will not transfer the patient to a hospital for emergency resuscitation procedures.

Though laws vary from state to state, in general, patients can request of their doctors that they be made a "DNR." If the PWA is too sick, confused, comatose, or is otherwise deemed incompetent, a family member or significant other can decide on his behalf whether heroic measures are to be taken. This is facilitated if the relative or significant other is named as the person who holds the PWA's health care proxy or durable medical power of attorney.

In the case of a PWA who has no close friends or relatives, some states provide for DNR orders if two doctors conclude that CPR would prove medically useless. A court can approve a DNR order if a request is filed on behalf of a patient.

DNR orders can be revoked at any time by the patient, simply by withdrawing consent and informing the doctor of this change. A DNR order **does not affect your treatment.** All tests, procedures, medications, surgeries, and so on will be performed as needed and as usual. A DNR order is only a decision about initiating resuscitation.

Decisions regarding DNR status are best made by the PWA early in the illness and should be made known to caregivers, friends, relatives, and medical personnel. The decision not to resuscitate must be restated at the time of each hospital admission, and in most states, consent forms must be signed to that effect.

The advantages and disadvantages of CPR and other resuscitation measures must be carefully weighed. Full explanations should be provided by the doctor. In general, when successful, CPR restores the heartbeat and breathing. At its best, it allows the person to resume his or her previous state of health. CPR allows the person to extend his life in most cases. However, there are situations when CPR will fail to restore pulse and respirations, leading to death.

If CPR *is* successful, often breathing or heartbeat can be maintained with support from machines, such as respirators, and through the use of drugs. This sometimes leaves the individual brain damaged or with new medical problems. After CPR, with or without the use of medications or machinery, persons are transferred to the intensive care unit for treatment and observation.

For the most part, the success of CPR depends on the person's overall medical condition and level of functioning before this emergency occurred, as well as how quickly emergency procedures were initiated.

In an emergency, if no DNR order is in place, all patients are "coded" (i.e., CPR and advanced life support measures are initiated), because it is assumed that all patients would consent to and desire CPR.

Any adult in a hospital or nursing home can consent to DNR status by informing his physician. In some states, this must be done in the presence of witnesses. Often, consent forms must be signed by the PWA, the doctor, and a witness; these documents are always made part of the medical record (see Figure 26.2). It is also possible to specify DNR orders under certain limited circumstances. For example, you can mandate that you do not want to be resuscitated only if you are in a coma. You can also direct that specific procedures such as mouth-to-mouth resuscitation and closed chest compressions be done, but that no other measures, such as intubation, be performed.

In most states, you are presumed by law to be mentally competent to decide about DNR status unless two or more physicians or a court determine that you are incapable. If this occurs, or if you are comatose and have not left directions in advance (usually a living will), a DNR order can be issued with the consent of someone previously chosen by you and noted in a health care proxy or durable medical power of attorney, or by a close family member. In some states, someone who is not related to you by blood, but who has a close personal relationship with you (such as a lover), can also make this decision.

Patient Name _____

Decision-Making Capacity

1. This patient _____ does, _____ does not have decision-making capacity for the purpose of providing informed consent regarding his/her resuscitation status. (Patients with capacity can understand the relevant information needed to make a decision, appreciate the situation and its consequences; explain the basis for consent or refusal.)

2. This patient has a terminal condition as defined by:

_____ injury, disease, or illness for which there is no reasonable probability of recovery.

_____ a persistent vegetative state characterized by a permanent condition of unconsciousness in which there is an absence of voluntary action or cognitive ability.

Examination of the patient has been completed and documentation of objective data is recorded which meet the above criteria by:

_____	_____
Patient's Attending Physician	Date
_____	_____
Patient's Consulting Physician	Date

Life-Sustaining Procedures/ Resuscitation

Regarding artificial life-sustaining procedures and resuscitation measures, the undersigned patient requests and consents to:

_____ withdrawal _____ withholding _____ both

Regarding artificial life-sustaining procedures and resuscitation measures, the undersigned _____ legal guardian, _____ parent, _____ sibling, _____ spouse, _____ child, _____ medical health care proxy holder of patient requests and consents to:

_____ withdrawal _____ withholding _____ both

I/We have had an opportunity to discuss the patient's medical condition in detail with the attending and consulting physicians and all questions have been answered to my/our satisfaction.

Name	Relationship	Signature	Date & Time
Attending Physician	Signature	Date & Time	
Witness Name	Signature	Date & Time	
Witness Name	Signature	Date & Time	

Note: Two witnesses must sign. Neither may be a spouse or blood relative of the patient.

FIGURE 26.2 **Sample DNR (Do Not Resuscitate) Form**

A person other than yourself can consent to a DNR order only when you are unable to decide for yourself and only if you are at the end stage of a terminal illness, are permanently unconscious, or if a doctor deems CPR to be futile.

What to Do

- Consider all of your options carefully before deciding. Ask questions of your doctor and be sure you get clear answers.
- Discuss your options with those whom you trust and who are closest to you.
- Seek out counseling from clergy, social workers, therapists, support groups, and so forth.
- Make your opinions known to all significant others, orally and in writing.
- Make your decision known to your doctor and ensure that a DNR consent form and doctor's order to this effect are placed in your medical records upon each hospital admission.
- Ask your doctor how he feels about DNR orders. If he tells you that he is unable to comply with your wishes, consider changing physicians.
- Read all you can about your right to make these decisions. Know the laws in your state and make certain that any necessary legal documents have been properly completed. Draft a living will.
- Consider giving health care proxy or durable medical power of attorney to a person of your choice if you haven't already done so. Let your doctor and all concerned know whom you have chosen to avoid confusion in the future.

PART V

Appendixes

Directory of Laboratory Tests

This section provides a brief explanation of the laboratory and diagnostic tests that are most commonly involved with the diagnosis, evaluation, and treatment of AIDS. The list is not all-inclusive, as it would be impossible to explain all of the tests that might be conducted during the course of AIDS infection within the confines of this book. Included for each entry are an explanation of how the test is done, the meaning and accuracy of the results, the cost (when known), any special preparations that need to be made, the recovery period from the test procedure itself, and any other relevant considerations.

Blood Tests

HIV Testing

An HIV test is performed by taking a small sample of blood from a vein in your arm. A positive test means that you have been infected with the virus at some time in your life and have antibodies to the virus in your blood. It is believed that once these antibodies are present, infection is lifelong. **Having the antibodies to HIV in your system, however, does not necessarily mean you have AIDS. It *does* mean that you can transmit the virus to another person**, through sexual intercourse, through sharing intravenous drug paraphernalia, through pregnancy, or through blood and organ donation.

A negative HIV test means that you are not currently infected. Note, however, that you may not be truly negative unless you have waited approximately four to six months past your last potential exposure to be tested. This is the *window period* during which an infected person may still test negative. **The only way to be sure that a negative test is accurate is to avoid all risky behaviors for four to six months before you are tested.** Note also that a negative HIV test **does *not* indicate immunity, that is, whether you can become infected in the future.** The only way to prevent infection is to practice the safe behaviors outlined in this book.

There are at present two principal tests for the presence of HIV.

Enzyme-Linked Immunoabsorbent Assay (ELISA). In this test, a plate consisting of blood serum is mixed with HIV viral antigens (proteins). If antibodies to HIV are present in the blood being tested, the sample turns yellow. Although the test is more than 99 percent accurate, another ELISA test is performed if the blood tests positive. If both tests are positive, the lab goes on to do a second, more specific test called a *Western Blot.*

Western Blot. This tests uses an *electrophoresis* technique. The person's blood serum is placed in contact with strips of paper that have been treated with antigens from two structures on the virus—the core and the envelope. When a dark line appears on the paper at certain specific locations, this indicates an antigen-antibody reaction between the person's blood and the commercially prepared viral antigens, and the test is positive.

The main factor in obtaining false negative results is premature testing. As explained previously, **there is a window period during which time an infected individual will still test negative**. This is generally within the first six months after exposure. A false positive test, however, is more likely to be the result of human error. According to the CDC, fewer than 1 to 5 of every 100,000 persons tested will be falsely told that they are infected with the AIDS virus. In other words, if you are informed that your HIV test is positive, you may be assured that the test has been done three different times, by two separate methods, and that in 99 out of 100 cases, the test result is accurate.

If your ELISA test is positive and the Western Blot is negative, the ELISA result is likely to have been a false positive. This is because the ELISA test is highly sensitive, but it is not as specific to the virus as is the Western Blot. People with *autoimmune* diseases (such as *lupus* or rheumatoid arthritis), people with disturbances in their liver function (e.g., chronic hepatitis or alcoholism), people who have certain *leukemias* or lymphomas, or people who have had multiple blood transfusions may test falsely positive to HIV on the ELISA test but not to the Western Blot. If your ELISA test is positive and the Western Blot is indeterminate (meaning that your blood reacts with a nonspecific pattern of bands on the treated paper), further medical evaluation and repeat testing after time has elapsed are needed to determine if the test was falsely positive or if testing was performed early on in the infection, during the window period.

The only reason for a false positive Western Blot is poor laboratory technique and human error. The Western Blot can be falsely negative if it is conducted during the window period, or during the end stage of AIDS. People with terminal AIDS may become so immunosuppressed that they lose their ability to produce certain antibodies to HIV.

The approximate cost of the ELISA and Western Blot tests is $35 each, but many sites around the country provide this test free of charge. To locate a test site near you, consult your doctor, local hospital, STD clinic, community AIDS support group, and/or refer to the hotlines listed in Appendix G.

Caregivers who have been intimately exposed to the blood or body fluids of an infected person should certainly be tested for HIV; however, you cannot become infected with HIV by casual contact. Intimate contacts should get a baseline test with a follow-up test in six months; however, additional testing is individualized according to risk and exposure. Therefore, household contacts need not be tested, unless they want to know their HIV status or have other

---

> ## Anonymous versus Confidential AIDS Testing
>
> *Anonymous* testing means that you are known to the counselor only as a number, not a name. *Confidential* testing means that your name will be known to at least one person at the facility where you receive the test. Laws governing medical confidentiality vary from place to place. Some facilities require that the information be noted in your chart; thus, it can be released to anyone who has a valid reason to review your medical record (such as another doctor or nurse). It may also be available to the courts should your chart be subpoenaed for any reason. Finally, some states require that results be reported to their departments of health for statistics, tracking, casefinding, and so on. Know to whom, when, and why your positive result might become available before consenting to a confidential test. Discuss the possibilities with a doctor, counselor, or lawyer before being tested.

---

reasons to suspect that they might have been infected. According to statistics compiled by the Johns Hopkins AIDS clinic and based on estimates made by the U.S. Public Health Service, only two persons who were home health care providers for AIDS patients developed the disease, and it is not known exactly how they contracted it.

Consider anonymous rather than confidential testing if you suspect that your test result is likely to be positive and you fear repercussions should the fact become known (see box above).

Find an accredited test site where you will receive pre- and posttest counseling and sign an informed consent before having your blood drawn. Counseling should cover:

- an explanation of HIV and AIDS.
- an assessment of your particular risk of acquiring the infection.
- the meaning of the test results.
- the accuracy of the testing procedure.
- whether the testing is anonymous or confidential.
- practices to reduce the risk of transmission of the virus if you are positive or to reduce the risk of acquiring the infection if you test negative.
- medical/legal/discrimination issues surrounding testing.
- information as to whether it will be necessary to retest in the future; what resources are available to you in terms of emotional support and medical care if you are positive.

T Cell Subsets

This test requires two tubes of blood to be drawn from a vein in one's arm. Changes in the proportions of various subsets of T lymphocytes is one of the earliest indicators of advancement from HIV positivity to AIDS. In PWAs, there is generally noted to be a decrease in the numbers of T4 (CD4 or T helper) cells, an increase in the numbers of T8 (or T suppressor) cells, and an overall reversal of the ratio of T4 to T8 lymphocytes. **The lower the overall numbers** of T4 cells and the lower the ratio of the T cell subsets, the more severe is the clinical picture.

Healthy, seronegative (HIV negative) people have CD4 counts averaging 1,100 per cubic milliliter. (This number can vary greatly depending on the particular person and the specific lab. Therefore, trends are more important than absolute numbers in tracking whether an HIV-infected person is becoming sicker with her disease.) People who are well but HIV positive may have normal or near normal T cell counts; people who are experiencing some of the earliest signs of the disease have lower counts, and those individuals with T4 cell counts of less than 200 per cubic millimeter generally have either Kaposi's sarcoma or an opportunistic infection. If not, **a CD4 count of 200/mm³ or less is a reliable indicator that some manifestation of AIDS will soon emerge.** Indeed, the new CDC definition of AIDS includes people with CD4 counts of 200 or less. HIV positive persons generally lose 85 to 100 cells/mm³ per year. Thus, T cell depletion to critical levels may take an average of ten years (although this varies widely from person to person).

The cost of this test ranges from approximately $30.00 to $75.00; it is often covered by health insurance. (T4/T8 ratio calculations are more costly, at $110–$150.)

Complete Blood Count (CBC) with Differential and Platelet Count

Blood is composed of various types of cells including primarily: red blood cells (which help transport vital oxygen needed for cells to survive), white blood cells (necessary to the body's defenses as described in Chapter 1), and platelets (useful in blood clotting so that we don't bleed to death when we are injured). People with AIDS frequently have anemia (a reduction in the number of red blood cells) from many causes. Viruses (like Epstein-Barr, cytomegalovirus, and *parvovirus*), inflammation, malnutrition (e.g., iron or vitamin B_{12} deficiency), cancers (both KS and lymphomas), and the drugs used to treat AIDS (AZT, pentamidine, Bactrim, and other antibiotics) may all cause serious anemias, frequently by suppressing the bone marrow where these cells are produced.

Monitoring PWAs for anemia requires drawing periodic blood specimens to check the complete blood count (CBC), differential count, and platelet count. The CBC refers to a count of the total numbers of red cells present, as well as measurements of the relative amounts of hemoglobin they contain based on their size and shape. Pale, small, or misshapen red blood cells interfere with oxygen transport and can cause illness. Included within a CBC are also the hemoglobin and hematocrit—measures of the relative degree of anemia present.

The CBC also provides the number of the total white blood cells present. The differential white count gives the proportions of the various types of white cells present, such as: lymphocytes, granulocytes, and monocytes (see Chapter 1). All of these may be altered in AIDS. For example, the total numbers of granulocytes are generally suppressed, whereas a specific type of white blood cell called an *eosinophil* may be elevated when the PWA is infected with a parasite or is being treated with the drug dideoxycytidine.

TABLE A.1   ***Typical Blood Values of Healthy Adults and PWAs***

	Healthy Adult	**PWA**
Total Red Blood Cell Count	Approx. 5 million/mm^3	Approx. 5 million/mm^3
Total White Blood Cell Count	5,000–10,000/mm^3	<3,500/mm^3
Total Platelet Count	150,000–400,000/mm^3	<80,000–150,000/mm^3

Finally, platelets are usually low for people infected with HIV. Early on, the reasons for this are unclear, but late in the infection, it appears to be due to suppression of the bone marrow (the site of platelet formation) from drugs used to fight AIDS. Table A.1 compares normal blood values with values typical of PWAs who are not affected by medications or other therapies.

The CBC test is generally inexpensive (less than $20) and requires no special preparation.

Erythrocyte Sedimentation Rate (ESR)

An *ESR* is sometimes performed as an adjunct to the CBC. Here, the same blood is used that was obtained for the CBC. The rate at which the red blood cells settle by gravity to the bottom of a tube gives a nonspecific measurement of inflammation and other pathology. Thus, an elevated ESR indicates illness. In PWAs, ESRs (also called "sed rates") are sometimes used as a marker of an improved or deteriorating condition. AIDS-related cancers and tuberculosis in particular elevate the sed rate.

A normal ESR is generally less than 20mm in one hour. The test may be run on the CBC specimen for an additional cost of about $5 to $10.

Chemistry Panel

The chemistry panel (SMAC, SMA6, SMA12 are other names for this type of test) uses a machine that measures a multitude of body substances, including enzymes and electrolytes, from a single small quantity of blood obtained by drawing a small tube of blood from a vein in the arm. Depending on what in particular is being checked, it may be necessary to avoid eating or drinking for a number of hours prior to having the blood obtained. It's best to check with your doctor before having this test performed.

A typical chemistry panel will measure glucose (blood sugar), calcium, phosphorus, various electrolytes (like sodium and potassium), liver enzymes, kidney function (blood urea nitrogen [BUN] and creatinine), cholesterol and triglycerides, and proteins, like albumin and globulin. People with AIDS must be monitored for abnormalities in their chemistry panel to detect the early signs of HIV-related kidney disease, liver disease, diabetes, lung infections, wasting, and dehydration—just to name a few instances in which these tests can be critical. Furthermore, many of the drugs used to treat AIDS can upset the chemical balance within the body or cause an inflammation of the liver. Here again, the chemistry panel is useful in identifying a drug reaction so that the medication can be discontinued, if necessary.

Chemistry panels vary in cost, depending on what is included in the test. Prices range from about $10 to $20 for standard enzymes and electrolytes.

Syphilis Screening Tests (RPR, VDRL, FTA)

PWAs are sometimes also infected with other sexually transmitted diseases. This can place an immunocompromised person in a perilous state of health; therefore, it is imperative to ensure that she is infection-free.

Syphilis may cause only minor symptoms in its earliest stages (a genital ulcer or a mysterious body rash). Left untreated, the sores and rashes will eventually disappear, but the bacterium that causes the disease remains in the blood, where it may progress to cause extensive damage to the heart and brain tissue. For PWAs, syphilis can be fatal.

Individuals who have no symptoms of syphilis are sometimes found to be infected through various screening tests that involve mixing a small blood sample with various chemicals; clumping of the serum indicates a positive result. The *VDRL* (venereal disease research laboratory) or *RPR* (rapid plasma reagin) will detect a case of syphilis from 70 percent to 100 percent of the time, depending on the stage the disease is in. However, other conditions may cause the test to be falsely positive. These include rheumatoid arthritis, autoimmune diseases such as lupus, liver damage, narcotic addiction, and certain viral infections.

To help confirm the presence of the disease and eliminate false positive results, a more specific test called the *FTA* (fluorescent treponemal antibody) is conducted, using the same blood. Though a false positive result is still possible, the FTA correctly diagnoses syphilis in 85 percent to 100 percent of cases, depending on the stage. If a person has a positive VDRL or RPR and a negative FTA, she is considered to have a biological false positive result.

In a pattern that is very similar to that of the HIV test, syphilis serologies are most commonly falsely negative in the earliest and latest stages of the disease. They may also be negative if the person had alcohol before being tested.

Syphilis tests are free in many states, through the Department of Health.

Other Blood Tests

Other blood tests may be ordered by the doctor, if they are relevant to the PWA's case. These may include Hepatitis B and C profiles, glucose tolerance tests, serologies for toxoplasmosis, cryptococcal antigens, blood cultures, *erythropoietin* levels (a hormone from the kidneys that stimulates production of red blood cells), and levels of vitamin B_{12} and folate to assess anemias.

The PWA should always ask the doctor about the purpose, reliability, cost, preparation, and outcome of any exam she undergoes.

Microbial Cultures of Stool, Sputum, and Urine

Feces (Stool)

A specimen of fecal material is grown in a culture medium whenever an intestinal infection is suspected. This method is useful when looking for bacteria (salmonella, *shigella*), viruses (rectal herpes), or parasites (*giardia*, cryptosporidium). Either a small amount of stool is collected, or the rectum is swabbed with an ordinary cotton-tipped applicator to obtain potentially infectious material, although a sample of stool is more likely to give a reliable result than is a swab.

If the doctor or laboratory requires a stool specimen, the best method of collecting one is to use a bedpan or to place plastic wrap over the top of the commode to collect the stool without mixing it with water or urine. You can then use a small wooden stick, a tongue depressor, or a plastic spoon to transfer the specimen into the proper container.

If the rectum is swabbed, make sure that visible fecal material is present on the applicator, and be sure to follow any instructions given to you about handling the specimen.

Freshly passed stool is needed for bacterial examination, whereas frozen stool cultures may be used to examine for viruses. Stools for parasites should be warm when examined, and therefore it is usually necessary to collect these at the laboratory.

Cultures may also be taken of the blood, urine, sputum, spinal fluid, of wounds, the eye, throat, *urethra*, vagina, and cervix to check for a variety of infectious agents involved in AIDS. For example, sputum may be cultured for tuberculosis. A throat swab may reveal oral candidiasis (thrush). Urethral, vaginal, or cervical swabs may isolate herpes or other sexually transmitted diseases. Though it is not a culture per se, a related and specialized cervical swab, called a PAP smear (see page 282), properly fixed on a glass slide, checks for human papilloma virus, a type of STD that is a precursor of cervical cancer in some PWAs.

Cultures are usually painless to obtain. The method varies according to the particular site and infectious agent being examined. Often your health care provider will obtain the actual specimen. Following, however, are two common exceptions to that rule.

Sputum Culture

This specimen is most commonly used to isolate tuberculosis. Remember that saliva is not sputum. **It is essential that the PWA cough deeply, to ensure that the material comes from the lungs, not the mouth.** The best time to do sputums for tuberculosis testing is in the morning. Generally three separate specimens collected on three separate mornings are the standard for this test.

Urine Culture

Urine cultures are used to determine if the PWA has an infection of the urinary tract. **If the PWA is a woman,** the best method of obtaining a urine specimen that is not contaminated by vaginal secretions is to insert a tampon before beginning the procedure. Then use special moistened towelettes or wipes to cleanse the vaginal area from front to back. Next, the woman should urinate a small amount into the toilet first, and then catch the middle of the stream in the sterile container provided. She should take care not to touch the top or inside of the sterile container during the process. Be sure to seal the container immediately after collection and refrigerate it if it is not turned in to the laboratory at once.

If the PWA is a man, the procedure involves retracting the foreskin if he is uncircumcised, then wiping the tip of the glans with a towelette. He urinates a small amount into the toilet first, and then collects the middle of the stream in the sterile container. The longer the specimen is allowed to stand before testing, the more likely it is to become contaminated by environmental microbes, so refrigerate if advised and turn it in promptly to the lab.

Results, costs, and preparation are highly variable, depending on the particular culture. Again, discuss these factors with health care personnel.

Skin Tests

Mantoux Test for Tuberculosis

Tuberculosis is a major public health problem that has resurfaced in the era of AIDS. The problem is twofold: PWAs contract atypical and virulent strains of the bacteria, which seem to resist traditional drug therapy; and *tuberculosis is the only opportunistic infection of AIDS capable of extending beyond the borders of PWAs to the general public.* Because of this, if you are a PWA, a caregiver, or a close contact, it is important to get a Mantoux test, which screens for TB exposure.

The Mantoux test (also called a *ppd*) is performed by injecting a very small amount of tuberculin protein derivative under the skin of the forearm. If the person has been exposed to TB at some time in her life, an antigen-antibody reaction will take place, causing the site of the injection to become a hard, red lump.

Having a positive reaction to a Mantoux test does not automatically mean that the person has active TB at the present time. However, it raises a red flag to the doctor to check carefully for symptoms and to do a chest X ray to gain additional information about the person's state of health. Even if no active TB is found, it is usually necessary for the individual to take antibiotics for a period of time to ensure that the small amount of tuberculin germs present in her body do not activate at a future time into full-blown illness.

Because of their severe state of compromised immunity, PWAs don't necessarily show the normal antigen-antibody reaction to the Mantoux test. They may not have sufficient immune "strength," so to speak, to produce the traditional lump measuring at least 10 millimeters. Thus, criteria for PWAs are different from those for the non–HIV positive population. For persons with HIV infection, a reaction of 5 millimeters or more is considered positive. The CDC emphasizes that PWAs who have clinical signs and symptoms suggestive of TB should *never* have the possibility excluded, even if their test is completely negative. This is because PWAs may be *anergic,* meaning that their immune system is so weakened that they fail to show exposure to even the most commonplace antigens, or proteins. To check for *anergy,* another skin test, appropriately called an "anergy panel," is often administered to PWAs.

Anergy Panel An anergy panel is administered in exactly the same manner as the ppd. However, here small amounts of three or four common proteins from viruses and fungi (e.g., mumps and candida) are introduced. An adult with an intact immune system will show evidence of having been exposed to these proteins by forming the characteristic red lump at each injection site. Those who are immunosuppressed from HIV will not.

Costs for both Mantoux and anergy tests are minimal, and the procedure will be performed by either a doctor or a nurse. **You will need to return to the clinic, hospital, or doctor's office in 48 to 72 hours for health care personnel to correctly read the test. It is very important to adhere to these guidelines, as premature or late interpretations are unreliable.**

Pulmonary Tests

Chest X Ray It is likely that a PWA will be exposed to numerous chest X rays during the course of her illness—for diagnosis, to monitor the success of treatment, even to check the placement of intravenous lines or chest tubes, should they be used. A chest X ray is capable of revealing the lungs; the bones surrounding them (the *sternum*, or breastbone; the ribs and *clavicles*, or collarbones); the heart; the diaphragm; and some of the lung linings and soft tissues surrounding the chest cavity.

When film is exposed to X rays, it turns black. Thus, any black area on an X ray indicates an area where the ray passed through the body unimpeded. Since healthy lungs are filled with air, the lung tissue on a normal chest X ray usually shows up black or very dark. If fluid or infection are present within the lung, the diseased area will appear gray instead of black. Denser materials absorb more of the radiation, thus the film in contact with bones and soft tissues will be lighter on the developed X ray, with soft tissue (like the heart) being lighter than lung, and bone tissue being the lightest of all.

A radiologist (a doctor trained to read X rays) can see many things in those black and white shadows. She can diagnose the presence of fluid (from cancers, heart failure, infections); *infiltrates* suggestive of pneumonia; tumors, fractures, bone diseases, enlarged lymph nodes (as in PCP and TB), a collapsed lung, or blood in the chest cavity. Old injuries and inactive TB can also be identified and distinguished from active problems. The opportunistic infections most commonly diagnosed by chest X ray include PCP, bacterial pneumonia, KS of the lung, and tuberculosis.

No special preparation is necessary for a chest X ray, although any kind of metal object (like jewelry) should be removed; X rays won't penetrate beyond it and underlying abnormalities won't be revealed. If she is able, the PWA will be asked to stand unassisted, remain still, and take a deep breath when told to do so by the technician. However, if this is not possible, portable machines can be taken to the PWA's bedside.

Costs and reliability of results are variable, according to the facility where the X ray is taken.

Bronchoscopy

Sometimes, not enough information can be gathered from sputum cultures, skin tests, and chest X rays alone. The doctor may wish to perform a bronchoscopy, possibly with a *transbronchial* biopsy. This is a direct examination of the insides of the air passages leading to the lungs. It is accomplished by passing a rigid metallic tube or a flexible fiber-optic scope through the mouth.

If the rigid bronchoscope is used (rarely today), the procedure is performed in the operating room under sterile conditions and general *anesthesia*. More and more, the flexible fiber-optic scope is used instead, as it allows the procedure to be performed more comfortably and easily, often in a procedure room on the hospital floor and under local anesthesia. In addition, because it is so flexible, it can be manipulated by the doctor with greater ease to see more of the tracheobronchial tree and to diagnose more accurately.

Regardless of the type of bronchoscope chosen, a biopsy or tissue sample may be taken for laboratory analysis to establish the presence of an opportunistic infection (PCP, tuberculosis, *Cryptococcus neoformans,* CMV infection, and others). Bronchoscopy can also be used therapeutically to drain secretions and abscesses from severe infections.

Bronchoscopy cannot be performed on PWAs who have active asthma, a bleeding disorder, or a heart condition or on those who have active TB or hepatitis B (because of the risk of spreading it to others). Therefore, careful preparation and testing are required to rule out any possible *contraindications* to the procedure. Furthermore, the doctor performing the bronchoscopy should carefully explain the procedure step-by-step beforehand, including information on preparations, the recovery period, and all the risks involved. All of this information should be included on an informed-consent form, which should be signed before the procedure is carried out.

After the procedure, if general anesthesia is used (rarely today), the PWA will be observed in the recovery room to monitor her reactions to the test and the anesthesia. In all cases, PWAs will be watched to ensure that vital signs are stable and that they are able to swallow. Often they will be given oxygen to breathe for several hours postbronchoscopy, until the body's own oxygen levels (which may become lowered during the test) return to normal.

Bronchoscopy is done in a hospital setting. Costs may include doctor fees, use of the operating room, anesthesia, and laboratory analysis of biopsy specimens. These are generally covered in full by health insurance plans.

Note: The biopsy procedure was mentioned here within the context of the bronchoscopy. You should be aware, however, that a biopsy refers to the removal of a small amount of tissue from any body site for the purpose of laboratory analysis. Usually done via the scalpel, laser, or insertion of a needle to draw out a small amount of fluid, the goal is generally to look for either a cancer or an infection. Common biopsy sites for PWAs include the skin and bone marrow as well as the lung.

Techniques and preparation are as variable as the organ being biopsied, so it is best to check with your doctor for details.

Gastrointestinal Tests

Barium Swallow/ Barium Enema

A barium swallow, also known as an *esophagram,* is a procedure performed on PWAs who are experiencing difficulty swallowing, or when a tumor or lesion of the esophagus is suspected. Sometimes it is performed in conjunction with an *upper GI series.* Here, X rays are taken to examine the esophagus, stomach, and first portion of the small intestine.

If the person can tolerate it, the optimal position for a barium swallow and upper GI series is sitting upright. She is then given a mixture of barium (the contrast medium) to drink as the pictures are being taken. This fluid can be unpleasant to drink, and sometimes causes constipation or diarrhea afterward, depending on your particular constitution. However, other than this, very few discomforts or risks are associated with this procedure.

Barium also may be instilled into the lower tract by means of an enema, following a clear liquid diet and the administration of laxatives to cleanse the bowels. The PWA is positioned on her side on the examining table while the contrast medium (the barium) is slowly administered under the guidance of the radiologist, who is watching the procedure on the fluoroscope (an instrument used to see inside the body).

The purpose of the barium enema, like the upper GI series, is to diagnose malignancies, such as KS of the intestinal tract, or infections, such as cryptosporidium and *Isospora belli.*

Although not painful, these tests can be uncomfortable, embarrassing, and tiring, so it is important for caregivers to provide emotional support and encouragement, and to allow the PWA to rest afterward.

Endoscopy/ Colonoscopy

These diagnostic tests are similar to bronchoscopy in that they use a flexible fiber-optic scope, but the site examined in this instance is a portion of the intestinal tract. When the scope is passed through the mouth, down the esophagus and into the stomach, the procedure is known as an *endoscopy.* When the scope is inserted into the rectum to view the lower portion of the tract, the procedure is known as a colonoscopy.

Both endoscopy and colonoscopy require the PWA either to fast after midnight the night before the test or to eat a special (usually clear liquid) diet beforehand. Colonoscopy usually requires the administration of an enema or oral medication to ensure that the bowels are sufficiently empty to allow the doctor a good look. Depending on the situation, these tests may be performed in an outpatient or hospital setting, at the bedside or in an operating room, under general or local anesthesia.

Endoscopy and colonoscopy permit the physician to diagnose causes of upper and lower gastrointestinal bleeding, pain, and diarrhea. It will identify malignancies, ulcers, and inflammatory bowel disease. In the case of AIDS, these conditions most commonly include candidiasis, herpes, CMV colitis, and Mycobacterium Avium Intracellulare.

Costs vary and include physician fees, use of the operating room, and hospital room, when hospitalization is necessary, in addition to the fee for the actual test. Most of the time, health insurance covers the procedure.

Tests of the Brain and Spinal Cord

Lumbar Puncture (Spinal Tap)

The prospect of undergoing a *lumbar puncture,* or spinal tap, can be a frightening one for the PWA. Sometimes it helps to ease anxieties to know that no pain will be felt, and that there is virtually no risk of paralysis. Even so, PWAs may need help to cooperate with the exam, especially if it is being done because they are confused or experiencing other neurological symptoms.

A lumbar puncture is done at the bedside under sterile conditions by a doctor, sometimes an anesthesiologist, trained in this procedure. The PWA must be able to hold completely still in a fetal position while a needle is inserted (after local anesthesia has been administered) to withdraw a small sample of the *cerebrospinal fluid* (the fluid that bathes the brain and spinal cord).

The fluid is then analyzed to determine the presence of various opportunistic infections, (most commonly *Cryptococcus neoformans,* toxoplasmosis, cytomegalovirus, MAI, tuberculosis), lymphoma of the central nervous system, and encephalitis.

It is recommended that the PWA lie flat for 6 to 12 hours after the procedure to prevent a so-called "spinal headache." Taking fluids can also minimize the chances of this occurring.

Costs vary and are covered by health insurance.

Computerized Axial Tomography (CAT Scan) and Magnetic Resonance Imaging (MRI)

CAT scans and MRIs have become popular in recent years because they afford the opportunity to view structures inside the body in great detail and in three dimensions. They can diagnose suspected brain infections and can differentiate cancerous from noncancerous masses, often precluding the need for more invasive tests or exploratory surgery.

CAT scans use X ray technology, often with the injection of a contrast medium. Pictures are taken in a series of cross-sectional slices. The PWA remains stationary, while the scanning machine moves around him to achieve the different angles necessary for the complete series. CAT scans are painless and noninvasive. They may take 30 to 60 minutes to complete; the worst effect may be a sense of claustrophobia.

MRI scans are the latest achievement in diagnostic testing. They use absolutely no radiation, relying instead on a strong magnet to excite the particles within the human body. Depending on how these particles react, a picture will be produced, revealing different densities that correspond to bone and soft tissue. MRIs require that the person be completely enclosed within a narrow tube while a series of loud banging noises are heard, for a period of 30 to 60 minutes. As with CAT scans, claustrophobic fears are probably the most unpleasant aspect to the test, which is otherwise painless and noninvasive.

CAT scans and MRI imaging require no special preparation, no hospitalization, and no anesthesia (so long as the PWA is able to cooperate during the test). However, they are among the most costly of exams, with fees for MRIs sometimes exceeding a thousand dollars. Most of the expense will be defrayed by insurance.

Ultrasound

Ultrasound is a type of diagnostic imaging that uses the patterns of echoes and sound waves as they bounce off tissues to determine if those tissues are normal and what their densities are. For example, an ultrasound might be performed to detect or determine if a mass is solid or semisolid in nature. In PWAs, ultrasound is frequently used to diagnose abdominal pain and liver or kidney problems for which an underlying cause has not been found.

Ultrasound involves no harmful ionizing radiation or injection of a contrast medium, and it is completely safe, painless, and noninvasive. It can be done both as an outpatient (e.g., in a doctor's office or radiology facility) or in a hospital. There is usually no special preparation needed, and costs vary according to the type of test done and the facility where it is performed.

Gallium Scan

In a gallium scan, a contrast medium called gallium is introduced intravenously. Often, the contrast medium will cause a hot flash or burning sensation as it is introduced into the site, which disappears after the injection is completed. Forty-eight to 72 hours later, after the contrast has had time to circulate throughout the body, a scan is done. The contrast medium will localize to the site of a tumor or concentrate in an area of acute or chronic inflammation.

A gallium scan will not provide information as to whether a tumor is cancerous or not; it merely shows the location and approximate size of a tumor. The concentration of contrast media in a specific location is called "increased uptake." Gallium scans are often used to look for inflammation in the lungs and to detect pneumonias, tuberculosis, and KS. These scans can be performed for a specific area of the body or for the body as a whole.

Gallium scans require no special preparation other than intravenous access; an informed-consent form, however, must be completed and signed. This test does not require hospitalization. Cost varies depending upon which body part is to be scanned.

Pap Test

Invented by Dr. George Papanicolou in 1928, the Pap test is a method of detecting cervical cancer. During a *pelvic exam,* a device called a speculum is inserted into the vagina to separate its muscular walls, allowing the examiner to view the cervix, which is the lowermost portion of the uterus. The doctor or nurse practitioner then uses a wooden spatula, cotton swabs, and/or soft brushes (called cytobrushes), which feel a little like pipe cleaners, to collect cells from the cervix and vagina. These are then transferred to a glass slide and sent to a laboratory where a trained physician called a pathologist looks at the cells to determine if there is any evidence of infection, cancer, or precancerous tissue.

Pap tests are only *screening* tests that depend on the examination of material that has been shed from the uterus. Therefore, the accuracy of the test depends on many factors, including whether the person performing the exam was able to collect an adequate sample, and the expertise of the pathologist. In addition, it must be kept in mind that Pap tests don't reliably screen for any other type of female cancer or disease (e.g., ovarian or endometrial cancer).

Pap tests are mentioned here because the latest definition of AIDS considers invasive cervical cancer an AIDS-defining diagnosis in HIV positive women. In other words, not all women with abnormal Pap tests have AIDS—only those who are HIV positive and who have indications on their Paps that the cancer has spread beyond the cervix.

Routine Pap tests are performed at a doctor's office and cause little or no discomfort. Generally, they are done in conjunction with other tests to screen for sexually transmitted diseases, vaginitis, and so forth. It is recommended that Pap tests not be done just before, during, or just after menstruation, as the presence of blood can make the interpretation of the slides more difficult. It is also suggested that you refrain from having intercourse and using douches, feminine hygiene products, or vaginal medications for at least 48 hours prior to getting tested, as these can either wash out the cells or otherwise adulterate them.

The cost is twofold: The doctor or nurse practitioner may charge for the office visit (which often also consists of a routine complete physical exam) and the lab charges for the reading of the slide. Prices vary, ranging anywhere from $25 to over $100. Some organizations, such as Planned Parenthood and women's health care clinics, may offer these services for free or on a sliding scale based on one's ability to pay.

APPENDIX B

Medication Guide

PWAs and their caregivers are confronted with literally dozens of different medications during the course of the illness. Many of these interact with one another, or with food, alcohol, or with over-the-counter preparations. To add to the complexity of the situation, drug therapies for the various opportunistic diseases and cancers are changing constantly, which makes it impossible to provide information about specific medications that would remain current or useful. Instead, this section provides general information about medications, and their administration. For resources to refer to for information about a specific medication, see Appendix H, "The Caregiver's Bookshelf."

What You Need to Know about Medications

To ensure that medications are used properly, PWAs and their caregivers need to be aware of the nature and purpose of each medication, as well as of potential danger signs during their administration. See the box on page 284 for questions to ask your doctor, as well as Table B.1 for how to distinguish side effects from allergic reactions.

Types of Medications

Because of the complexity of AIDS and the multitude of associated complications (e.g., opportunistic infections, cancers, pain, nausea, diarrhea, neurological disease, psychological manifestations), many categories of medications may be prescribed. These include:

- *antibiotics* to combat infections from bacteria, viruses, fungi, and parasites.
- *antiemetics* to minimize or eliminate nausea and vomiting.
- *antidiarrheals* to combat loose stools.
- *chemotherapeutic agents* to fight cancer.
- *analgesics* to decrease or eradicate pain.
- *antipyretics* to fight fevers.
- *sleeping aids, antidepressants,* and *antianxiety medications* to help allay some of the emotional symptoms of AIDS.
- *antihistamines* for itching, hiccups, nausea, and/or insomnia.
- *vitamins and minerals:* drugs prescribed when other medications deplete or interfere with the absorption of these essential substances and when a PWA becomes malnourished because of his illness.

What to Ask About Your Medications

Be sure to ask your health professional (doctor, nurse, or pharmacist) the following questions before you begin to take (or administer) **any** drug.

- What is the purpose of this medication?
- How does it work?
- What are the advantages versus the disadvantages of being on this drug?
- Is this still considered an experimental therapy? How successful has it been in the past? What are the odds that it will help my condition?
- What are the side effects that I might expect to experience and how are they managed? Will I experience them right away?; if not, then when can I anticipate a side effect? Are there any long-term side effects? Are there any effects that I need to report immediately? How will I be monitored for adverse reactions?
- Are there any interactions with other medications, with food, or with alcohol? (*Caution:* PWAs should always avoid alcoholic beverages, although some medicines may contain small amounts of alcohol as part of their formulations.)
- Will I be administering this medication myself at home, or will I be receiving it at the hospital?
- When should this medication be taken relative to food (e.g., with meals or on an empty stomach)?
- How is this medication administered (e.g., injected intramuscularly or taken orally)? What is the dose and schedule of this medication? (E.g., four times daily is not exactly the same as every six hours—get clarification as to whether you must be awakened to take the medicine.)
- How long will it be necessary to take the medication?
- How expensive is this drug, and are there any less costly alternatives? Is there a way to get the cost of this medicine reduced or to receive it for free via a government or drug company–sponsored program? (See Appendix G for additional information about these programs.)
- What should I do if I vomit the medication?
- What should I do if I miss taking a dose?
- Is there any activity I should avoid while on this medication?
- What is an allergic reaction versus a normal side effect for this drug?

- *anticoagulants* to interfere with blood clotting.
- *corticosteroids* to reduce inflammation and/or replace the hormone manufactured by the adrenal glands if they are not working properly.
- *antacids:* generally, over-the-counter formulations to combat excess stomach acid and heartburn. Also used when another medication is irritating to the stomach.
- *anticonvulsants* to control seizures.
- *appetite stimulants* to assist PWAs in their attempts to eat food.

TABLE B.1   *How to Differentiate a Side Effect from a True Allergic Reaction*

Is This Symptom ...	... An Allergic Reaction?	... A Side Effect?
Rash	yes	no
Wheezing*	yes	no
Shortness of breath*	yes	no
Chest tightness*	yes	no
Sensation of throat closing	yes	no
Facial or body swelling	yes	no
Loss of consciousness	yes	no
Palpitations/racing pulse	no	yes
Nausea	no	yes
Vomiting	no	yes
Diarrhea	no	yes
Abdominal pain	no	yes

*Note: Never assume that a symptom is an allergic reaction without discussing it with your doctor first. For example, symptoms like wheezing, shortness of breath, and chest tightness are common in respiratory diseases like pneumonia. Therefore, if you have these problems while on a drug for the treatment of pneumonia, you need the help of your doctor or nurse to decide if the cause is the disease or the medication.

Responsible Use of Medications

What to Do

- Inform your doctor of any adverse reactions to a drug. If you consult a reference book about side effects, be aware that not everyone will experience every side effect. Many people have none at all.
- Implement any treatments the doctor suggests to manage side effects.
- Take your medication as prescribed even if you are experiencing side effects, but then notify your doctor of the problem as soon as possible.
- Keep a schedule or calendar and/or set the beeper on your watch to remind you to take your medications.
- Check with your doctor or pharmacist before crushing pills or diluting them in liquids, as sometimes this interferes with their efficacy.
- Make sure you notify your doctor before taking **any** medicine she has not prescribed—even an over-the-counter drug—as it can interact with prescription drugs.
- Store medications as ordered or directed by your pharmacist. Generally, all medications should be kept in a dry place out of the direct sunlight. (The bathroom medicine cabinet is *not* a good choice, because of the humidity in the atmosphere there.) Some may need to be refrigerated, kept in light resistant bottles, and so on.

- Be sure that you keep up your supply of the medication as well as any associated paraphernalia (e.g., syringes, alcohol wipes, etc.).
- Take your medicines with you whenever you leave your house, whether for a brief outing or a long trip, to ensure that you don't miss a dose. When traveling, make sure that you carry extra drugs and supplies and/or prescriptions that will be honored at your destination. Carry the medicine onto the plane with you when flying, rather than allowing it to go into the baggage compartment; then, if your luggage is lost, you will not be without your drugs.
- Tell your doctor if you know that you are allergic to a medication.
- If a medication is making you nauseated, and you only need to take it once a day, find out if you can take it at bedtime so you'll sleep through the nausea. Otherwise, try eating small, frequent meals throughout the day instead of three large meals. Drink liquids after instead of with your meals. Try taking a walk before eating, if you feel up to it. Rest, in a seated position, for as long as you are able after eating.
- If a medication causes a loss in appetite, nausea, or a metallic taste in the mouth, use marinades to improve the flavors of meats and poultry. Switch from metal to plastic utensils.
- Keep all scheduled appointments for checkups while on a particular medication, as it may be vital to monitor your body's reaction to the medication.
- If your vision has been affected by your illness, make sure that you have someone assist you in taking medications. PWA or caregiver should always double-check the label for the proper name, dosage, and expiration date (if appropriate) before the medicine is taken.
- When pouring liquid medicines, the correct dose is arrived at by having the bottom of the curve of the liquid lined up with the *calibration* line on the measuring cup or dropper when observed at eye level.
- If you are involved in mixing or diluting solutions for tube feedings or intravenous administration, make sure you prepare substances exactly as ordered and instructed using sterile equipment, the correct diluent (diluting agent), in the proper concentration, and at the directed rate. Make sure to discard used needles, syringes, and partially used *ampules* of medications carefully.
- Take the medicine only for the problem for which it is prescribed.
- Remember to keep all medicines out of the reach of children and confused individuals.

What Not to Do

- Never transfer drugs from their original containers, as this can lead to confusion and may reduce the shelf life of the medication.
- Do not take a drug that appears adulterated; for example, if its color is off or if there is an unusual odor or precipitate present.
- Do not assume that if your dosage of a particular drug is different from what appears in a reference book, it was prescribed incorrectly. Doctors prescribe

medication regimens in a highly individualized manner. Ask for specifics about the regimen prescribed for you.

What to Discuss with Your Doctor

- If you experience any difficulty breathing, including a tightness in your throat or chest, shortness of breath, or wheezing after taking a prescribed drug, **CALL AN AMBULANCE**. If you have an allergic reaction to a drug, call your doctor immediately.
- The purpose and effects of any new medication. Refer to the list of questions in the box earlier in this section.
- A recommendation for a good reference book to consult about your medications. You can also read the package inserts that accompany some drugs. These are generally directed at medical personnel and so may be technical, but they are excellent sources of information. Ask your doctor or pharmacist to explain anything that is unclear.

Advice on Administering Medications

The following sections provide guidelines to the administration of drugs by the routes PWAs and caregivers are most likely to encounter during the course of the illness. There are other methods of giving medicines that are not covered here, and that should be taught to you by your home care nurse before you attempt them on your own. These include administration via *nebulizer* (a machine that administers medications in aerosol form), gavage tubes, and central venous access devices. For general information on gavage tubes and central venous access devices, see Chapter 23.

Pills and Liquids

What to Do

- Give pills with food and beverages to minimize stomach upset, unless doing so will interfere with the absorption and effectiveness of a drug.
- Find out if the medicine is available in liquid form and ask your doctor to prescribe it that way if a person has difficulty swallowing pills. If not, find out if the drug may be crushed and placed in food (e.g., cereal or applesauce) or diluted in a liquid and injected into the mouth with a syringe (minus the needle!). If a tablet is scored (indented down the middle to facilitate breaking), break it in half and place it on the back of the tongue for easier swallowing.
- Have the PWA sit up for 30 minutes after taking a pill, if he can, to minimize the potential for choking and/or gastric upset.

- Make sure that capsules and coated pills are swallowed intact—not chewed, broken in half, or crushed—unless you are advised by a pharmacist that altering them will not interfere with their absorption and effectiveness.
- Be certain that pills that are supposed to be placed under the tongue or between the cheek and the gums are not chewed or swallowed. They are designed to be absorbed directly into the body through the mucosa; if chewed or swallowed, the digestive process might destroy them.
- Shake liquid medications well before pouring.

What *Not* to Do

Never give oral medications to a vomiting or comatose person.

When to Consult Your Doctor

If the PWA is unable to swallow the medication in an oral form or if he repeatedly vomits after administration.

Injections

Subcutaneous injections are the type most commonly given at home. The medicine is injected under the skin, but not deep enough to penetrate the muscle layer (as one would with an *intramuscular* injection). Both intramuscular and subcutaneous injections can be given at home when called for. Injections are used because of their ability to have a rapid onset of the medication's effect, and because it is the best method of medication delivery for the unconscious or uncooperative patient or for the person who is unable to swallow for any reason. Often a medication, for example, insulin, is available only in an injectable form—this is because sometimes a drug is destroyed if permitted to come in contact with the digestive tract and its strong gastric juices.

No one can be taught to give a "shot" simply by reading instructions in a book. It takes practice, guidance, and willpower to stop your hands and knees from shaking! What follows are simple instructions on how to give intramuscular (IM) and subcutaneous (SQ) injections. **Remember to follow what is taught to you firsthand by a doctor or registered nurse; practice; be patient with yourself; and use these instructions as a refresher.** Keep in mind the thought that there isn't a doctor or nurse alive who was born able to give an injection. We all had to learn and conquer our fears. You can, too!

Finally, realize that no injection is completely pain-free. Sometimes helping someone means hurting them just a little. Intramuscular injections, in particular, can hurt, and the area injected often remains sore for hours after the injection. This is normal, unless the area is particularly red or swollen, or feels warm to the touch.

What to Do

- Ascertain the type of injection to be given. Learn from a physician or registered nurse how to give IM and SQ injections properly.

- Practice—using an orange as a model is a tried and true method.
- Keep well stocked with your drug and necessary supplies. Always renew your prescription and reorder supplies before you run out.
- Always use the type of syringe and the needle size prescribed by your doctor.
- Keep alcohol, needles, syringes, medications, and disposal containers out of reach of children and confused adults.
- As with all medications, observe the medication's effects and store properly—often, this means in the refrigerator.
- **If you are accidentally pricked with a used needle, allow the wound to bleed, then wash thoroughly with soap and water, and apply an adhesive bandage, if necessary.**

   Report the incident to your doctor as soon as possible. There are measures that can be taken to monitor you for HIV exposure as well as other bloodborne diseases, such as hepatitis. You should know that it is highly unlikely that you will contract HIV from a small needle stick; hepatitis is much more contagious, however, but illness from this potentially (but rarely) fatal disease can be minimized if caught early.

Preparing a Medication for Injection

What to Do

(Follow along with Figure B.1.)

- Gather all the supplies you will need, including: gloves, alcohol wipes, gauze pads, syringe, needle, and medication vial.
- Check the name and expiration date on the vial.
- Wash your hands thoroughly (Figure B.1*a*).
- Sometimes it is necessary to *reconstitute* a powdered medication with a diluent, such as normal saline or sterile water. Do this now, as you have been taught, mixing it with the proper amount of fluid and rotating the vial until the powder has completely dissolved in the fluid (Figure B.1*b*).
- Most medication vials for injection have a hard plastic cap, under which is a rubber stopper. Once the hard plastic cap is removed, it cannot be replaced. With multiple-dose vials (vials used more than one time), it is necessary to wipe the rubber top of the vial with alcohol **each and every time** before you give an injection to maintain sterile technique (Figure B.1*c*).
- After the top of the vial has been wiped with alcohol, pull back the plunger of the syringe until the amount of air in the syringe equals the desired dose of medication (Figure B.1*d*). Inject the air into the vial (Figure B.1*e*). (*Note:* For reconstituted medicines, it is not necessary to inject air into the vial. Simply pull back on the plunger to withdraw the desired amount of the drug into the syringe as described.)
- Turn the vial, needle, and syringe upside down, still holding the needle in place inside the vial, so that the vial is situated above the needle and syringe. (Do not remove the needle from the vial during this process.) Pull the needle out just far enough so that the tip of the needle is present in the fluid in the

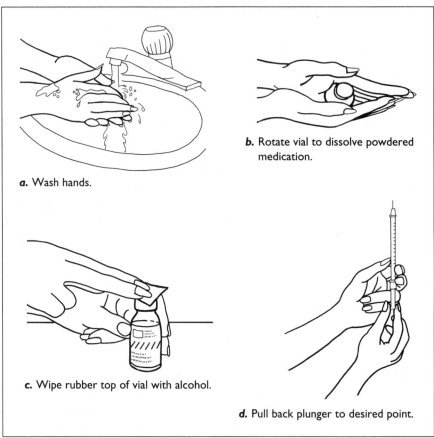

a. Wash hands.

b. Rotate vial to dissolve powdered medication.

c. Wipe rubber top of vial with alcohol.

d. Pull back plunger to desired point.

(continued)

FIGURE B.1
Steps in Preparing a Medication for Injection

vial, and pull on the plunger to allow fluid to enter the syringe (Figure B.1*f*).

- Draw up the desired amount of medication into the syringe and withdraw the needle from the vial. *Note:* If air is present in the syringe, inject the medication back into the vial and try again. Be sure that the needle is below the fluid line and pull back on the plunger slowly, to allow medication to enter the syringe.
- Remove any remaining small air bubbles by tapping the syringe until they rise to the top of the syringe and slowly easing the plunger up, making sure that only the air and not any medicine is expelled (Figure B.1*g*).
- Make sure the amount of medicine in the syringe equals the amount prescribed, and that none of the space within the syringe is filled with air.
- If the medication is in a glass ampule, break the neck of the glass to access the medicine. The best method of accomplishing this is to wrap an alcohol pad (in its package) around the neck of the ampule. Hole one end of the ampule with one hand and the end covered by the alcohol pad with the other

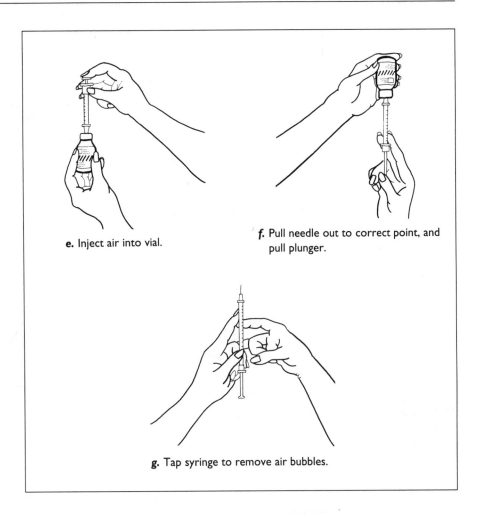

e. Inject air into vial.

f. Pull needle out to correct point, and pull plunger.

g. Tap syringe to remove air bubbles.

**FIGURE B.1
(continued)**

hand. With a quick, firm movement, break the ampule, holding it away from you as you do so. Dispose of the glass in the hard plastic container you maintain for this purpose.

- Remove medication contained within an ampule by inverting it and placing the needle inside, taking care not to touch the sides with the needle. Pull the plunger back as before, drawing up the desired amount of medication into the syringe and discarding any air bubbles in the manner previously described.

Giving an Intramuscular or a Subcutaneous Injection

The information here is in no way intended to take the place of one-on-one and step-by-step instructions taught to you in person by a trained doctor or nurse. It is designed merely to refresh your memory when that individual is not there to guide you. If our instructions digress from those that have been given to you, always follow the advice of your doctor.

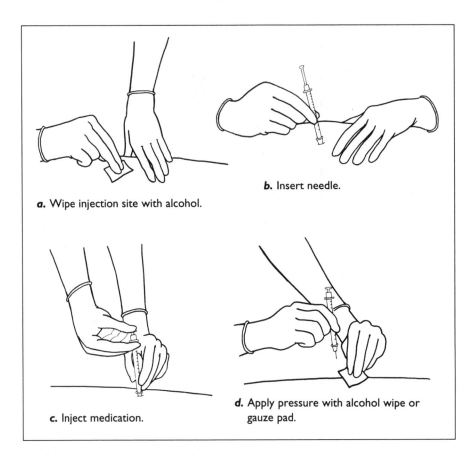

FIGURE B.2
Steps in Giving an Intramuscular Injection

a. Wipe injection site with alcohol.

b. Insert needle.

c. Inject medication.

d. Apply pressure with alcohol wipe or gauze pad.

What to Do

(Follow along with Figure B.2.)

- **Always wash your hands and don gloves** if you are giving an injection to another person. If you are injecting yourself, it is not necessary to wear gloves, but you should wash your hands before and after the procedure.
- Choose the site to be injected. For an IM injection, choose the
   — upper arm;
   — upper outer aspect of the leg between the knee and thigh; or
   — upper outer aspect of the buttock near the hip.

   For a subcutaneous injection, choose the
   — upper outer arm;
   — outer thigh; or
   — abdomen and flanks (between the nipples and hip bones and avoiding the area surrounding the navel).

Note: **Check with your doctor or nurse, or read the medication package insert to determine where the injection should be administered.** Some medications have a preferred site for injection.

- Remember to rotate sites as explained in Chapter 17.
- Assess the skin of the person to be injected. Look for redness, swelling, scarring, pain, and other abnormalities of the skin. Do not inject into a damaged or painful area of skin.
- Position the person for comfort. Relax the muscle area to be injected, if possible. For example, if you are giving a shot into the buttock area, it is preferable to have the person lying on his stomach, rather than bending over, as this permits greater muscle relaxation.
- Wipe the area to be injected with an alcohol pad (Figure B.2*a*).
- For an IM injection, stretch the skin beneath the site selected between your gloved thumb and index finger.
- Dart straight in, quickly, at a 90-degree angle (Figure B.2*b*).
- For an SQ injection, the procedure is almost identical to giving an IM injection except for the following: Do not stretch the skin as for an IM injection. Instead, pinch the skin between your thumb and index finger, forming a "tent." Enter the pinched area of skin at a 45-degree angle. (You may release the tent once you have completed the injection.)
- Check to make sure that you have not inadvertently entered a blood vessel by gently pulling back on the plunger to check for a blood return. If blood does *not* enter the syringe, then inject the medication (Figure B.2*c*). If blood does enter the syringe, remove the syringe, discard the medication, prepare another injection, and reinsert a new needle at another site. Aspirate (pull back on the syringe) again and inject the medication once you are correctly in the muscle or subcutaneous tissue, and not a blood vessel.
- Pull out the syringe and needle in one fluid movement after the medication is injected.
- Apply pressure to the injection site with an alcohol wipe or gauze pad (Figure B.2*d*). Massage the site gently to help spread the medication and ease the discomfort.

Dispose of the needle and syringe carefully, by placing it in a hard plastic container with a screw-on lid. These are provided by most home care companies and are for sale in surgical supply houses. For a homemade version, use an empty coffee can with a lid or a used bottle of liquid detergent. Label the container. When full, tape the lid shut and dispose of it according to your doctor's instructions or those of your locale. (State laws vary. You should also check with your local health department or department of sanitation.)

What Not to Do

- Never give any kind of injection over a bony area (e.g., hip, shoulder, knee).
- **Never recap a used needle.** You stand a good chance of pricking yourself if you do!

When to Consult Your Doctor

- If the PWA experiences swelling of his face, becomes extremely short of breath, and/or complains of a suffocating or choking sensation, this may signal a severe allergic reaction to the medication being injected. **CALL AN AMBULANCE.**
- If you are a caregiver and **accidentally get stuck by a contaminated needle.**
- If you have **any** questions regarding injection techniques or you need to discuss a medication.
- For renewals of prescriptions for syringes, needles, or medications. **Insulin is the only injectable medication available without a prescription.** Syringes and needles, however, require a prescription.
- If you think an injection site feels hot or looks red, swollen, or in any way inflamed or infected.

Eye Drops

Refer to Chapter 12.

Rectal Suppositories

Rectal suppositories are useful when a PWA is unable to swallow medications or is nauseated, vomiting, or comatose.

What to Do

- Keep suppositories refrigerated unless you are instructed to do otherwise.
- Always wear gloves when inserting a suppository.
- Position the PWA on his left side and have him take slow, deep breaths, to relax the *sphincter*. (Have him remain in this position for about 15 to 30 minutes after insertion to ensure that the suppository has had time to melt and does not get accidentally expelled.)
- Lubricate the suppository with petroleum jelly. Slowly and gently insert the lubricated suppository into the rectum, pushing it upward about 2 inches.
- Watch for accidental expulsion of the suppository.

What Not to Do

Do not attempt to administer a suppository to a person with diarrhea.

Adjunct Therapies

We want to begin this appendix by stating very clearly that we believe conventional medical therapy to be the *best approach* to the treatment of AIDS. With your doctor's approval, a decision to enter a clinical trial and use an experimental medication or treatment protocol can also be very beneficial. This appendix is about adjunct therapies aimed at reducing stress, boosting your immune system, inducing a state of relaxation, alleviating pain, improving your outlook, and maintaining hope. All of these goals are of paramount importance in the battle against AIDS. The critical point we wish to emphasize is that these therapies are mentioned here as *adjunct, meaning in addition to, not instead of, conventional medical treatments.*

Considering Adjunct Therapies

There are many kinds of adjunct therapies. Some boast of spiritual and psychological benefits, others of physical benefits. Some offer a cure by claiming to reduce stress and boost the immune system. Others state that they can improve a person's outlook and induce a feeling of serenity that helps alleviate some symptoms. Remember: Adjunct therapies should not hurt you (except for the minor pain sometimes involved with massage). They should not contain "secret ingredients," be extremely expensive, or promote the exchange of or exposure to blood or body fluids.

We include some adjunct therapies that have been tried by PWAs and caregivers who want to feel that they are doing something positive and creative to help themselves instead of passively sitting on the sidelines and watching the days slip by.

It is not unusual for those with illnesses not yet curable to become desperate. Often they believe that "miracle cures" will work for them. They leave the arena of conventional medicine and try anything that promises a cure. If you decide to try these or other adjunct therapies, remember that you should **never discontinue your present medical treatment to try them**, nor should you allow yourself to be taken in by those who would take advantage of people who so urgently seek a cure.

How to Avoid Adjunct Therapy Rip-Offs

- Beware of claims to cure or other too-good-to-be-true pronouncements. To date no cure for AIDS has been proven.

- Do not be fooled by credentials. Names followed by impressive-sounding initials do not guarantee that the treatments offered are safe or effective.
- Be aware that credentials other than "M.D.," such as "N.D." (naturopathic doctor), are licensed and monitored differently from state to state (see the box below). Try to investigate the doctor to make sure that he is currently legally permitted to practice and that no complaints have been filed against him by former patients or the authorities.

What Kind of Doctor Are You Seeing?

Allopathic Doctor (M.D.). This is a physician who treats illness and injury with active treatments, such as the prescription of drugs or the performance of surgery. All U.S. M.D.s are graduates of allopathic medical schools.

Doctor of Osteopathy (D.O.). This type of doctor is a fully licensed physician in the United States, able to prescribe medications and perform surgery in all 50 states. D.O.s usually practice in hospitals, offices, clinics, and medical centers, much as their allopathic counterparts do. However, their training focuses more intently on a holistic approach. They are taught to treat the patient and not the disease, with an emphasis on the musculoskeletal system, including study about how nerves, muscles, and bones interact with other systems of the body. They undergo additional training in physical manipulation of bone and tissue.

Homeopathic Doctor (H.O.). Usually this is a licensed physician with additional training via national study groups and/or exchange of information from one person to another. Few states license practitioners strictly for homeopathic medicine.

Naturopathic Doctor (N.D.). These practitioners are licensed in only a few states. They complete four years of graduate training at one of only two accredited U.S. colleges that have a curriculum similar to that of conventional medical schools. They learn to perform minor surgery in addition to taking classes in homeopathy, botanical medicine, spinal manipulation, natural childbirth, oriental medicine, and stress management.

Chiropractic Doctor (D.C.). Chiropractors emphasize the active pursuit of health, believing that it can be improved not only by restoring spinal function but also by improving the habits of lifestyle: good diet, fresh air, exercise, and good sleeping and working practices. Chiropractors expect and require *involvement and active participation* by their patients—as for example, by following a prescribed dietary or exercise regimen. Although chiropractors may order tests (generally X rays and an occasional blood test) and may suggest vitamins or other nutritional supplements, their method is very low-tech and natural. Chiropractors have the same premedical undergraduate education as prospective physicians. They go on to a graduate level of training in one of only about 15 schools nationwide, which lasts from three to five years. Then graduates serve a 15-month internship under a practicing doctor of chiropractic. Chiropractors must be licensed and board-certified.

- Always ask to see studies published in respected journals that back up the use of the therapy in question. Never rely solely on testimonials.
- Beware of promises that seem too good to be true and big promotions for products or treatments.
- Remember that therapies offered in other countries may not be covered by consumer protection laws in the United States.
- Be suspicious of costly therapies.
- Research all therapies thoroughly, because education is the best protection. Read, ask questions, and take notes for future reference.
- Be wary of "mega" anything. An excessive amount of a product or treatment of any kind is probably worthless at best, and potentially harmful at worst.
- Be cautious of those who would try to talk you out of seeking a second opinion about a particular therapy.

Deciding on an Adjunct Therapy

What to Do

- Carefully and thoroughly investigate the adjunct therapy you feel inclined to participate in. (Refer to the preceding section on avoiding rip-offs.)
- Ask questions and read everything you can on the subject.
- Discuss the adjunct therapy with your loved ones. Get their opinions and enlist their help, if necessary.
- Consider your options, cost, the time necessary, and so forth before choosing a therapy.
- Dedicate yourself to learning and practicing the therapy if this is appropriate.
- Monitor your progress.
- Remember that you can stop and change to another therapy at any time.

What Not to Do

- Do not be afraid to discuss adjunct therapies with others, including health care personnel. Don't feel embarrassed or shy even if you meet disapproval. It is your right to seek adjunct therapies.
- Do not fall prey to extreme forms of therapy (e.g., fasting if you have diarrhea and malnutrition) or those that make outrageous claims.
- Do not practice any adjunct therapy that involves the exchange or introduction of blood or body fluids.
- Do not stop conventional medical treatment.

When to Consult Your Doctor

- To seek approval for any therapy that is invasive, painful, involves taking any kind of "medicines" or substances, or is in any way questionable. Be sure that she feels there is no contraindication to the therapy in your case. (For example, if you have phlebitis, you cannot undergo massage therapy because the kneading of a blood clot may cause it to break off from the vessel in which it is located; it could then travel to a vital organ where it might cause a stroke or a heart attack, or it might exacerbate the inflammation in an already irritated area.)

Types of Adjunct Therapies

Following are discussions of adjunct therapies. Every day a new one is created or is being developed. Each person must decide for himself what to try according to what is suited to him and his unique situation.

Current thinking indicates that standard medicine is only half right. Lifestyle changes, new ways of reducing stress, exercising, and eating right may be just as important to the mind/body connection.

Acupuncture

Used mostly to aid in pain relief, acupuncture involves the use of presterilized, disposable needles of varying lengths, which are passed through the skin at specific points according to charts derived from Eastern medicine. The free end of the needle is then twirled, or can be used to conduct small electrical currents to the preselected point, thereby inducing a type of anesthesia, which in turn causes pain relief or reduction. It is thought that acupuncture may accomplish this by triggering the release of *endorphins,* which are substances produced by the brain and believed to be the body's natural painkillers.

A person undergoing acupuncture is awake at all times. It is said to be painless, but an individual response is possible (i.e., some people feel discomfort, which may or may not be psychological in nature). Treatments can take place once or twice a week for months or can be limited to a single visit. The length of each session also varies.

Some states require a license to practice acupuncture; others require certification by the National Commission for the Certification of Acupuncturists. Costs vary greatly. If performed by an M.D., acupuncture may be covered by some medical insurance policies.

Biofeedback

Biofeedback is a process of monitoring certain bodily functions, such as blood pressure, muscle tension, sweat production, and skin temperature, to learn to actively control them and therefore control stress. The PWA is connected to various machinery, none of which is invasive or painful. For example, muscle tension is gauged by placing a Velcro band around the forehead; skin temperature is monitored using a band worn on the finger. Each monitoring device tells a person when his stress is reduced by reflecting a change on the device.

The practitioner of biofeedback is taught to reduce his blood pressure, regulate his skin temperature, and so forth by means of learning a series of breathing techniques, muscle relaxation exercises, and skin temperature regulation techniques that must be practiced for 15 to 20 minutes twice a day. The person's practice is aided by audiotapes; home monitoring devices register physiological responses.

Biofeedback requires a time commitment to practice the techniques. Change does not happen overnight. Biofeedback can be costly, although if your biofeedback instructor is a doctor, you may be covered by your medical insurance. Credentials, like costs, vary greatly.

Colonic Irrigations

Caution: This adjunct therapy is noted to be of questionable safety due to the presence of fecal material.

During the process of normal digestion, food passes from the mouth down the esophagus, into the stomach, and through the small and large intestines before it is expelled from the rectum. Water is added to food by the stomach and small intestine during the process. The colon is the part of the large intestine that extends to the rectum. It transports the contents of the small intestine and moves them to the rectum by contracting spasmodically. The colon reabsorbs most of the water through its walls, yielding firm feces.

In *colonic* irrigation, a large amount of fluid is introduced into the colon via the rectum (in a process similar to receiving an enema) to fill the colon and flush it out. It is not intended to induce defecation, but rather to wash out materials and cleanse the walls of the intestines as high as the fluids will reach. Those who practice colonic irrigations believe that this washes their bodies clean of poisons.

There are two methods of performing colonic irrigations. In the first, a single tube is inserted into the rectum, filling the colon to capacity and then allowing the liquid to run out through the same tube. A second method uses two tubes, one for infusion of fluid and one for outflow. Sometimes a machine is used to provide water pressure to introduce the fluid. All tubes should be disposable—used once and then thrown away.

Colonic irrigations are not licensed. Some practitioners claim to be certified by various organizations that are self-regulated. Costs, length of time per treatment, and frequency of irrigations all vary.

Crystals

A crystal is a solid, inorganic substance with atoms or molecules in a regular, repeating, three-dimensional pattern. The exact pattern is what marks the shape of the crystal. Believers in the power of crystals say that different crystals represent help for different problems. For example, amethyst is said to help those with headaches and aid in balance, concentration, and calm. Clear quartz is said to be an all-around healer. Many believe that a crystal can be programmed by the owner to emit healing powers via their belief in it.

Crystals are sold as jewelry, or by the weight and quality of the particular stone. They can be worn, carried, or kept in the presence of the believer. Cost and quality vary.

Herbal Remedies

These folk recipes often have been passed down through families from generation to generation. Usually one must make a tea or a poultice out of the substance and then drink it or apply it to a specific area of the body. In excessive or inappropriate quantities, herbal remedies can sometimes cause untoward side effects—they can even be poisonous. Therefore, if you decide to try an herbal remedy, be sure to consult someone with expertise in this field (such as a nutritionist or a homeopathic doctor) and, as always, to check with your regular doctor to ensure that these substances won't harm you or interact with another treatment you may be undergoing.

Homeopathy

Homeopathy is a system of healing based on the theory that "like cures like." A specific substance is diluted to achieve the smallest amount of the substance that can be used to control a symptom. Only one substance or medicine is used at a time. Homeopathy is based on principles designed to bolster a body's natural protective mechanisms using "medicines" made of very dilute solutions of herbs, minerals, and animal and plant extracts. Homeopaths believe that physical symptoms are the body's way of trying to cure itself. For example, to homeopathic thinking, a runny nose and sneezing are the body's way of curing its own cold. Thus, if you cause the nose to run, you help the body to cure itself.

No school is accredited to teach homeopathy exclusively. Education is generally via national study groups. Some homeopaths are medical doctors with added training.

Hypnosis

Named for Hypnos, the Greek god of sleep, hypnosis is the passive, trancelike state that in some ways resembles sleep. During hypnosis, a person's perception of reality and memory are changed, increasing his responsiveness to suggestion. Hypnosis is usually induced by monotonous repetition of words or gestures while the PWA is completely relaxed. The ability to be hypnotized varies from person to person. Those who are unable to be put into a trance are usually very rigid, anxious, mistrusting, and uninventive personality types.

Self-hypnosis is easily learned, and through this technique, one can be taught to reduce stress, increase relaxation, overcome pain, and stop smoking. To learn self-hypnosis, seek out a psychiatrist, psychologist, or other therapist who is knowledgeable in this technique.

Often, insurance will pay for treatment by these professionals. The number and length of each session varies as does the cost. Many of those who teach and use hypnosis are not licensed or certified, nor are they physicians. Ask for qualifications.

Laughter/ Humor

Laughter and humor are known to defuse anger, decrease depression and stress, and act as a natural tranquilizer (i.e., laughing makes you tired, causing sleep). A good, strong belly laugh causes you to breathe deeply and expand your lungs and thus to take in more oxygen—in other words, it acts as a miniature *aerobic* workout. It is also believed that laughter can activate endorphins and thus relieve pain. It can cause beneficial changes in blood pressure, pulse, and skin temperature. All in all, laughing makes people feel more alive!

You can create a humor kit for laughter therapy complete with jokes, gags, and cartoons. Compile a humor library of your favorite funny books, videotapes, and audiocassettes. Keep a humor journal in which you record situations in which humor entered your life; what you and others have done to make you laugh; what you think is funny; and the funniest story, joke, or cartoon of the week. This therapy believes in aimless playfulness for its own sake.

Massage

This adjunct therapy involves the manipulation of soft tissue via stroking, rubbing, kneading, or tapping. Massage can increase circulation, improve muscle tone, and induce relaxation. Massage is performed either with bare hands or by mechanical means. Inflamed areas, open wounds, rashes, and tumor sites are avoided. Caution must also be exercised in cases of cardiac illness, diabetes, skeletal muscle conditions, and *phlebitis.*

There are many different types or schools of massage. They include:

- Rolfing. This is a form of deep manipulation using the elbows, knuckles, and fingers on the PWA's skin. It is said to be physically strenuous and can cause some minor pain.
- Shiatsu. Here, finger pressure is applied along specific points, as in acupuncture. This often causes minor discomfort.
- Swedish. This school of massage uses long, slow strokes and kneading friction on superficial muscle layers. It is said to be not painful.
- Reflexology. Performed mostly on the palms of the hands and the soles of the feet, this type of massage applies pressure to specific points to relax many areas of the body. It may cause some minor pain.
- Acupressure. This is an oriental form of massage that uses pressure on specific sites to help relax tense areas.

Cost, number of massages, length of sessions, and the abilities of masseuses vary. Some use oils or lotions to augment the effects of their work. Research the type of massage therapy you wish to try and find a reputable practitioner. Licensure varies from state to state. Some chiropractors are also kinesiologists, that is, specialists in the study of muscles and movement.

Meditation

Meditation is a state of consciousness in which the individual tries to stop his awareness of his surroundings and his internal dialogue so that his mind can focus on a single sound, word, thought, or image. Meditation is a self-induced state of rest and relaxation without sleep, during which you temporarily turn off the outside world. It is also an attempt to quiet a chattering mind.

Through meditation, after time, you improve your ability to handle stress, lower your blood pressure, normalize your pulse, increase your pain threshold, relax your breathing, and center yourself. You are capable of reaching a place that is peaceful, silent, and calm within yourself.

To meditate, you close your eyes and sit or lie quietly in a quiet, comfortable atmosphere. You breathe deeply and become aware of your heart beating and your breaths coming calmly and regularly, as you focus on one sound or word.

Meditation must be practiced at home and takes time to become adept at. Learning meditation can be accomplished through a center or an instructor. Practitioners are not licensed. There is no regulation of costs, number of sessions, or length of sessions.

Paced Breathing

This is a method of breathing akin to what is taught to expectant mothers in childbirth education classes. It is easily done and can induce a state of relaxation.

Paced breathing involves sitting comfortably and closing your eyes. You then slowly breathe in through your nose for three to four seconds, hold the breath for less than a second, and then breathe out through your mouth or nose for another count of three to four seconds. This is repeated for as many cycles as is desired.

Once this is mastered, the next step is to attempt diaphragmatic breathing. Place your hand on your abdomen near your belly button. Slowly breathe in and out as before, but using this technique, your chest should not rise and fall. Instead, your abdomen will move in and out with each breath, as singers are trained to do.

Eventually, this type of breathing will permit you to feel calm and relaxed, as you concentrate on your breathing and clear your mind of its worries.

Relaxation Exercises

Here are some examples of relaxation exercises that combine paced breathing with meditation techniques:

1. Sit quietly in a comfortable position in a place where there should be few distractions. A good time of day to attempt this is before breakfast or dinner, when digestion won't interfere. Make sure to take off your glasses, loosen your clothing, and attend to any physical needs that might be distracting—an itch, a need to go to the bathroom, and so on. If distractions do occur, try to ignore them by not dwelling on them.
2. Close your eyes.
3. Relax all of your muscles.
4. Breathe naturally, in through the nose and out through the mouth. Inhale and exhale, counting silently after each exhalation—"one" ... "two" ... "three"—up until ten, then begin counting again.
5. Set a limit on the time you'll meditate, say, 20 minutes, but don't use an alarm clock to end the session. It may cause you to tense up again. Once you are finished, sit quietly for a few minutes before resuming your activities.

Religion

It is impossible to explain religion in just a paragraph or two. In general, religion describes the ability to believe in something or someone—a power greater than ourselves—that can be called upon for answers and strength when life becomes difficult. Those who have abandoned the religious or spiritual side of their lives often may find that they want to return to it for comfort when confronted with immense problems.

In prayer we seek out the all-embracing relationship by expressing what we feel (anger, doubt, fear, joy, and our needs). We are assured that we are heard and loved. We pray for guidance and to know the will of a supreme being. We listen for answers, for a message, for statements of truth and enlighten-ment. We read and memorize. Some who are religious embrace symbols of their beliefs (pictures, prayer books, a crucifix, rosary beads, tefillin, a tallis, or a mezuzah). Through religion, we seek out clergy to talk, to gain support, and to offer service to help others.

Those who are religious believe that our psychological and physical beings are also interwoven with a spiritual being, and that the strength of the individual is directly related to the strength of the weave.

Therapeutic Touch

Therapeutic touch is a healing modality that is performed by rearranging the energy patterns of the ill person via the concentration and meditation of the PWA and the person trained to perform the therapeutic touch. The performer of therapeutic touch keeps her hands approximately 6 inches above the PWA's body *never touching* it as she works from the problem area outward in an attempt to cast away the pain. Therapeutic touch is said to reduce pain and muscle tension in the ill individual.

Although there are no formal licenses or state regulations, one can sometimes be certified in therapeutic touch by organizations who hold all-day or weekend seminars in this type of therapy. Cost for training varies, as does cost for receiving treatment.

Visualization/ Guided Imagery

Visualization and guided imagery are not exactly the same, but are often mistaken for each other. With visualization, you might form a mental picture of your ideal self—how you want to be: healthy and free of disease. You can also picture yourself killing off your illness or guiding the hands of your physician toward a cure. Other visualizations might include picturing an alter ego who can be ill in place of your true self, or pictures of your blood cell counts rising to normal range. You might visualize a particular treatment working for you.

The idea is to create a self-fulfilling prophecy. Your body is not supposed to be able to distinguish between the vivid mental picture you have conjured up and the actual reality. Thus, the images chosen must be of your own creation and must be believed by you to be possible. (See example in the box below.)

Guided imagery is used to induce a state of calm and relaxation. It takes one on a mental journey to a safe, comfortable, peaceful, and soothing place.

An Exercise in Visualization

1. On a white piece of paper held vertically, draw a crayon picture of yourself, your treatment, your disease, and your white cells eliminating the disease. Use all the colors of the rainbow as well as black, white, and brown. This picture is to be used to help in healing yourself.
2. On a second piece of white paper, held horizontally, draw a picture of any scene taken from your reality or your dreams. Again, use crayon to bring out all of the colorful images in your imagination.
3. A third picture can be drawn of your home, your family, loved ones, or other additional images that call forth material from the unconscious.
4. Concentrate on these pictures to aid in your visualization process.

Guided Imagery: A Guide to a Safe Place

1. Find a quiet place and sit or lie down in comfort.
2. Close your eyes.
3. Breathe slowly and quietly. Listen to the sound of your own breathing.
4. After a few minutes, picture that your mind is a black screen with nothing on it—like a screen in a movie theater with no picture. No one and nothing is there. Just darkness.
5. Continue to breathe slowly. As you see the blackness, you will eventually stop listening to the sound of your breathing.
6. On the black screen, picture a place from your past, any place that makes you laugh and feel safe and happy. Picture this place in detail—be it the mountains, the sea, a room, a house, a car, or the beach. Picture it with no people at first.
7. Now put yourself in the picture. See yourself looking around. See the shapes and colors in this picture. Experience how vivid they are. Feel the textures and temperatures within the scene. Take your time. Run your hands over the objects in the place you picture. Imagine whether they feel hot, cold, smooth, rough, soft. Remember this place in all its detail and slowly remember how it felt to be there.
8. After a few minutes, hear the sounds of where you are: the trees rustling in the wind, the birds or crickets chirping, water rushing to the shore, or the music of a symphony orchestra lulling you.
9. Now smell its odors: flowers, grass, salt water, home-baked cookies.
10. Take it all in: the sights, the sounds, the textures, the tastes, and the smells.
11. Let the feeling of peace, calm, and joy wash over you from your head down your neck; to your shoulders, chest, back, hands, fingers, stomach, thighs; down your legs and to your feet and toes.
12. Slowly become aware of your breathing again, rhythmic and calm. Experience the sensation of peace and serenity.
13. After a few minutes, open your eyes and stretch in place as you slowly stop listening to the sounds of your breathing.

It calls upon the right hemisphere of the brain, which is believed to be responsible for your visual life, and uses your imagination to create a safe haven.

Guided imagery techniques may also be used to picture disease and attack it; however, in this case the PWA opens his eyes to a tense feeling rather than a peaceful one. (See the box above for an example of a guided imagery exercise.)

In both guided imagery and visualization audiotapes, purchased or made by yourself or a friend, may be used to deliver instructions or guidance. Classes are also taught in these techniques. Information about them is often available through local AIDS service organizations. Costs, lengths of classes, and availability of instruction and tapes vary. Often tapes can be purchased at book, music, or video stores.

Home Safety, Comfort, and Hygiene Checklist

This checklist has been adapted from tools used by occupational therapists to evaluate the homes of their clients for safety and equipment needs. We suggest that the PWA and caregiver use it to inspect the PWA's living space (and working space, if applicable) so that the necessary changes to these environments can be made to maximize safety and comfort.

Instructions: Assess each of the following factors in the PWA's environment. Then work with health care personnel and other resources in the community to make any necessary changes.

I. Access to the Home/Office
   A. Main Entrance
      1. Steps?
         Number of steps ————
         Height of steps ————
      2. Ramp?
      3. Handrails?
      4. Elevator accessible?
      5. PWA able to open all doors and locks?

II. Living/Working Area
   A. Floor Plan and Furniture Arrangement
      1. Hallways and walkways free of obstructions?
      2. Loose carpeting tacked down?
      3. Doorsills even with the floor?
   B. Lighting
      1. Adequate lighting, including night-lights?
      2. Light switches accessible?
   C. Furniture: Sofa, chair, and desk comfortable for PWA to sit in, work in, and rise from?
   D. Electrical Appliances
      1. Electrical cords in good condition?
      2. Electrical cords stowed behind furniture or tacked down?
      3. Electrical sockets not overloaded?
      4. Television, radio, telephone, clocks accessible?

E. Climate Control
   1. PWA able to open/close windows?
      a. For confused PWAs, windows locked and/or window guards installed?
   2. PWA able to operate thermostat for central heating and/or air conditioning?
   3. Steampipes/radiators insulated?
   4. Asbestos present?

III. Bedroom
  A. General
    1. Doorways and walkways passable?
    2. Carpets, rugs, heavy draperies, and other dust collectors removed if the PWA has respiratory illnesses?
    3. Night table/lamp/telephone/television controls accessible?
    4. PWA able to open dresser drawers and closets?
    5. PWA able to dress and change linens?
  B. Bed
    1. Stable bed?
    2. Height of bed appropriate?
    3. Mattress comfortable with good support?
    4. Hospital bed necessary?

IV. Bathroom
  A. General
    1. Entrance and walkway passable?
    2. Rugs and bathmats properly secured against slipping?
    3. Light switch accessible?
  B. Commode
    1. Toilet seat accessible?
    2. Toilet paper within reach?
    3. PWA able to flush?
  C. Sink
    1. PWA able to reach basin?
    2. PWA able to turn faucets?
    3. Hot water turned down for confused or diabetic PWAs?
    4. PWA able to reach soap and towels?
    5. PWA able to wash, brush teeth, shave, comb hair, trim nails?
  D. Vanity/Medicine Chest
    1. PWA able to reach medicine chest?
    2. For confused PWAs, childproof locks on medicine chest and bottles?
    3. PWA able to reach mirror, comb, toothpaste, etc.?
  E. Bathtub/Shower
    1. PWA able to climb in and out of tub?
    2. PWA able to sit down and stand up in tub?
    3. Shower present?

    4. Shower chair or bathtub chair necessary?

    5. PWA able to turn faucets, drain and fill tub?

    6. For confused or diabetic PWA, hot water turned down?

    7. Nonskid rubber mats present?

    8. Grab bars present?

    9. PWA able to reach soap, towels, shampoo, face cloth?

V. Kitchen

  A. Stove/Oven

    1. PWA able to reach and manipulate oven interior, burners, and controls?

    2. For confused PWAs, safety devices in place?

    3. PWA able to reach and manipulate pots and utensils?

    4. Special implements necessary?

  B. Sink

    1. PWA able to reach basin (to the bottom) and faucets?

    2. Dishwashing supplies accessible?

    3. Dishwasher accessible, PWA able to load, empty, and operate?

  C. Cabinets

    1. PWA able to reach, open, and close cabinets?

    2. For confused PWAs, childproof locks present?

    3. Dishes, glasses, utensils, and other commonly used items within reach?

    4. Knives and other sharp items safely stored away?

  D. Refrigerator/Freezer

    1. PWA able to open, close; remove and replace food?

    2. Stale food removed?

    3. Nutritious food available?

    4. Temperature settings adequate to maintain coolness?

  E. General

    1. Dining area accessible?

    2. Cutting boards, countertops, and other food areas clean?

    3. Floors clean and uncluttered?

VI. Laundry/Cleaning Facilities

  A. Washer/Dryer

    1. Washer/dryer present within the home?

    2. PWA able to open, close, load, empty, and operate?

  B. General

    1. Detergent, fabric softener, carts, and baskets available?

    2. PWA able to carry, sort, fold, and/or iron garments?

    3. PWA able to dust, sweep (or vacuum), mop, empty trash, etc?

VII. Fire/Emergency Provisions

  A. General

    1. Telephone and emergency numbers accessible?

    2. PWA able to call for assistance?

      3. Extra key with reliable friend, relative, neighbor?

      4. Police, fire department, and utilities know homebound and/or confused person lives there?

  B. Physical Safety

      1. PWA able to exit home two different ways (doors, windows, fire escapes)?

      2. Smoke detectors present (with fresh batteries)?

      3. Fire extinguisher present and able to be operated?

      4. Locks operate from both sides of the door?

Special Needs/Comments:

How to Move People Safely

Changing the position of an immobile PWA is key to maintaining good skin integrity as well as decreasing the possibility of muscle *atrophy* (wasting) and contractures (locking) of the joints. Position changes should take place every one to two hours. Even minor changes in position can help relieve pressure on areas of the body most prone to skin breakdown.

Special care must be taken not to injure yourself or the PWA when attempting a position change. Proper body mechanics (see the following section) for the caregiver are just as important as proper body alignment is for the PWA. Each move must be thought out before it is attempted, and all equipment must be within reach to minimize the chance of injury. When the PWA can move on his own but is too weak to do this all the time, the caregiver must encourage the PWA to be as independent as possible without being unsafe.

Proper positioning of a weak or immobile person takes practice; it is most easily accomplished when you are working with an alert, cooperative person. Remember to discuss all moves with the individual before you attempt them and to enlist his aid, if he is able. It is always more difficult to move and position someone who is lethargic, confused, or comatose. At the very least, for comatose, confused, or lethargic persons, inform them of the need for repositioning and explain each step along the way.

Be patient with yourself and with the PWA. Moving another human being is not easy, but it is possible. As you perform this task repeatedly, you will develop your own methods of mastering it, your own tricks and shortcuts. Share them with others to make the job of caregiving easier.

Proper Body Mechanics for the Caregiver When Lifting

What to Do

- Use the strength in your legs and thighs to lift. Bend at the knee. Lift the object and then straighten your legs.
- Avoid bending at the waist and lifting, as this places all the stress on your back and can cause injury.
- Use the strength in your arms to pull by grasping the item, backing up a few steps, and gradually moving closer while holding the new position. This technique utilizes your arms and legs rather than your back.

- Avoid twisting your back to one side or the other by facing the object or person to be moved. Jerking movements and/or sharp turns to the side can cause you pain and injury.
- Always place your feet comfortably apart to provide a stable base of support.

General Guidelines for Moving People

What to Do

- Begin any move by first discussing it with the PWA to be moved or repositioned.
- Move the PWA little by little, if necessary, until he is safe and comfortable. Don't attempt a move in one maneuver if it is difficult for you or uncomfortable for him.

What *Not* to Do

- Never move someone who is capable of moving himself. Offer assistance only.
- Do not attempt to move someone who is obviously too heavy for you. Get help if you are able. If no help is available, make the PWA as comfortable as possible without attempting to lift him.
- Do not attempt to move or reposition someone if he is fighting you. You will wind up injuring either yourself or him, or both of you.
- Do not begin moving until you have decided what the final position will be.
- Do not start until you have all of the necessary equipment within reach.

Equipment

To properly position someone, any or all of the following items may be necessary:

- Pillows. Soft ones are easier to work with because they conform to the curvatures of the PWA's body.
- Wheelchair or sturdy chair with two arms.
- Foot stool or footrest.
- Chuck or flat sheet. Used to make a "pull sheet" to help pull the PWA up in bed or to turn him from side to side.

Repositioning a PWA

When repositioning someone, first decide where he is moving to. Is he turning from one side to the other in bed? Is he going from a sitting to a reclining position? Is he moving from the bed to the chair?

Basic Positions

- *Flat on the back with legs slightly separated.* In this position, the head may be slightly elevated, flat, or turned to one side. The feet may also be slightly elevated or the knees bent.
- *Turned on one side.* Here, the knees may be straight, slightly bent, or bent as in a fetal position. The arms may be out in front; one may be positioned along the body or slightly behind it. The head may be flat or slightly raised.
- *Sitting upright in bed.* The feet extend straight out in front or are slightly elevated.
- *Sitting with the legs dangling over one side of the bed.* This should only be attempted when a PWA can sit without support to his back for a period of time.
- *Sitting in a chair or wheelchair.* The legs dangle or are elevated.

Pulling a PWA Up in Bed

Assess the need for the PWA to be pulled up in bed by determining his comfort level and by observing whether he is slumped over or hanging over the edge of the bed.

What to Do

With Only One Caregiver

1. Have a pull sheet in position under the PWA. If it is not already in place, do so now (follow the instructions in the box below).
2. Encourage the PWA to bend both knees and plant his feet flat on the bed if he is able.
3. Position yourself behind the head of the bed. Reach down and grasp the pull sheet on either side of the PWA at shoulder level.

Placing a Pull Sheet under a PWA

1. Roll up a flat sheet or chuck halfway and place it alongside the PWA's body with the rolled-up side nearest to him and the still open side closest to you.
2. Turn the PWA to one side, carefully protecting his head and neck. **The best method is to place one of your hands at his shoulders and the other at his sacrum or buttocks.** Now, gently push him onto his side.
3. Balance the PWA by supporting him with one hand. With the other hand, push the pull sheet partially under him as far as it will go.
4. Assist the PWA back into a flat position, then move to the other side and again help him onto his opposite side while pulling the pull sheet out from under him and unrolling it. The pull sheet is now in position under his body and you are ready to move him up in bed.

4. Have the PWA push with his feet on the count of "three" while you pull the sheet up to the head of the bed. Be careful not to hurt your back!

Note: In the event that a PWA cannot get out of bed to allow the linens to be changed, the procedure for making an occupied bed is the same as for placing a pull sheet except that you can layer a pull sheet on top of a regular full-sized flat sheet before rolling them under the PWA's torso. Tuck in the sheet corners as you normally would do.

With Two Caregivers

One caregiver stands on each side of the bed and grasps the pull sheet at the PWA's midsection. Jointly, they pull toward the head of the bed, lifting if possible, and taking care not to allow the PWA's head and neck to hyperextend (in other words, tilt backward).

Other Variations

- *If no pull sheet is available.* Stand behind the head of the bed and grasp the PWA under the armpits while he holds onto your arms (if able). This method, however, is not preferred, because the PWA will be sliding his bare skin along the bedsheets, thereby creating a shearing force that can damage skin integrity.
- *If the bed has side rails.* Always encourage the PWA to lift himself up in bed if able, while you offer assistance. He can grasp the top of the mattress to lift or use the side rails if he has a hospital bed. The PWA raises both arms over his head, grasps the side rails, and pulls himself up while pushing with his feet.
- *If there is a trapeze.* A strong PWA can grasp a trapeze and then lift his torso completely off the bed. Then, he can push himself up with his feet and lower himself back down in the new position. (A trapeze is a triangular piece of metal that is suspended above a hospital-style bed on a metal frame.)

Centering a PWA in Bed

Assess the need to center the PWA in bed; for example, when he is too close to the edge or when you wish to turn him to his other side.

What to Do

1. Place a pull sheet under the PWA. Then, move the PWA's legs in unison to the center of the bed.
2. Next, move the PWA's head and shoulders, either by placing one hand under the PWA's head or under his pillow. Reach the other hand across the PWA's chest and grasp him under the shoulder. Then move head, neck, and shoulders to the center of the bed as far as is comfortable for the PWA.
3. Now grasp the pull sheet and pull toward the caregiver until the PWA is centered in bed.
4. Repeat these steps as frequently as is necessary until the PWA is centered.

If no pull sheet is available, proceed as described except instead of grasping the pull sheet, either slide both hands under the PWA's torso or slide one hand under his torso and reach the other hand across his chest or abdomen to maneuver him to the center of the bed. **Remember that sliding along the sheet can cause shearing force and subsequent redness of the skin, so avoid this if possible and assess the PWA's skin frequently.**

Turning a PWA from His Back to His Side

Assess the need for repositioning. For example, is the PWA uncomfortable? Has he been in the same position for two hours or more? Do you need to move him to clean him?

What to Do

- Decide, with the PWA, into which position he will be moved.
- Encourage the PWA to move on his own while he directs you about how to help him.
- Have all necessary equipment handy, such as pillows to place behind his back for support.
- Place a pull sheet beneath the PWA's torso if one is not already in position (see the box describing how to do this).
- Place the PWA flat in bed without any pillows under his head.
- Choose one of the following methods for turning the PWA from his back to one side.

Method 1: Pulling

1. Stand on the side the PWA wishes to turn onto. Reach across his torso to grasp the pull sheet from the other side. Pull it toward your body until the PWA is on his side.
2. Hold the PWA in position with one hand while placing a pillow behind his back for support.
3. Next, comfortably position a pillow under his head and the shoulder that is against the mattress. Always take special care to protect the head and neck. Be sure that the arm closest to the mattress is not trapped beneath the PWA's body. Prevent him from rolling back by tucking the pillow slightly beneath his back. Two or three pillows may be needed for support and comfort.
4. Now attend to the PWA's legs. Either place them straight (but separated to prevent pressure sores) or bend them slightly at the knees with a pillow between the legs.

Method 2: Pushing

1. Stand on the side opposite the one that the PWA will face when turned.
2. Grasp the pull sheet and push the PWA onto his side, placing pillows behind the back and buttocks for support. Position him as described in Method 1.

Method 3: If No Pull Sheet Is Available

1. Stand on the side opposite the side to which the PWA will be turned. For example, if turning from the back onto the left side, the caregiver stands on the PWA's right.
2. Place the PWA's right leg over the left and the right arm across the chest. Turn the PWA's head to the left. Encourage the PWA to do this himself if able. If you have a bed with side rails, have the PWA grasp the left rail with his right hand.
3. Now place one of your hands at the shoulder blades and one under the buttocks or hips. Push the person to the left side.
4. Place pillows behind the back for support and carefully position the PWA's head, arms, shoulders, and legs.

Assisting a PWA from a Bed to a Chair or a Chair to a Bed

What to Do

- Decide which chair will be used. It is advised that you use either a wheelchair or a sturdy nonmobile chair with arms. Place it alongside the bed facing the foot of the bed. If you are using a wheelchair, apply its brakes.
- Decide if padding such as a pillow or foam seat cushion will be placed on the chair seat. In addition, consider putting a waterproof pad or chuck on the seat to protect it from soiling.
- Place a flat sheet over the chair, to be used to lift the PWA back into bed if you suspect that the PWA will be too weak to return to bed and more than one caregiver is present to lift him. (See information for two or more caregivers.)
- To begin the process, have the PWA try to get into a sitting position on his own with you assisting as needed.
- Have the PWA sit on the side of the bed with his legs dangling for a few moments before attempting transfer into a chair. This permits him to gain balance and avoid lightheadedness from a sudden shift in blood pressure. You may have to assist him in moving his legs over the side of the bed by grabbing them in unison with one of your hands while keeping the PWA upright with the other. If the PWA has an electric hospital-style bed, use the controls to raise the head of the bed until the PWA is in a sitting position. Then help him to turn by moving both of his legs in unison as described above.
- Help the PWA to the edge of the bed until his feet are flat on the floor but he is still seated.
- Apply the brakes on the wheelchair if you are using one.

With Only One Caregiver

- Place your feet comfortably apart but firmly on the floor to give you balance and a secure stance. Place one leg on the side of the PWA's nearest the chair and the other leg between his legs. This will give you a base of support if the PWA's knees buckle.

- Have the PWA place his arms around your neck and shoulders. Place your arms around his torso in a bear hug. Bend your knees slightly.
- Lift the PWA up from a sitting to a standing position by straightening your knees and holding the PWA tightly. This allows your legs and thighs to carry the burden rather than your back.
- Pivot yourself and the PWA until the backs of his knees are against the chair.
- Bend your knees until the PWA is in a sitting position.
- Have the PWA place his feet flat on the floor in front of him to help him sit farther back into the chair. Stand behind him and grasp him under his arms. Have him push back while you pull up.
- Always leave the PWA with a method of calling for assistance and check him frequently.
- Have frequently needed items within reach. For example, have tissues, the telephone, and urinal nearby.
- Encourage the PWA to shift positions within his chair often, and assist him in doing so.
- To return to bed, make sure the chair's brakes are applied, then simply reverse the procedure. In other words, have the PWA slide to the edge of the chair with his feet planted firmly on the ground. Position yourself in front of him, feet comfortably apart and firmly on the ground. The PWA's arms should be around your neck and shoulders. Your arms should be around his chest in a bear hug and your knees should be bent. When you are ready, straighten your knees while holding them tightly. Stand, pivot toward the bed, and when the bed is touching his knees, bend your knees until the PWA is sitting on the edge. Make sure he is seated securely before letting go. Assist the PWA in lifting his legs onto the bed if necessary, and guide his upper body comfortably onto the mattress.

With Two or More Caregivers to Return the PWA to Bed

- Use a flat sheet that has been previously placed in the chair under the PWA. Have him place his legs together (cross his ankles) and his hands in his lap.
- One caregiver stands behind the chair and grasps the sheet on either side of the PWA's shoulders. The other caregiver grasps the sheet at the level of the PWA's thighs. Together, in unison, they lift the PWA using the sheet and place him in bed.
  Note: This is *not* the preferred method of transferring from chair to bed, because of the possibility of injury to the caregivers' backs, the risk of dropping the ill individual, and the clumsy manner in which one must lower the PWA into bed. However, it is often a necessary alternative to pivoting.

What Not to Do

- Never sit a comatose or very lethargic PWA in a chair.
- Never leave a confused, lethargic, or otherwise unsafe PWA in a chair unattended. Use a vest restraint (sometimes called a posey) to prevent falls.
- Do not leave the PWA in a chair for periods of time that exceed his ability to sit up. Assist him back to bed if he gets sleepy or is uncomfortable.

APPENDIX F

Preparing for Hospitalization

What to Take to the Hospital

1. A bag or small suitcase packed with
   - glasses or contact lens supplies
   - toothbrush and toothpaste
   - comb, brush, and shampoo
   - makeup, if desired
   - disposable razor, charged shaver (some hospitals do not allow you to use electrical outlets), and battery
   - pajamas, nightgown, robe, slippers, socks and underwear
   - books to read
   - a small amount of money for purchasing newspaper, renting a television, etc.
2. A list of all medications you are currently taking, including doses and schedules for each.
3. A list of all of your allergies to foods, medications, and contrast dyes.
4. The name and telephone number of your health care proxy, medical power of attorney, or someone to be contacted in the event of an emergency.
5. A copy of your health care proxy and/or durable medical power of attorney.
6. A brief description of your medical history (it's good to keep this with you wherever you go).

Whom to Tell, and What to Tell

1. Inform your *significant other* and ask that he call others who you feel need to know of your hospitalization. Provide the primary caller with the necessary names and telephone numbers.
2. Be sure to inform the person who holds your health care proxy and/or durable medical power of attorney, if applicable.
3. Notify your employer or supervisor.
4. Let the insurance company know you are in the hospital, if applicable.

For all persons to be informed, include the name of the hospital, the address and telephone number for the facility, and your room number. Be sure you convey to those who will know about your hospital stay how you feel about receiving calls and visitors. Encourage your visitors to follow the hospital rules for visiting hours and for the number of visitors allowed at the same time (usually two). Remember: Most hospitals don't allow children to visit you in your room, but some will permit you to visit with them in a patient lounge or in the lobby.

Hospital "No-Nos"

1. Never bring large amounts of cash or expensive jewelry with you. Hospitals assume no responsibility for these items when left in your room. Consider placing these things with the admissions or cashier's office. You will be given a receipt and can get your items back upon discharge. Think about sending these items home with your significant others for safekeeping.
2. Leave your cigarettes at home. Most hospitals do not allow smoking.
3. Most hospitals don't permit you to bring in and use electrical items, such as blow dryers, shavers, or fans. Battery-powered ones are fine.
4. Do not bring or take any medications, even Tylenol, without permission from your doctor. Let your nurse know if you do so.

APPENDIX **G**

Where to Seek Additional Help

This section lists national and international organizations that have services relating to AIDS. There are also many organizations at the local level, particularly in areas where AIDS is prevalent, such as the east and west coasts and major cities. Call or write to the health department, gay organizations, and government offices in your city and state for additional contacts and information.

Most of the telephone numbers in this section are 800 (toll-free) numbers. For all others, the state is given after the number.

AIDS (General)

The American Association of Physicians for Human Rights
To locate a physician who is HIV positive or who is interested in and willing to treat gays and PWAs, contact:
(415) 255-4547 (California)

American Foundation for AIDS Research (AMFAR)
(800) 392-6327

Centers for Disease Control and Prevention National AIDS Clearinghouse
(800) 458-5231
For the deaf: (800) 243-7012

Hyacinth Foundation
(800) 433-0254
This group sponsors the following confidential programs: a hotline, buddy services, support groups, individual and family therapy, legal and advocacy services, and general AIDS education.

National AIDS Hotline
Prerecorded general information: (800) 342-2437
Spanish: (800) 344-7432
Hearing impaired: (800) 243-7889

PWA Coalition Hotline
(212) 645-4538 (New York)
This group provides current information on traditional, holistic, and alternative treatments, support groups, meal programs, and counseling from one PWA to another. The PWA Coalition also puts out printed materials, including their *Newsline* and *SIDAhora* (in Spanish).

Blindness

American Council of the Blind
(800) 424-8666
This group maintains a clearinghouse of information on where to obtain low-vision devices, treatment, large-print educational materials, and so on.

American Foundation for the Blind
(800) 232-5463
New York State residents: (212) 620-2147
This organization provides services to the blind and their families and publishes a catalog of free publications and products.

National Association for the Visually Handicapped
(212) 889-3141 (New York)
This group distributes more than a thousand free book titles in large print and provides referrals to low-vision services in your area.

National Library Services for the Blind and Physically Handicapped
(800) 424-8567

Cancer

American Cancer Society
(800) ACS-2345
The American Cancer Society funds cancer research; it also offers support groups, provides information, helps to arrange transportation, and supplies home care items.

National Cancer Institute
(800) 4-CANCER
This governmental agency provides free printed and telephone information on the latest developments in cancer research and treatment.

Death and Dying

American Association of Suicidology
(303) 692-0985 (Colorado)
This organization provides information concerning suicide prevention.

Choice in Dying (formerly the Society for the Right to Die)
(212) 366-5540 (New York)
This group focuses on issues related to the care of the terminally ill and the rights of the dying to make decisions concerning life support and similar issues. It will send you a living will appropriate for your state.

Hemlock Society
>(503) 342-5748 (Oregon)
>This group was founded to campaign for the right of the terminally ill to end their lives peacefully, painlessly, and legally. It also provides copies of living wills and durable powers of attorney for health care for a small fee.

Make Today Count, Inc.
>(314) 346-6644 (Missouri)
>This organization provides information and emotional support to people with life-threatening ailments and to their loved ones and caregivers. It runs workshops and a buddy system, arranges home and hospital visits, helps with transportation, and publishes a newsletter with information for caregivers.

Diabetes

American Diabetes Association
>(800) 232-3472
>This national organization provides information about the disease as well as practical tips, such as recipes for food that complies with your exchange diet.

The Diabetic Food Emporium
>To order a catalogue: (800) 285-3210
>This is a New Jersey-based mail order company that specializes in foods for diabetics. All products are sugar-free; many are low salt as well. The concept is to allow diabetics more variety and more exotic foods than they would normally find in the local supermarket. Included are jams, cake mixes, salad dressings, prepared foods, and esoteric seasonings.

National Diabetes Information Clearinghouse
>For a list of free publications: (301) 468-2162 (Maryland)
>This is a branch of the National Institute of Health, offering information to people with diabetes and their caregivers.

Drug and Clinical Trials Information

AIDS Drug Assistance Program
>(800) 542-2437
>Applicants are eligible for free AZT, pentamidine, alpha interferon, Bactrim, leucovorin, dapsone, fansidar, acyclovir, DHPG, nystatin, fluconazole, clotrimazole, and ketoconazole.

AIDS Prescription Project
>(800) 227-1195
>Call this number to find out how to eliminate prescription costs by obtaining medications free of charge if you are in financial need.

Government-Sponsored Drug Trials
>AIDS Clinical Trials Information Service (ACTTS)
>(800) TRIALS-A Call Monday-Friday 9 A.M.-7 P.M. EST
>Bilingual: (800) 874-2572

Project Inform
>(800) 822-7422
>This group maintains information for and from PWAs concerning conventional medical treatment and experimental therapies.

Gay and Bisexual Organizations

Gay Men's Health Crisis (GMHC)
>(212) 807-6655 (New York)
>Hearing impaired: (212) 645-7470 (New York)
>This organization develops and distributes materials addressing the various aspects of AIDS; it also conducts seminars for health professionals and the general public. GMHC provides counseling, buddy programs, and support groups for PWAs and partners; addresses pediatric issues; and offers advice on legal and financial matters. GMHC is open to all—whether you are gay or straight and whether you have AIDS, are HIV positive, or are just interested in learning more about this illness.

Hemophilia

Hemophilia Association of New York
>(212) 682-5510 (New York)
>The AIDS program exists to serve hemophiliacs affected by HIV and their families. Services include advocacy, counseling, support groups, patient networking, camps for children and teens, financial assistance, and information and referral via this 24-hour hotline.

National Hemophilia Foundation
>Hemophilia and AIDS Network for the Dissemination of Information (HANDI): (212) 431-8541 (New York)
>Maintains a library of research materials, resources, and literature concerning AIDS and hemophilia.

Insurance and Government Assistance

Medicaid
> Check the Blue Pages of your phone book under "State Government."

Medicare
> (800) 638-6833

State Insurance Department
> Handles grievances, questions, and concerns about health insurance coverage. Specific numbers vary from state to state. Check your phone book under "State Government."

U.S. Social Security Administration
> Check the Blue Pages of your phone book under "Federal Government Agencies" for the regional office nearest you.
> Social Security Information: (800) 772-1213

Veteran's Administration
> Check the Blue Pages of your phone book under "Federal Government Agencies" for the appropriate number for your area.

International AIDS Organizations

AIDS Committee of Toronto
> c/o Hessle Free Clinic
> 556 Church Street—2nd Floor
> Toronto, Ontario
> Canada M4V 2E3
> (416) 340-2437

AIDS Network of Edmonton
> 11303 102nd Ave.
> Edmonton, Alberta
> Canada T5K 0P6
> (403) 426-1516

AIDS Policy Coordinator
> Jon Kvan Wigngaarden, MD
> Buro G.V.O.
> Prins Hendriklaan 12
> 1075 BB
> Amsterdam, Netherlands
> 011-31-20 671-2815

Association des Gais Medecins
45 rue Sedaine
Paris, France 75011
011-33-1-48-058171

Capitol Gay
38 Mount Pleasant
London, England MC1XOAP
011-44-71-738-7010

Centretown Community Resources
100 Argyle Avenue
Ottawa, Ontario
Canada K2P 1B6
(613) 741-6025

Comite SIDA du Quebec
3757 rue Prud'homme
Montreal, Quebec
Canada H4A 3H8
(514) 282-9991

Dying With Dignity
175 St. Clair Ave. West
Toronto, Ontario
Canada M4V 1P7
(416) 486-3998

Gay Social Services Project
5 rue Weredde Park
Montreal, Quebec
Canada H3A 145
(514) 931-8668

Vancouver PWA Society
1447 Hornby Street
Vancouver, British Columbia
Canada V6Z 1W8
(604) 683-3381

Lobbying Groups, Legal Services, and Discrimination Issues

AIDS Coalition to Unleash Power (ACT/UP)
(212) 564-AIDS ([212] 564-2437) (New York)

Lambda Legal Defense and Education Fund, Inc.
   (212) 995-8585 (New York)
   This New York-based organization provides legal aid and referrals.

Mental Health

The Humor Project
   (518) 587-8770 (New York)

The Society for Psychological Study of Gay and Lesbian Issues Association of Gay and Lesbian Psychologists
   (202) 336-5500 (Washington, D.C.)

Stress Regulation Institute
   (212) 288-9309 (New York)
   Staff are available Tuesday and Thursday from 9:30 A.M. to 6:00 P.M. and Wednesday from 2 to 6 P.M. At other times, an answering service picks up and will pass along your message so that someone from the Institute will call you back.

Minorities

National Minority AIDS Council
   (800) 669-5052

Nursing and Home Care

Hospice Education Institute
   Hospice link: (800) 331-1620

National Association for Home Care/Foundation for Hospice and Home Care
   (202) 547-7424 (Washington, D.C.)
   This organization assists people in setting up home care and makes referrals to hospices. It offers printed materials for consumers and provides names of home health care agencies.

National Hospice Organization
   (800) 658-8898
   This organization provides information about hospice services available in your area.

Visiting Nurses' Association of America
        (800) 426-2547

Nutrition

National Association of Meal Programs
        (202) 547-6157 (Washington, D.C.)
        This Washington-based association provides home-delivered meals and/
        or will refer you to an organization in your community that provides this
        service.

National Center for Nutrition and Dietetics of the American Dietetic
        Association
        (800) 366-1655
        This is the professional organization of all registered dietitians. Call their
        Consumer Nutrition Hotline at the number above to speak to a nutrition
        specialist about food and health, to receive brochures related to nutrition,
        or for a directory of registered dietitians in your locale.

Safety

American Heart Association
        (800) 242-8721
        This group offers CPR training courses and certification.

American Red Cross
        (202) 737-8300 (Washington, D.C.)
        The American Red Cross is a national service organization focusing on
        health and safety issues. It offers classes in CPR and stress management
        as well as publishes many brochures on a variety of subjects of interest to
        PWAs and their caregivers. These includes AIDS-specific information and
        leaflets on more general subjects, like safety in the home. **The Greater
        NY Chapter offers a home nursing course for AIDS caregivers. Call
        for information at:** (212) 787-1000, ext. 8200.

The Safety Zone
        (800) 999-3030
        This company carries products for safety in the home or car, while trav-
        eling, and so on, items that might be difficult to find in surgical supply,
        department, or discount stores. Call the number above to obtain a cata-
        logue, to order from the catalogue, or for the location of a store near you.

Sexuality

National Sexually Transmitted Disease Hotline, American Social Health Association (a division of the Centers for Disease Control and Prevention)
(800) 227-8922

Sex Information and Education Council of the United States (SEICUS)
(212) 819-9770 (New York)
This organization serves as an advocacy group and a clearinghouse for information that includes an annotated bibliography, publications, lists of organizations providing referrals to qualified sex therapists, and a unique research library and database.

Spiritual and Religious Guidance

Check your local telephone directory for appropriate organizations in your area.

Substance Abuse

Alcoholics Anonymous
Check your local telephone directory for chapters in your area.

Narcotics Anonymous
24-hour hotline: (800) 992-0401

Women and AIDS

Boston Women's Health Book Collective
(617) 625-0271 (Massachusetts)
This is a public information center that contains national and international publications concerning women's health and other issues pertaining to women. It has prepared packets of information on women and AIDS, which are available for a small fee.

Holistic Health for Women and AIDS Testing Service (formerly the Women's AIDS Project)
(213) 650-1508 (California)

National Women's Health Network
>   (202) 347-1140 (Washington, D.C.)
>   A national organization devoted exclusively to women and health, it publishes a newsletter as well as special news alerts concerning issues that require immediate attention. Both are available to members.

The San Francisco AIDS Foundation (formerly the Women's AIDS Network)
>   (415) 864-5855 (California)

The Caregiver's Bookshelf: Suggestions for Further Reading

Books

About AIDS

Callaway, C. Wayne, M.D., with Catherine Whitney. *Surviving with AIDS: A Comprehensive Program of Nutritional Co-Therapy*. Boston: Little, Brown, 1991.

Johnson, Earvin "Magic." *What You Can Do to Avoid AIDS*. New York: Random House, 1992.

Mikluscak-Cooper, Cindy, R.N., and Emmett E. Miller, M.D. *A 12 Step Approach for a Person Living in Hope: At Risk or Infected with HIV*. Berkeley, CA: Celestial Arts, 1991.

Moffatt, Bettyclare. *When Someone You Love Has AIDS*. New York: Penguin, 1986.

Rudd, Andrea, and Darien Taylor, eds. *Positive Women: Voices of Women Living with AIDS*. Second Story Publishers, 1992.

About Relationships

Brown, Marie Annette, and Gail M. Powell-Cope. *Caring for a Loved One with AIDS: The Experiences of Families, Lovers, and Friends*. Seattle: The University of Washington Press, 1992.

Isensee, Rik. *Love between Men: Enhancing Intimacy and Keeping Your Relationship Alive*. Englewood Cliffs, NJ: Prentice-Hall, 1990.

About Medications

The Physician's Desk Reference—47th ed. Oradell, NJ: Medical Economics Company, 1993.

About Adjunct and Experimental Therapies

Abrams, Donald, M.D., et al. *AIDS/HIV Treatment Directory*. Compiled and Published by the American Foundation for AIDS Research [AMFAR], 1993.

LaCroix, Nitya. *Learn Massage in a Weekend*. New York: Alfred A. Knopf, 1992.

About Practical Matters

Appel, Jens C., III, and F. Bruce Gentry. *The Complete Will Kit*. New York: John Wiley & Sons, 1990.

Barnett, Terry J. *Living Wills and More: Everything You Need to Ensure That All Your Medical Wishes Are Followed*. New York: John Wiley & Sons, 1992.

Enteen, Robert, Ph.D. *Health Insurance: How to Get It, Keep It, or Improve What You've Got*. New York: Paragon House, 1992.

About Dying

Ahrohheim, Judith, M.D., and Doron Weber. *Final Passages: Positive Choices for the Dying and Their Loved Ones*. New York: Simon & Schuster, 1992.

Froman, Paul Kent, Ph.D. *After You Say Goodbye: When Someone You Love Dies of AIDS*. Chronicle Books, 1992.

Humphry, Derek. *Final Exit: The Practicalities of Self-Deliverance and Assisted Suicide for the Dying*. New York: Dell Publishing, 1992.

Kübler-Ross, Elisabeth. *On Death and Dying*. New York: Macmillan, 1969.

Newsletters

AIDS Treatment News
(John James, Publisher)
P.O. Box 411256
San Francisco, CA 94141

The Body Positive
2095 Broadway—Suite 306
New York, NY 10023

GMHC's Treatment Issues
Department of Medical Information
129 West 20th Street
New York, NY 10011

PWA Newsline
PWA Coalition
31 West 26th Street–5th Floor
New York, NY 10010

Treatment Alternatives Project
  c/o the PWA Health Group
  150 West 26th Street
  Suite 201
  New York, NY 10003

Sources for Pamphlets, Videotapes, and Cassettes

The American Red Cross

Centers for Disease Control and Prevention National AIDS Clearinghouse

Gay Men's Health Crisis

State and Local Health Departments

Glossary

acquired immunodeficiency syndrome (AIDS)   A complex of opportunistic diseases, malignancies, and/or physical signs and symptoms indicating a malfunctioning of the immune system.

acupuncture   A therapy for relieving pain: fine needles are inserted into the skin at certain predetermined locations.

acute   Severe; having a rapid and intense onset.

aerobic   Referring to the presence or need of air or oxygen, as in exercise.

alopecia   Baldness or hair loss.

ampule   A vial or container for a liquid, solid, or gaseous substance.

analgesic   Drug that relieves pain.

anemia   Decreased number of red cells within the blood.

anergy   Lack of activity; an immune defect in which the body does not fight off foreign substances effectively.

anesthesia   The lack of normal sensation or awareness, especially to pain.

ankylosis   The "freezing" of a joint in place—often in an abnormal position and usually due to a destruction of cartilage or bone.

antibiotic   Any natural or synthetic substance that inhibits the growth of or destroys microorganisms; used to treat infections.

antibody   A substance that defends the body against bacteria, viruses, and other foreign bodies; developed in response to an invader; part of the immune system's antigen-antibody reaction.

anticoagulant   Usually a medication, this substance prevents or delays blood clotting.

anticonvulsant   A drug or treatment that prevents seizures or makes a seizure less severe.

antiemetic   A drug or treatment that stops or lessens nausea and/or vomiting.

antigen   A substance (usually a protein) that is foreign to the body and that induces the formation of antibodies; part of the antigen-antibody reaction of the immune system.

antihistamine   A substance that reduces the effect of chemicals called "histamines" that are made by the body in response to something it is allergic to.

antipyretic   A drug or treatment that reduces fever.

antiviral   A substance that destroys or weakens viruses.

anxiety　A feeling of apprehension, worry, uneasiness, or dread—especially of the future.

aphrodisiac　An agent or substance that increases sexual desire.

ARC (AIDS related complex)　An outdated term used to describe a pre-AIDS condition.

arrhythmia　Irregular rhythm; any change in the normal pattern of the heartbeat.

aspiration　Removal of fluids or gases by the application of suction (e.g., pulling back on a syringe to remove air bubbles before injecting).

asymptomatic　Without symptoms.

atrophy　A failure to grow or a withering.

autoimmune　A condition in which the body reacts against its own tissue—usually mounting an immune response against it.

autopsy　Examination of a corpse to determine the cause of death.

axillary　Referring to the underarm area.

barium　A contrast medium often used in X ray examinations.

benign　Not malignant; noncancerous.

biofeedback　A process of monitoring certain bodily functions—often with the goal of learning how to control them through learned relaxation techniques.

biopsy　Excision or removal of a piece of living tissue for microscopic examination; usually done to help establish a diagnosis.

bolus　An amount of a substance taken quickly and all at once, as in a dose of a drug that is injected intravenously.

bone marrow　The soft tissue inside the center of bones where red blood cells are made.

bronchi　Air structures in the lungs.

bronchodilator　A drug that relaxes airway structures (bronchi and bronchioles) within the lungs to improve breathing.

bronchoscopy　An examination of the lungs and bronchial tree; often used to diagnose lung problems, obtain sputum, tissue samples, and to remove foreign bodies.

calibration　Scale of measurement.

candidiasis　Infection of the skin or mucous membrane with a yeastlike fungus called *Candida albicans.*

CAT scan (computerized axial tomography)　A diagnostic test that uses X rays and a contrast dye to view the body in a series of cross-sectional slices.

catheter　A hollow, flexible tube that can be inserted into a blood vessel or other space in the body for the purpose of either removing or adding fluids.

cerebrospinal fluid　The fluid that bathes the brain and spinal cord.

cervical dysplasia　A precancerous condition with abnormal changes in the tissues covering the cervix.

cervix　The lowermost portion of the uterus; the part that extends into the vaginal cavity.

chemotherapy The use of chemicals or drugs in the treatment of disease, as in cancer.

chiropractor A person with the degree of Doctor of Chiropractic (D.C.); trained in the manipulation of the spinal column, physiotherapy, and nutrition. Chiropractors avoid the use of drugs and surgery.

chuck A disposable or reusable absorbent pad used for placement under an incontinent person (one who cannot control her bladder or bowels) to absorb body wastes.

clavicle Collarbone.

clone A group of cells or organisms with identical genes; an exact duplicate.

coinsurance A second insurance policy—usually from your spouse; also may refer to the portion of a fee that the subscriber pays because it is not covered by insurance.

colonic Pertaining to the lowermost portion of the large intestine (colon) that extends to the rectum.

colonoscopy A diagnostic test involving the passage of a scope into the rectum and up into the lower intestinal tract so that it may be viewed.

complement Complex proteins in the blood that bind with substances (antibodies) that defend the body against foreign invaders (antigens); part of the immune system response.

complete blood count (CBC) Microscopic examination of a sample of blood to discover the total number of red blood cells present and to measure the relative amount of hemoglobin they contain based on their size and shape.

condom A device made of latex rubber or lambskin and placed on the erect penis before sex; acts to prevent pregnancy and/or the spread of disease.

consumption The act of eating; also an outdated term for tuberculosis.

contagious Easily spread from one person to another, as in disease.

contaminated No longer clean or sterile.

contraceptive Any process, device, or drug that prevents conception and pregnancy.

contracture An abnormal condition of a joint caused by a shortening or wasting away of muscle fibers and/or by excessive scar tissue formation over a joint.

contraindication A factor that prohibits a certain activity or treatment for a specific person.

convulsion A sudden, violent, uncontrollable contraction of a group of muscles; also called a "seizure."

corticosteroid Any hormone made in the outer layer of the adrenal gland of humans that influences or controls key bodily functions; also made synthetically.

cryptococcosis A fungal infection that can involve any organ of the body but is most often seen in the brain.

cryptosporidiosis A type of parasite.

cyanosis Bluish discoloration of skin, lips, and nailbeds due to diminished oxygen in the blood under certain medical conditions.

cytomegalovirus (CMV)   One of a group of species-specific herpes viruses that can cause many diseases, including CMV colitis and CMV retinitis.

decubitus ulcer   Pressure sore or bedsore; an ulcer resulting from pressure to an area of the body from being sedentary in a bed or a chair.

defecate   To have a bowel movement.

dehydration   The removal of fluid (water) from a substance; a condition resulting from a lack of or loss of body fluid.

delirium   A temporary mental disturbance involving confusion, disorientation, hallucinations, and restlessness; usually brought on by disease states or toxic states (as from the influence of drugs or alcohol).

dementia   The absence of or loss of intellectual ability; similar in some of its symptoms to delirium, but not reversible.

dental dam   A 6-inch-square piece of latex used to cover the vaginal area when oral sex is performed to prevent contact with body fluids.

diabetes   A disorder of blood glucose (sugar); the two types are Type I (also called juvenile onset or insulin dependent) and Type II (adult onset or noninsulin dependent).

diaphragm   The muscle wall separating the chest and abdomen; also a contraceptive device made of rubber and shaped like a cup or dome, which is inserted by the woman to block her cervix from the entry of sperm.

dietitian   A person trained and experienced in the field of nutrition.

differential   A blood test showing the breakdown of the various types of white blood cells present in a sample.

dilate   To widen or expand.

dildo   An artificial penis used to produce sexual pleasure.

dilute   To water down or thin out.

directive   Instruction or order.

DNR (Do Not Resuscitate)   A term used in hospitals to indicate the PWA is not to have CPR performed or be placed on life-sustaining machines in the event that cardiac or respiratory activity stops.

douche   A procedure in which fluids are flushed into the vagina under low pressure and allowed to flow out again; usually for cleansing or medication purposes.

dysphagia   Inability to swallow or difficulty in swallowing.

dyspnea   Air hunger due to labored or difficult breathing; shortness of breath.

echocardiogram   A noninvasive diagnostic technique that uses sound waves to view cardiac structures.

eczema   Skin disease marked by dry, reddened patches.

edema   Swelling.

ejaculate   Ejection of seminal fluid from the male urethra; male orgasm.

electrocardiogram (EKG)   A diagnostic test used to record the electrical activity of the heart.

electrolyte   Ionized salts, such as calcium, potassium, and sodium, in blood, tissue, and cells.

electrophoresis   Diagnostic tests based on the movements of charged particles through a medium because of changes in electrical potential.

ELISA (enzyme-linked immunoabsorbent assay)   One of the two tests used to detect HIV in the blood.

embolus   A mass of undissolved matter present in a blood or lymphatic vessel; bits of tissue, tumor, fat cells, or air bubbles carried to the vessel by the blood or lymph current.

encephalitis   An infection of brain tissue.

endorphin   A brain chemical that functions as the body's natural painkiller.

endoscopy   A diagnostic test in which a scope is passed from the mouth into the stomach.

enteral   By way of the intestine.

Epstein-Barr   A herpeslike virus.

erythropoietin   A kidney hormone that stimulates production of red blood cells.

esophagram   A diagnostic test involving the swallowing of barium and taking of X rays to study the esophagus.

esophagus   The muscular canal extending from below the tongue to the stomach; the narrowest part of the digestive tube.

ESR (erythrocyte sedimentation rate)   A blood test that measures the rate at which red blood cells settle out in a tube of unclotted blood; indicates inflammation in the body from a variety of diseases.

expectorate   Spit out.

extravasation   Passage or leakage of fluid (usually blood) out of the vein into the tissue; usually occurs in conjunction with intravenous therapy.

finger cot   A piece of latex that covers a single finger; used when touching your partner's genitals to prevent contact with body fluids.

flatus   Expelled gas from the digestive tract.

fungi   A division of plantlike organisms that includes molds and yeasts.

gallium scan   A diagnostic test involving the injection of contrast media and X rays.

gastric   Pertaining to the stomach.

gavage   Feeding via a stomach tube or nasal tube leading to the stomach.

giardia   A protozoal parasite.

glaucoma   A disease of the eye sometimes leading to blindness if left untreated.

glucagon   A hormone that stimulates the production of glucose in the body when blood sugar is low; can be injected to treat hypoglycemia.

glucose   A simple sugar.

health care proxy   A person chosen to speak for you if you are unable to do so for yourself in matters of health care.

hematocrit   A measure of the number of red cells found in the blood, stated as a percentage of the total volume.

hemoglobin   A complex blood protein containing iron and responsible for carrying oxygen to the cells.

hemophilia   A group of hereditary bleeding disorders in which there is a lack of one of the factors needed in the clotting of blood; a hemophiliac is one who suffers from hemophilia.

hepatitis   An inflammation of the liver, which may be caused by diseases, medications, toxic chemicals, or other substances.

herpes simplex   An infectious disease characterized by painful sores—usually on the lips, gums, or genitalia.

heterosexual   One who is sexually attracted solely to the opposite sex.

histoplasmosis   An infection caused by breathing in spores of the fungus histoplasma capsulatum.

holistic   Having to do with the whole; as in the philosophy of healing that focuses on the whole body.

homeopathy   A system of healing based on the notion that "like cures like."

homosexual   One who is sexually attracted solely to members of one's own sex.

hormone   A complex chemical substance produced in one organ of the body that influences the activity of another organ or group of cells in another part of the body.

human immunodeficiency virus (HIV)   The virus thought to cause AIDS.

hyperalimentation   The intravenous infusion of a solution that contains nutrients (amino acids, glucose, vitamins) and electrolytes to sustain life.

hyperglycemia   Too much glucose in the blood; high blood sugar.

hyperventilation   An increased rate of breathing in excess of what is needed.

hypoglycemia   Low blood sugar; less glucose in the blood than is necessary for normal functioning.

hypoxia   Too little oxygen in the cells; characterized by cyanosis.

immunocompromised   Having a weakened immune system.

immunodeficiency   An abnormal state of the immune system in which the resistance to infection is decreased.

implanted   Embedded or inserted into tissue.

impotence   Male sexual dysfunction marked by an inability to achieve an erection or, less commonly, to ejaculate.

incentive spirometer   A device used to encourage deep breathing (inspiration) to help maintain lung capacity and prevent pneumonia in bedridden and other susceptible individuals.

incontinent   Inability to control urination or defecation.

infertility   Inability to conceive a child.

infiltrate   Areas where fluid has passed into tissue.

infusion   The introduction of a substance, usually a medicine, directly into a vein.

insomnia   Chronic inability to fall asleep or remain asleep.

insulin A medicine used to treat diabetics to help lower their blood glucose level and maintain it within the normal range; types include regular and NPH.

intercourse Coitus; the sex act.

intramuscular Into a muscle.

intrathecal Into the spinal canal.

intravenous Into a vein.

intubation The passing of a tube into a body opening—most commonly putting a breathing tube down the trachea to provide an airway.

irradiate Administer a dose of radiation.

irrigation The process of washing out a body cavity or wound area with a stream of water or another fluid.

Isospora A type of parasite.

jaundice A yellow discoloration of the skin, eyes, and mucous membranes common in certain diseases of the liver.

Kaposi's sarcoma (KS) A common cancer of AIDS that begins as a soft brown or purple spot on the skin that spreads.

ketoacidosis An excessive level of acid in the blood accompanied by an increase in ketones. It is a complication of diabetes.

ketones Substances produced in the body via a normal change that fats undergo during their digestion; used as fuel by muscles.

labia Fleshy liplike structures at the opening to the vagina.

lactose A sugar found in milk and other dairy products.

lethargy A state of sluggishness or drowsiness.

leukemia A cancer of the blood-forming organs characterized by the replacement of bone marrow with immature white blood cells.

leukocyte White blood cell responsible for destroying bacteria, fungi, and viruses. There are five types: lymphocytes; monocytes; neutrophils; basophils; and eosinophils.

libido The drive and desire for sexual activity; sexual urge.

lipid Fat or fatlike substance in tissue; stored in the body and serves as an energy reserve.

living will Written document stating the wishes of the author regarding resuscitation and other life-sustaining measures.

lumbar puncture Spinal tap; the introduction of a hollow needle into the spinal canal for therapeutic or diagnostic purposes.

lumen A cavity or channel within any organ or structure; the space within an artery, vein, intestine, or tube.

lupus (systemic lupus erythematosus; SLE) A chronic, progressive disease of the skin and/or other bodily organs thought by many to be autoimmune in nature.

lymphadenopathy Swollen glands; a disease of the lymph nodes causing their enlargement.

lymphocyte   Lymph cell or white blood cell. (Examples of these are B cells, T cells, null cells, and natural killer or NK cells.)

lymphoma   A tumor of lymphoid tissue; usually cancerous. (Examples are Burkitt's Lymphoma, Hodgkins disease, and non-Hodgkins lymphoma).

macrophage   A large white blood cell capable of surrounding and digesting foreign substances.

malignancy   A tumor that is cancerous; also called a neoplasm.

malnutrition   A condition of poor nutrition due to poor dietary intake, under- or overeating, or improper use of food by the body; may also be caused by excessive loss of nutrients, as from diarrhea, dehydration, or vomiting.

mammography   X ray examination of the breasts to check for cancerous growths and other disease states.

Mantoux test (ppd)   Test for tuberculosis exposure.

Medicaid   A federally funded state-run program of medical assistance to those with low incomes.

Medicare   Federally funded national health insurance plan mainly for eligible persons over 65.

melena   Black, tarry stools indicative of internal bleeding.

meningitis   An infection or swelling of the membranes covering the brain and spinal cord.

menstruation   Monthly bleeding experienced by women between puberty and menopause during which the uterine lining is shed.

microbe   A microorganism; a tiny, one-celled form of life.

microbiologist   One who studies microbes.

migraine   A specific type of vascular headache, usually characterized by intense, throbbing pain localized to one side of the head and accompanied by other symptoms such as visual disturbances or vomiting.

molecule   The smallest unit of a substance that has the properties of an element or compound; made up of two or more atoms that are chemically combined.

MRI (magnetic resonance imaging)   A diagnostic test that uses strong magnets to scan the body and that can identify different densities of tissue to detect tumors and other abnormalities.

mutation   An unusual change in genes that occurs spontaneously—with or without the influence of mutagens such as X rays or certain drugs; the change causes a difference in the physical trait determined by that gene.

Mycobacterium avium intracellulare (MAI)   A species of mycobacterium causing disease; a form of tuberculosis.

nasogastric   Referring to the nose and stomach, as, for example, a nasogastric tube that is passed through the nose into the stomach.

nebulizer   A device for making a fine spray or mist to be inhaled, usually for the purpose of administering medication.

necrosis   Death of tissue as a result of disease or injury.

neurological   Referring to the nervous system.

neurosyphilis   Syphilis infection of the central nervous system (brain and spinal cord).

nucleus   Core or center, as in the nucleus of a cell.

occlusion   A closure, covering, or blockage.

oncology   A branch of medicine dealing with tumors and cancers.

ophthalmologist   A physician specializing in the eye.

opportunistic infections   Infections with any organism—especially fungi and bacteria—that occur due to the opportunity afforded by an altered or weakened immune system.

oral hairy leukoplakia   Spots or patches on the tongue or in the mouth that appear hairy; an AIDS opportunistic infection.

organism   A life-form; a living being.

otolaryngologist   A physician specializing in the treatment of the ears, nose, and throat; an ENT doctor.

ovulation   Monthly release of an egg from a woman's ovary.

palliative   Pertaining to a measure taken to relieve or lessen pain and other uncomfortable symptoms, but not to cure.

pallor   Paleness.

palpitations   Pounding or racing of the heart.

pancreas   A gland in the body that releases insulin, glucagon, and some other enzymes of digestion.

Pap smear   A screening test for cervical cancer and human papilloma virus (a precursor to cervical cancer, in some cases) performed by scraping the superficial cells from the cervix during a pelvic examination and subjecting them to laboratory analysis.

parasite   An organism that lives within, upon, or at the expense of another organism known as its host, without contributing to the survival of the host.

parenteral   A route outside of the digestive tract.

pathogenic   Referring to the ability of an organism to cause disease.

pelvic examination   A physical examination of the internal and external female genitalia.

periodontal disease   Disease of the tissues (e.g., the gums) around a tooth.

phagocyte   A cell that is able to surround and digest small living things (such as bacteria) and cell wastes.

phagocytosis   The process by which the engulfment and digestion of foreign bodies takes place.

phlebitis   Inflammation of a vein.

pitting edema   Swelling in which indentations can be made into the swollen area when it is pressed with a finger to displace the fluid.

placebo   An inactive substance given as if it were an actual medication; a "sugar pill."

platelet   A component of blood responsible for clotting.

***Pneumocystis carinii* pneumonia (PCP)** A common pneumonia found in AIDS.

postural drainage Use of various body positions to help gravity to drain secretions from the lungs and enable it to be coughed up and eliminated from the body.

power of attorney Legal document granting another person the power to make decisions for you.

progressive multifocal leukoencephalopathy (PML) A rare, rapidly spreading disease of the central nervous system.

prophylaxis Rules or procedures followed to prevent disease.

prostate A gland present in the male that contributes to the production of semen.

protocol A list of requirements or procedures to follow, as in an experiment.

protozoan A single-celled living thing that is the lowest form of animal life.

psychiatrist A physician who specializes in the study, treatment, and prevention of mental disorders.

psychologist One who is trained in methods of psychological analysis, therapy, and research; usually with a Ph.D. degree; a nonphysician.

psychotherapist One who provides therapy for a variety of mental conditions; levels of training and education are variable.

PWA Person with AIDS.

radiation Process by which energy is sent through space or matter and used to treat or diagnose diseases such as cancer.

radiologist A physician who studies and practices radiology (radiation).

reconstitute Returning a substance from powder form (altered for preservation during storage) back to a usable, liquid form by the addition of sterile water or saline.

regimen A plan, a system to be followed, as in a medication regimen.

resuscitation Revival or attempt at revival after apparent death.

retina A structure of the eye that receives images formed by the lens.

retrovirus A virus that contains RNA as its genetic material instead of DNA.

rubella German measles.

salmonella A type of bacteria that often produces abdominal illness.

seizure Types include grand mal, petit mal, focal, tonic/clonic, and partial; see convulsion.

septicemia A disease marked by the presence of pathogenic bacteria in the blood.

serology A diagnostic test performed on the noncellular portion of the blood called serum.

seronegative Negative result of a serologic test.

shigella A type of bacteria.

sigmoidoscopy A diagnostic test examining the final portion of the colon, called the sigmoid colon, performed by inserting a rigid or flexible tube into the rectum.

significant other   A spouse, partner, relative, close friend, or other loved one.

silicone   An organic compound used in adhesives, lubricants, prostheses, and other medical equipment.

spasm   An involuntary, sudden movement; a convulsive muscular contraction.

spermicide   A chemical agent that kills sperm.

sphincter   A circular band of muscle fibers that narrows a passage or closes a natural opening in the body, as in the anal sphincter.

sternum   Breastbone.

stomatitis   Painful inflammation of the mouth.

subarachnoid hemorrhage   Bleeding in the brain.

subcutaneous   Beneath the skin.

sucrose   A sugar derived from sugar cane; table sugar.

sulfonylureas   A group of oral diabetes medicines.

suppositories   Easily melted cylinders of material containing medication to be administered via the rectum, urethra, or vagina.

syncope   Sudden loss of consciousness.

T cell   A type of circulating lymphocyte (white blood cell) made in the bone marrow instrumental in the body's defense against foreign invaders; two types important in AIDS are *T4* or *T helper* cells and *T8* or *T suppressor* cells.

thrush   An infection caused by *Candida albicans*; a yeast infection.

toxin   Poison.

toxoplasmosis   A disease caused by infection with the protozoan *Toxoplasma gondii*.

trachea   Windpipe.

transbronchial   Across the bronchi.

trapeze   Triangle-shaped metal device suspended above a bed to help the PWA change her position.

tuberculosis   Infectious disease caused by the tubercule bacillus, *Mycobacterium tuberculosis*.

tunneled   Regarding a route deep under the surface, as in a tunneled venous access device.

ultrasound   Diagnostic imaging test utilizing sound waves to view the body's internal organs.

urethra   A small, tubelike structure that drains urine from the bladder.

venous access device   An IV for long-term use; patients are often sent home with one in place. Types include nontunneled, tunneled, and implanted. May also be known as a Hickman catheter or a portacath.

vertigo   A form of dizziness; a spinning sensation.

virus   A minute organism not visible by ordinary light or microscopic techniques; a parasite that can grow, thrive, and reproduce only by taking over the cellular functions of another living thing that it infects.

Western Blot   One of two common blood tests that detect the HIV virus.

window period   The time after exposure to a disease during which the test for that disease will still be negative.

Bibliography

Abrams, D. I., et al. "Routine Care and Psychological Support of the Patient with Acquired Immunodeficiency Syndrome." *Medical Clinics of North America* 70, No. 3 (1986): 707–720.

Ahronheim, Judith, and Doron Weber. *Final Passages: Positive Choices for the Dying and Their Loved Ones*. New York: Simon & Schuster, 1992.

American Psychiatric Association: Diagnostic and Statistical Manual of Mental Disorders. 3d ed., rev. Washington, D.C.: American Psychiatric Association, 1987.

Barrett, Douglas. "The Clinician's Guide to Pediatric AIDS." *Contemporary Pediatrics* 5 (January 1988): 24–47.

Bartlett, John G. *1992–1993 Recommendations for the Medical Care of Persons with HIV Infection: A Guide to HIV Care from the AIDS Care Program of the Johns Hopkins Medical Institutions—Second Edition*. Baltimore: Critical Care America, 1992, pp. 1–86.

Bartlett, John G., and Ann K. Finkbeiner. *The Guide to Living with HIV Infection*. Baltimore: The Johns Hopkins University Press, 1991, p. 47.

Bates, Barbara. *A Guide to Physical Examination*. 2d ed. Philadelphia: J. B. Lippincott, 1979.

Berkow, Robert, editor-in-chief, et al. *The Merck Manual of Diagnosis and Therapy*. 16th ed. Rahway: Merck Sharp & Dohme Research Laboratories, 1992.

Boyle, Lynnette Z. "Legal Implications of the Patient Self-Determination Act." *Nurse Practitioner Forum* 3, no. 1 (March 1992): 12–15.

Brown, Marie Annette, and Gail M. Powell-Cope. *Caring for a Loved One with AIDS: The Experiences of Families, Lovers, and Friends*. Seattle: University of Washington Press, 1992.

Carr, Gary S. "AIDS and AIDS-Related Conditions: Screening for Populations at Risk." *Nurse Practitioner* (October 1986): 26.

Centers for Disease Control and Prevention. "AIDS in Women—United States." *Morbidity and Mortality Weekly Report* 39, no. 47 (November 1990): 845–846.

———. "Classification System for Human Lymphocytic Virus Type III/Lymphadenopathy-Associated Virus Infections." *Morbidity and Mortality Weekly Report* 35, no. 20 (May 1986): 335.

———. "The HIV/AIDS Epidemic: The First 10 Years." *Morbidity and Mortality Weekly Reports* 40, no. 22 (June 1991): 357–369.

———. "HIV/AIDS Surveillance—Year-End Edition" (January 1992): 3–22.

———. "Public Health Service Guidelines for Counseling and Antibody Testing to Prevent HIV Infection and AIDS" *Morbidity and Mortality Weekly Reports* 36 (August 1987): 31.

———. "Purified Protein Derivative (PPD)-Tuberculin Anergy and HIV Infection: Guidelines for Anergy Testing and the Management of Anergic Persons At Risk of Tuberculosis." *Morbidity and Mortality Weekly Reports* 40, no. RR-5 (April 1991): 29–33.

———. "1993 Revised Classification System for HIV Infection and Expanded Surveillance Case Definition for AIDS among Adolescents and Adults." *Morbidity and Mortality Weekly Reports* 41, no. RR-17 (December 1992): 1–19.

———. "Revision of the CDC Surveillance Case Definition for Acquired Immunodeficiency Syndrome." *Morbidity and Mortality Weekly Reports* 36, suppl. no. 1S (1987): 3S–15S.

———. "Update: Serologic Testing for Antibody to Human Immunodeficiency Virus." *Morbidity and Mortality Weekly Reports* (January 8, 1988).

Chemotherapy and You: A Guide to Self-Help during Treatment. Bethesda: U.S. Department of Health and Human Services, Public Health Service, National Institutes of Health, National Cancer Institute, 1988, NIH Publication No. 88–1136.

Chilnick, Lawrence D., editor-in-chief. *The Pill Book: The Illustrated Guide to the Most Commonly Prescribed Drugs in the U.S.* 3rd ed. New York: Bantam Books, 1986.

Conant, M., et al. "Condoms Prevent Transmission of AIDS-Associated Retrovirus." *Journal of the American Medical Association* 255 (1986): 1706.

Coping with AIDS: Psychological and Social Considerations in Helping People with HTLV-III Infection. Rockville: U.S. Department of Health and Human Services Public Health Service Alcohol, Drug Abuse, and Mental Health Administration, National Institute of Mental Health Office of Scientific Information, 1986.

Cousins, Norman. *Anatomy of an Illness.* New York: W. W. Norton, 1991.

Curran, J. W., et al. "The Epidemiology of AIDS: Current Status and Future Prospects." *Science* 229 (1985): 1352.

Dalgleish, A., et al. "The CD4 (T4) Antigen Is an Essential Component of the Receptor for the AIDS Retrovirus." *Nature* 312 (1984): 763–766.

Davidson, Bonnie. "Do You Wanna Trance?" Cosmo's Update on the Power of Hypnosis." *Cosmopolitan*, December 1992, 202–205.

DeVita, Vincent T., et al. *AIDS: Etiology, Diagnosis, Treatment and Prevention.* 2d ed. Philadelphia: J. B. Lippincott, 1988.

"Diabetes Management: The Team Approach." Indianapolis: Boehringer Mannheim Diagnostics, 1986, p. 15.

Doheny, Kathleen. "Exercise Benefits HIV-Positive Men." *The Sunday Star Ledger*, 22 March 1992, p. H-3.

Dorland's Illustrated Medical Dictionary. 25th ed. Philadelphia: W. B. Saunders, 1974.

Dreuilhe, Emmanuel. *Mortal Embrace: Living with AIDS.* New York: Hill and Wang, 1988.

Favero, Martin S., and Richard Sadovsky. "Office Infection Control, OSHA, and You." *Patient Care* (March 30, 1993): 117–134.

Flaskerud, J., and Peter Ungvarski, eds. *HIV/AIDS: A Guide to Nursing Care.* 2d ed. Philadelphia: W. B. Saunders, 1992.

Freidland, Gerald, et al. "Lack of Transmission of HTLV III/LAV Infection to Household Contacts of Patients with AIDS or AIDS-Related Complex with Oral Candidiasis." *New England Journal of Medicine* 314 (1986): 344.

Friedland, Gerald, and R. Klein. "Transmission of the Human Immunodeficiency Virus." *New England Journal of Medicine* 317 (1987): 1125–1135.

Friedman, H. Harold, ed. *Problem Oriented Medical Diagnosis.* 4th ed. Boston: Little, Brown, 1987.

Frohlich, Edward D. "A Portrait of the Immune System." *Modern Medicine* 40 (December 1987): 36–40.

Gallo, Robert. "The First Human Retrovirus." *Scientific American* 12 (1986): 88.

Glanze, Walter D., ed. *The Mosby Medical Encyclopedia: A Plume Book.* Scarborough, New American Library, 1985.

Goldfarb, Herbert A., and Judith Greif. *The No-Hysterectomy Option: Your Body, Your Choice.* New York: John Wiley & Sons, 1990, pp. 180–182.

Goldman, Erik L. "HIV-Infected Women Poorly Understood." *Internal Medicine and Cardiology News* 25, no. 18 (September 1992): 35.

———. "HIV Patients' Holistic Methods 'Seem to be Working.'" *Internal Medicine and Cardiology News* 25, no. 18 (September 1992): 1, 52.

Goldman, Peter, and Lucille Beachy. "The AIDS Doctor." *Newsweek* 21 July 1986, 38–50.

Gong, Victor. *AIDS: Facts and Issues.* New Brunswick: Rutgers University Press, 1986, pp. 15–89.

Gorroll, Allan H., et al. *Primary Care Medicine: Office Evaluation and Management of the Adult Patient.* 2d ed. Philadelphia: J. B. Lippincott, 1987.

Gostin, L., and Curran, W. "AIDS Screening, Confidentiality and the Duty to Warn." *American Journal of Public Health* 77 (1987): 361.

Haber, Judith et al. *Comprehensive Psychiatric Nursing.* 2d ed. New York: McGraw-Hill, 1982.

Hendrickson, Peter A. *Alive and Well: A Path for Living in a Time of HIV.* New York: Irvington Publishers, 1990.

"HIV & AIDS: The Basics." New York: GMHC, Inc., 1991.

Hoole, Axalla J., et al. *Patient Care Guidelines for Nurse Practitioners.* 3d ed. Boston: Little, Brown, 1988.

Humphry, Derek. *Final Exit: The Practicalities of Self-Deliverance and Assisted Suicide for the Dying.* New York: Dell, 1992.

Institute of Medicine National Academy of Sciences. *Confronting AIDS: Update 1988.* Washington, D.C.: National Academy Press, 1988.

Joneja, Janice Vickerstaff, and Leonard Bielory. *Understanding Allergy, Sensitivity and Immunity: A Comprehensive Guide.* New Brunswick, Rutgers University Press, 1990, pp. 8–11; 28–34; 48–51; 58–80; 110–114.

Kilo, Charles, and Joseph R. Williamson. *Diabetes: The Facts That Let You Regain Control of Your Life.* New York: John Wiley & Sons, 1987.

Kilo, Charles. *Educating the Diabetic Patient.* New York: Science & Medicine, 1982.

Klotzmann, D., et al. "Selective Tropism of Lymphadenopathy Associated Virus (LAV) for Helper-Inducer T Lymphocytes." *Science* 225 (1984): 59–64.

Kübler-Ross, Elisabeth. *On Death and Dying.* New York: Macmillan, 1969.

Learning to Live with Diabetes. Boston: Medicine in the Public Interest, Inc., 1984.

Loebl, Suzanne, et al. *The Nurses' Drug Handbook.* 3d ed. New York: John Wiley & Sons, 1983, pp. 21–35.

McCarthy, Laura Flynn. "Far From the Medical Mainstream." *Cosmopolitan,* November 1992, 262–266.

McFarland, Mary Brambilla, and Marcia Moeller Grant. *Nursing Implications of Laboratory Tests.* New York: John Wiley & Sons, 1982.

Michaels, Davida, ed. *Diagnostic Procedures: The Patient and the Health Care Team.* New York: John Wiley & Sons, 1983.

Milchovich, Suellyn K., and Barbara Dunn-Long. *Diabetes Mellitus . . . What's It All About?* Anaheim: Anaheim Memorial Hospital Community Health Education Center, 1986.

Moffet, Betty Clare, et al. *AIDS: A Self Care Manual.* Los Angeles: AIDS Project L.A., 1987.

Moore, C. Virginia. "Self-Determined Advance Directives: New Issues in Primary Care." *Nurse Practitioner Forum* 3, no. 1 (March 1992): 10–11, 35–50.

Moore, Ken. "Understanding HIV." *The Body Positive,* April 1989, 8–10.

Nichols, Eve K. *Mobilizing against AIDS.* Massachusetts: Harvard University Press, 1989, pp. 56–80.

O'Malley, Padraig, ed. *The AIDS Epidemic: Private Rights and the Public Interest.* Boston: Beacon Press, 1989.

Padus, Emrikas. *The Complete Guide to Your Emotions and Your Health: New Dimensions in Mind/Body Healing.* Emmaus: Rodale Press, 1986.

Phillips, A., et al. "Serial CD4 Lymphocyte Counts and Development of AIDS." *Lancet* 337 (1991): 389–392.

Physicians' Desk Reference. 47th ed. Oradell: Medical Economics Inc., 1993.

Pinch, Winifred J. "The Patient Self Determination Act: The Ethical Dimensions." *Nurse Practitioner Forum,* 3, no. 1 (March 1992): 16–22.

Rob, Caroline, and Janet Reynolds. *The Caregivers Guide: Helping Elderly Relatives Cope with Health and Safety Problems.* Boston: Houghton Mifflin, 1990.

"The Safer Sex Condom Guide—For Men and Women." New York: GMHC, Inc., 1987.

Safire, William, and Leonard Safir. *Words of Wisdom: More Good Advice.* New York: Simon and Schuster, 1990, pp. 48, 254.

Saumweber, Les J., and Carl E. Fasser. "HIV Infection: An Algorithmic Approach to Evaluation and Staging." *Clinician Reviews* (May, 1991): 57–77.

Sedlacek, Keith. "Biofeedback for Raynaud's Disease." *Psychosometics: The Journal of the Academy of Psychosometic Medicine* 20, no. 8 (August 1979): 535–541.

Sedlacek, Keith W. "Biofeedback: Valuable Treatment for Mind-Body Stress Problems." *Consultant* (January 30, 1985): 93–103.

Selwyn, Peter A. "AIDS: What Is Now Known." *Hospital Practice* (May 1986): 67–82.

———. "AIDS: What Is Now Known." *Hospital Practice* (June 1986): 127–164.

———. "AIDS: What Is Now Known." *Hospital Practice* (September 1986): 119–153.

Seymour, Lesley Jane. "Mom, I Have AIDS: Five Mothers' Stories." *McCall's*, January 1993, 85–87.

Shook, Mary. "Health Decisions: Maintaining Control of Health Care Choices." *Nurse Practitioner Forum* 3, no. 1 (March, 1992): 30–34.

Siegel, Bernie S. *Love, Medicine and Miracles.* New York: Harper & Row, 1986.

Snyder, Mariah. *A Guide to Neurological and Neurosurgical Nursing.* New York: John Wiley & Sons, 1983, pp. 277–281.

Sorensen, Karen Creason, and Joan Luckmann. *Basic Nursing: A Psychophysiologic Approach.* Philadelphia: W. B. Saunders, 1979.

———. *Medical-Surgical Nursing: A Psychophysiologic Approach.* 2d ed. Philadelphia: W. B. Saunders, 1980.

"Standards of Nursing Care in the Management of the Patient with an HIV Related Illness." *Professional Standards Review Council of America, Inc. AIDS Intervention Management System (AIMS), Under the Auspices of the AIDS Institute New York State Department of Health-ed I*, January 1990.

Tanne, Janice Hopkins. "To Test or Not To Test?" *New York*, 28 September 1987, pp. 40–46.

Tapley, Donald F., ed. *The Columbia University College of Physicians and Surgeons Complete Medical Guide.* Rev. ed. New York: Crown, 1989, pp. 452–453.

Thomas, Clayton L., ed. *Taber's Cyclopedic Medical Dictionary.* Philadelphia: F. A. Davis Co., 1982.

Thomason, Susan S. "Using a Groshong Central Venous Catheter." *Nursing 91* (October 1991): 58–60.

Tripp, Frederick, et al. "HIV: Fight Back with Nutrition-Nutritionists in AIDS Care." New York: The Greater New York Dietetic Association, 1992.

Ungvarski, Peter, and Joan Schmidt. "AIDS Patients Under Attack." *RN* (November 1992): 37–45.

Wallace, John, and Cathy Sears. "Fighting AIDS: Part 5—What Price Hope?" *American Health*, November 1987, 68–75.

Wallach, Jacques. *Interpretation of Diagnostic Tests: A Handbook Synopsis of Laboratory Medicine.* 5th ed. Boston: Little, Brown, 1992.

World Health Organization. "Global Programme on AIDS: The Current Global Situation of the HIV/AIDS Pandemic." (January 4, 1993), pp. 1–10.

———. "Global Programme on AIDS: Current and Future Dimensions of the HIV/AIDS Pandemic—A Capsule Summary." (January 1992), pp. 1–15.

Wickham, Sandra Purl, and Diane Welker. "Long-Term Central Venous Catheters: Issues for Care." *Seminars in Oncology Nursing* 8, no. 2 (May 1992): 133–147.

Wickwire, Peggy A. "Nutrition and HIV: Your Choices Make a Difference." Tennessee: Tennessee Department of Health and Environment, 1991.

"A Woman's Guide to AIDS." New York: New York City Department of Health, 1989, pp. 1–16.

Wood, Robert W., and Ann Collier. "Acquired Immunodeficiency Syndrome." *Infectious Disease Clinics of North America* 1, no. 1 (March 1987): 145–161.

Index

About the Authors

Judith Greif was born in Brooklyn, New York, and grew up in Wantagh, Long Island. She received a Bachelor of Science degree in microbiology from Cornell University and a Master's degree in nursing from Pace University. She is board-certified in Family Nursing Practice and is a certified HIV/AIDS counselor.

Ms. Greif practiced nursing in inner-city clinics, neighborhood family health centers, health maintenance organizations, occupational health, and, most recently, student health. She has also been an administrator and an educator, serving as an adjunct instructor at the Columbia University Graduate School of Nursing in New York City.

Ms. Greif has written for *New York Magazine* and *New Woman Magazine*. She has also contributed to medical publications, including *Emergency Medicine for the House Officer*, and most recently is a coauthor (with Herbert Goldfarb, M.D.) of the medical and science bestseller, *The No-Hysterectomy Option: Your Body, Your Choice.* She is currently collaborating on a book about infertility. Ms. Greif lives in East Brunswick, New Jersey, with her husband, Joe, and her daughter, Samantha.

Beth Ann Golden was born in Manhattan and grew up in the Bronx, New York. She received a Bachelor of Science degree in police science and criminal justice from John Jay College of Criminal Justice, a Bachelor of Science degree in nursing from Columbia University School of Nursing, and a Master's degree in adult primary care nursing from Columbia University Graduate School of Nursing. She is board-certified as an adult nurse practitioner by the American Nurses' Association.

Ms. Golden has worked as a bedside nurse in medicine and surgery, an AIDS specialist on the AIDS unit at St. Luke's–Roosevelt Hospital Center in New York City, and an adult nurse practitioner at Miller Institute for the Performing Arts. She is currently a clinical nurse specialist at Broward General Medical Center in south Florida. She is a member of many professional nursing organizations, including Sigma Theta Tau National Nursing Honor Society and the Association of Nurses in AIDS Care.